Disorders of Human Learning, Behavior, and Communication

Ronald L. Taylor and Les Sternberg
Series Editors

Louis Rowitz
Editor

Mental Retardation in the Year 2000

With 15 Illustrations

Springer-Verlag
New York Berlin Heidelberg London Paris
Tokyo Hong Kong Barcelona Budapest

Louis Rowitz, School of Public Health, The University of Illinois at Chicago, Chicago, IL 60680, USA

Series Editors: Ronald L. Taylor and Les Sternberg, Exceptional Student Education, Florida Atlantic University, Boca Raton, FL 33431-0991, USA

92-08282
0025764

Library of Congress Cataloging-in-Publication Data
Mental retardation in the year 2000 / Louis Rowitz, editor.
     p.   cm.—(Disorders of human learning, behavior, and communication)
     Includes bibliographical references and index.
     ISBN 0-387-97474-1 (alk. paper)
     1. Mental retardation—Forecasting.   2. Mentally handicapped—
Care—Forecasting.   3. Twenty-first century—Forecasts.
I. Rowitz, Louis.   II. Series.
RC570.M4168 1991
362.3′01′12—dc20   91-29807

Printed on acid-free paper.

W M 840

Production managed by Ellen Seham; manufacturing supervised by Jacqui Ashri.
Typeset by Best-set Typesetter, Ltd., Hong Kong
Printed and bound by Edwards Brothers, Inc., Ann Arbor, MI
Printed in the United States of America.

9 8 7 6 5 4 3 2 1

ISBN 0-387-97474-1 Springer-Verlag New York Berlin Heidelberg
ISBN 3-540-97474-1 Springer-Verlag Berlin Heidelberg New York

Foreword

When you look at the advances in the field of mental retardation over the past 30 years, it is hard to imagine that more change is inevitable. Yet, I think back to the time when, early in his presidency, President Kennedy called together the brightest scientists, researchers, doctors, and educators to develop a comprehensive plan for the nation to effectively care for, treat, educate, and house persons with mental retardation.

In the early 1960s the call for new research into the causes and the amelioration of mental retardation, the development of community-based programs, and the development of family care for appropriate education, vocational training, and jobs were seen as revolutionary. But, in the 30 years since then, we have seen time and time again that it is persons with mental retardation themselves who have led the way.

When the schools were opened to them, they learned more than any-one ever thought possible; when vocational training was provided, they learned skills that led to jobs; when employment became available, they proved to be good steady workers who earned money and paid taxes. When the playing fields were made available to them through programs such as Special Olympics, they showed the world they could train and compete and *WIN* in the sports of the Olympics. When communities welcomed them, they became our neighbors. They have earned the right to play on any field, to study in any school, to hold a paying job, and to be anyone's neighbor.

Perhaps one of the most visible changes has been the shift in the context of service from large, public institutions to small homes in community-based settings. Concomitant with this shift has been the attempt to improve the quality of lives for persons with mental retardation and developmental disabilities by promoting community and social integration.

Much of the change in public attitude during these years was brought about by the passage of 94–142, the Education for All Handicapped Children Act of 1975. Once schools were opened and a free and appropriate education was provided to these children in the least restrictive

vi Foreword

setting possible, everything else followed, including additional legislation, which expanded services, training, and recreational opportunities for these individuals and their families.

We have also witnessed many breakthroughs and advances in the scientific area over the past 30 years, including the elimination of mental retardation caused by the factor for Rh through the discovery of RhoGAM (D antigen immune globulin); the recognition that mental retardation can be caused by chromosomal abnormalities and inborn errors of metabolism and the prenatal diagnosis of these by amniocentesis; the description of Fragile X syndrome, one of the most common causes of mental retardation in males; the major breakthrough in the treatment of syndromes causing mental retardation through screening for phenylketonuria and hypothyroidism followed by medical treatment and prevention of mental retardation; prenatal diagnosis of Tay-Sachs disease and Lesch-Nyhan syndrome; prevention of the most common causes of mental retardation resulting from infection through the development of the measles and rubella vaccines; and, major reduction in retardation resulting from prematurity and low birthweight through new technologies for pregnancy management and treatment of prematurity. In addition, we appear to be on the threshold of a major breakthrough in the field of "gene therapy."

I am not a scientist, but I recognize the magnitude of these outstanding achievements and understand that new discoveries and advances will continue to be made—even if only in small increments—as our knowledge expands and better technology becomes available.

These achievements have resulted in fundamental changes in the location, structure, and funding base of services provided to persons with developmental disabilities, and where once only persons with mild or moderate levels of disabilities were served in community-based programs, it is now almost routine for persons with more severe levels of disabilities to be included.

As we look ahead to the year 2000, I think it is important to reflect on the major unaddressed issues in the field of mental retardation. In a very decentralized system, so much depends on local conditions: Are there adequate housing stocks? Will there be qualified and appropriate pools of labor? Will the human services sector attract, recruit, and retain enough workers by providing sufficient training, compensation, and recognition? Will the health-care system be responsive? As the economy continues to shift toward a service economy and as more technical competency is required, will there be enough jobs for persons with disabilities? Will research in these areas continue to be funded and attract new young scientists? The answers to these questions will say a lot about what the future will be like for persons with mental retardation in the year 2000.

Today, I see glimmers of hope. In New York City at the Albert Einstein College of Medicine, a pediatric acquired immune deficiency syndrome (AIDS) project works with families, schools, and staff. Also in New York, at Montefiore Medical Center and St. Luke/Roosevelt Hospital, a managed health-care initiative is underway for persons with mental retardation. At City University of New York, a new training program has been designed specifically for the direct-care providers of services and programs in the field of mental retardation. It is a college-level degree program that offers a new curriculum and education to enhance the career opportunities for these workers and to address the serious shortage and turnover problems in this important area.

Another unique program now operating successfully in 111 universities and colleges across the country is Best Buddies of America. Matching college students with a "buddy" with mental retardation, this program enables them to become friends, to build a relationship based on mutual needs and interests, and to participate together in social, recreational, and educational activities that enhance the life experiences of both. Best Buddies exemplifies community integration at the best level—friendship.

In Ohio, at the University of Akron, an innovative program for elderly persons with mental retardation was developed, which provides them with a "peer" companion—a nondisabled elderly friend. Both parties gain great benefits and enjoyment from this fine program.

In Charlottesville, Virginia, Planned Lifetime Assistance Network (PLAN) offers parents of persons with mental retardation the assurance that when they die the monitoring and advocacy efforts for their child will continue.

In the Sacramento, California, Public School System a program called the Community of Caring addresses the issues of teenage pregnancy, prevention of low birth weight babies, and care for pregnant and parenting teens.

At the Beach Center at the University of Kansas, a model "family"-centered program is currently under development.

At Johns Hopkins University in Baltimore, Maryland, researchers are working on the Down syndrome mouse model, moving ever closer to the time when it may be possible to "correct" the chromosomal problem that causes Down syndrome *before* birth.

New advances in technology, such as computer-enhanced learning assistance devices, also offer great potential and an enhanced quality of life for those with disabilities.

All of these examples give hope for the future. If we look at the most innovative efforts across the country, we will find many more outstanding examples of programs that are on the cutting edge of the field. They will lead us into the next century.

Mental Retardation in the Year 2000 offers us a glimpse into the future. Perhaps the most important question for all of us is "Will the condition that today is labelled mental retardation still exist in the year 2000 and beyond?" I raise this question because of the ethical implications of DNA screening and the potential for "gene therapy." In addition, the rethinking on the classification system and diagnostic procedures also raises important questions about the future. And finally, the lumping together and relabeling of various conditions into one large, "homogenized" category raise still other imperative questions for us all. All of the contributors to this book are experts in their fields. It is to them that we will look for help in addressing these questions and concerns now and into the next century.

One thing is certain, however; just as in the past, persons with developmental disabilities will continue to surprise us and to move beyond our expectations and the limits we set for them.

Eunice Kennedy Shriver
The Joseph P. Kennedy Jr. Foundation
Washington, D.C.

Contents

Epilogue

Contributors

Sharon A. Borthwick-Duffy, Ph.D., University of California, Riverside, Riverside, CA 92521, USA

David L. Braddock, Ph.D., Institute for the Study of Developmental Disabilities, The University of Illinois at Chicago, Chicago, IL 60608, USA

Robert H. Bruininks, Ph.D., Institute on Community Integration, University of Minnesota, Minneapolis, MN 55455, USA

Michael Chapman, M.Ed., University Affiliated Program, Johns Hopkins University, Baltimore, MD 21205, USA

Herbert J. Cohen, M.D., University Affiliated Program, Albert Einstein College of Medicine of Yeshiva University, Bronx, NY 10461, USA

Allen C. Crocker, M.D., Director, Developmental Evaluation Center, Children's Hospital & Medical Center, Boston, MA 02115, USA

Ione DeOllos, M.S., Arizona State University, Tempe, AZ 85287-2101, USA

Paul R. Dokecki, Ph.D., George Peabody College, Vanderbilt University, Nashville, TN 37205, USA

Richard K. Eyman, Ph.D., Lanterman Developmental Center, Pomona, CA 91769, USA

Bernard Farber, Ph.D., Arizona State University, Tempe, AZ 85287-2101, USA

Glenn T. Fujiura, Ph.D., Institute for the Study of Developmental Disabilities, The University of Illinois at Chicago, Chicago, IL 60608, USA

James F. Gardner, Ph.D., The Accreditation Council on Services for People with Developmental Disabilities, Landover, MD 20785-2225, USA

Laraine Masters Glidden, Ph.D., Human Development, St. Mary's College, St. Mary's City, MD 20686, USA

Penny Hauser-Cram, Ed.D., Department of Pediatrics, University of Massachusetts Medical School, Worcester, MA 01655, USA

Stanley S. Herr, J.D., Ph.D., University of Maryland, School of Law, Baltimore, MD 21201, USA

Matthew P. Janicki, Ph.D., State of New York, Office of Mental Retardation and Developmental Disabilities, Albany, NY 12229-0001, USA

Marty Wyngaarden Krauss, Ph.D., The Heller School, Brandeis University, Waltham, MA 02254-9110, USA

K. Charlie Lakin, Ph.D., Institute on Community Integration, University of Minnesota, Minneapolis, MN 55455, USA

Sheryl A. Larson, M.A., Institute on Community Integration, University of Minnesota, Minneapolis, MN 55455, USA

Frank J. Menolascino, M.D., Pediatrics Department, University of Nebraska Medical Center, Omaha, NB 68105, USA

Jane R. Mercer, Ph.D., University of California, Riverside, Riverside, CA 92521, USA

Hugo W. Moser, M.D., The Kennedy Institute, Baltimore, MD 21205, USA

Wendy Parent, M.D., Rehabilitation Research & Training Center, Virginia Commonwealth University, Richmond, VA 23284, USA

Louis Rowitz, Ph.D., School of Public Health, The University of Illinois at Chicago, Chicago, IL 60680, USA

Marsha M. Seltzer, Ph.D., University of Wisconsin-Madison, Waisman Center & School of Social Work, Madison, WI 53705, USA

Eunice Kennedy Shriver, The Joseph P. Kennedy, Jr. Foundation, Washington, D.C. 20005, USA

Jack A. Stark, Ph.D., Department of Psychiatry, Creighton-Nebraska Medical School, Omaha, NB 68108, USA

Gregg C. Vanderheiden, Ph.D., Trace Research & Development Center, University of Wisconsin, Madison, WI 53705, USA

Paul H. Wehman, Ph.D., Rehabilitation Research & Training Center, Virginia Commonwealth University, Richmond, VA 23284, USA

James F. White, Department of Developmental Services, State of California, Sacramento, CA 94244-2020, USA

Andrea G. Zetlin, Ph.D., California State University, Los Angeles, CA 90032, USA

Prologue

1
Mental Retardation in the Year 2000

Louis Rowitz

We are at an interesting time in history. We have entered a new decade, and we are only a few years away from a new century. This century is also the beginning of the third millennium, so this is an excellent time to evaluate our past. The last 30 years have seen major changes in the ways that we view ourselves as parents of children with disabilities or as professionals who have committed themselves to working with families who have children with mental retardation.

When we realize that *deinstitutionalization, normalization, least restrictive environments, community integration, supportive employment* and *integrated employment,* and *social support* were not terms or processes that we used before 1960, we become immediately aware of how far we have come. It would be interesting to have a time machine like the one in the H. G. Wells classic story and return to a conference in 1890 and see what our predecessors predicted for the 20th century. They probably predicted that there would be more institutions, expansion of special education services, and maybe even predicted the development of more psychometric measures like a test that would measure intelligence.

As we enter the 1990s, it is a good time to make some predictions about where the field of mental retardation seems to be headed during the last decade of the 20th century. Making predictions is fraught with all sorts of biases, yet the many predictions that grow out of the chapters in this book will lead to discussion, argument, disagreements, and eventually public policy that can either make the predictions come true or reverse them through conscious efforts. What this book will address are 19 major trends in the field of mental retardation from the vantage point of the early 1990s. Within the discussion of these trends, a number of predictions will be made that will impact the field of mental retardation throughout the 1990s and well into the first decade of the new century.

A *trend* refers to a general process that occurs over time. It builds on information from the past and uses this information of a more factual nature by adding intuition to it to make predictions about future directions. Thus, a trend is a sign in time.

A trend analysis has a number of functions, as follows:

1. It takes present information from a number of sources, combines the information, and synergistically comes up with a trend.
2. The trends taken together give a system perspective on a given area at one point in time.
3. The trends give information about a possible future.
4. The trends show present priority areas as well as emerging and diminishing ones.

There are several useful reasons for exploring trends. Trend analysis allows for the evaluation of a field at a particular point in time. It also allows the professional to determine goals and objectives for the future. These goals and objectives allow for the support of the present trend, reversal of the trend, change in the trend, and also a change in its priority in the grand scheme of things. There are also several negative aspects in a trend analysis. A significant proportion of the analysis may be subjective in nature in that the trends are formulated by one individual or group of individuals. Trends tend to be global, and the everyday problems of service delivery can become lost. The service picture in the United States often differs from the service picture in another country, although some of these differences are beginning to disappear.

I addressed a concern about where the field of mental retardation is headed in the 1990s in an article in 1989 (Rowitz, 1989). This preliminary article on trends in mental retardation for the 1990s listed 22 trends, which were determined on the basis of a review of major journals in the field, mental retardation convention programs, books, newsletters, and technical reports. The trends discussed in the article ran the gamut of concern related to a trend called "the homogenization factor," which pointed out that mental retardation was being affected by the tendency to include mental retardation under the generic terminology of "developmental disabilities," to the newly evolving concerns related to quality of life. The present book builds on the earlier article. Key people in the mental retardation field or related fields explored the trends outlined in the 1989 article. As this process evolved, the trends were greatly fleshed out. Many new dimensions were added. This book is the result of that activity and explores 19 major trends in the field. Within the discussion of each trend, many predictions are made about the field of mental retardation over the next decade and beyond. The final chapter of the book summarizes these predictions.

The Trends

The trends explored in this book relate to conceptual areas of prominence in the field, trends on family and life course, trends on health and service, and finally major trends on service and policy issues. The trends include the following:

Changing Paradigms of Disability

The way that disability is defined greatly affects the diagnostic process. Major changes are occurring in the methods of screening for mental retardation and other developmental disabilities. Although the cognitive approach to defining mental retardation is in an ascendancy, this will not remain the major diagnostic perspective. Standardized testing procedures will change, with intelligence tests playing lesser and lesser roles. Psychomedical models will predominate in the next decade, with more multidisciplinary paradigm models predominating by the year 2000. Social forms of diagnostic categories will decline. Concerns with generic definitions of disability will also need to be addressed.

Community Ethics

Ethicists see a shift in thinking toward ethical communities. This shift will address issues related to inequality that is due to biological or social factors. Future services for people with mental retardation will help these individuals and their families adjust to community living in an environment that enhances their chances for success. There will also be a shift in power relations that will see communities becoming the source of major decision making and not politicians. If the power relations do not change, it will be extremely difficult to bring a true community-based system into being. Pessimists have doubts about the reality of the ethical community model.

Increasing Concern With Quality of Life Issues

Quality of life and quality of care concerns, of interest to service providers in many countries, are now becoming more important in the United States. Definitional issues will be resolved during the 1990s. The subjective and objective determinants of quality of life will be explored. Research and methodologic issues will also be a major concern. The service implications of the issues in quality of life will also be a critical concern.

Expanding Research On Families

The U.S. National Institute on Child Health and Human Development funded five major research projects on the family in 1987. These studies should give us much new information on the family dynamics of mental retardation. More family research will occur throughout the 1990s. New research directions will occur. Research will concern such issues as the relationship between ordinary families and families with a disabled family member, study of the single parent with a child with a disability, the effect of a child with a disability on the working life of the mother, the impact of a changing service-delivery system on family adjustment, changing family paradigms and how these changes affect family adjustment, and the effect of disability on the lives of siblings.

Family Caregiving Across the Life Span

Concern for issues related to caregiving throughout the life span (Rowitz, 1988a) will continue. The changing age structure of the United States will mean that service providers will need to be concerned more with caregiving during the latter stages of life. For researchers, age and cohort effects will be investigated. A major push for more longitudinal research will be made. Because caregiving problems differ at different times in the life of persons with disabilities, more supportive and life-stage–specific services will need to be developed. There will be a continuing need for caregiver reeducation at each successive life stage. The sibling as caregiver will also be a concern in the 1990s and beyond.

Concern With Adolescents With Mental Retardation

Service providers will become increasingly concerned with the unique problems associated with adolescence and mental retardation (Rowitz, 1988b). A higher prevalence of adolescents with mental retardation will be living in community settings during the 1990s and beyond. A significant percentage of this population will be living in poverty or in low-income settings. Problems related to poverty will strongly impact on these adolescents. Labeling issues will be critical for this population. The risk of substance abuse in this population may be increased. Major research and service concerns will involve the issue of transition to adulthood.

Concern With Lifelong Disabilities

The numbers of older people with developmental disabilities are increasing. These individuals have had to deal with the problems of lifelong disability. Questions arise as to whether the aging service-delivery system, the mental retardation service-delivery system, or the generic health-care system is or will be responsible for the provision of service to this population. In the 1990s, there will be more interaction between these various service systems. Existing legislation and future legislation will be more responsive to these overlapping concerns for more effective service provision to older persons with mental retardation.

A number of major trends are related to health and service issues. The following trends address these issues:

HIV Infection and Mental Retardation

The issue of mental retardation and infection with human immuno-deficiency virus (HIV) has become one of the major concerns of the 1980s. Clearly, the issues of HIV infection will also be a major issue of the 1990s and beyond. During the 1990s, HIV infection will become the most common infectious cause of mental retardation and other developmental disability. There will be attempts to develop cures, but this will probably not become a reality during the early part of the 1990s. Special service programs and greatly improved treatment interventions will occur during the 1990s. Concern will exist over HIV-infected children whose parents are deceased because of the disease.

Prevention and Genetic Breakthroughs

During the 1990s, interest in prevention will continue, with major arguments over federal funding for prevention-related activities. Despite funding concerns, major advances will occur. DNA markers for all of the major genetic causes of mental retardation will be available by the year 2010. More effective therapies and interventions will be discovered and implemented. The possibility of large-scale screening for genetic disorders at affordable prices will become feasible during the 1990s. Major advances will also occur in human genome research, which will greatly increase the knowledge base about the genetic causes of mental retardation. Improvements in cytogenetic techniques and breakthroughs in chorionic sampling for early prenatal diagonsis will occur during the 1990s.

Increase in Concern About Mental Illness and Mental Retardation

Research on dual diagnosis will triple by the year 2000. During the 1990s, there will be major attempts to improve diagnostic procedures for people with mental retardation who also have a mental disorder. With the improvement in diagnosis, there will be an increase in the prevalence of people with both disorders. Breakthroughs in neuroanatomy will lead to improvement in treatment and interventions for this special population. Improvements in pharmacology will also benefit this group of people. Shortages of personnel capable of working with people with a dual diagnosis will be a major problem during the 1990s.

Expansion of the Health-Care Delivery System

With an increasing number of people with mental retardation and other developmental disabilities living in the community, the delivery of health-related services becomes a concern. An expansion of the current health-care system will be needed to accommodate the needs of adult community residents with a disability. During the 1990s, primary health care for people with mental retardation will be delivered primarily by general community-based physicians. Case management services will be expanded. Portable health and habilitative service records will accompany patients on their health-care visits. Funding mechanisms for these services will be a problem. Revisions in Medicaid will have to occur. Children with mental retardation will also receive health care from the generic medical care system. Funding here will also be an issue, although parents will have to bear the brunt of financing these services. Retraining of health-care providers to better serve patients with special needs will be a necessity during the 1990s.

Expansion of Programs for Infants and Toddlers With Mental Retardation

In 1986, amendments to the Education of the Handicapped Act related to programs for infants and toddlers created a situation that will affect programs in the 1990s in a significant manner. The 1990s will see an increase in early intervention programs that will use other family members in program and service planning for their children with disabilities. Other family members will also become recipients of care. An Individualized Family Service Plan will outline the dimensions of the services to be provided. More services will be provided to children, beginning at age 3. New methods of family assessment will be developed. New models of early intervention programs will evolve throughout the 1990s and well into the new century.

Changes in Residential Services

The commitment to community care will continue. Many more institutional closings will occur. However, many large residential institutions will still be around in the year 2000. Most people with mental retardation in an out-of-home placement in the 1990s and beyond will live in small community residences. Interstate variation in access and funding of community programs will still be a problem in the 1990s. Programs will be developed that will help people with disabilities to finance their own apartments or homes. There will be shifts from publicly provided residential and nonresidential services to privately provided residential and nonresidential services. Family-support programs will continue to expand.

Foster care programs will be difficult to maintain. Programs to improve the community living skills of people with mental retardation will expand.

The next several trends concern service and policy issues. An introductory discussion of these trends follows:

Changes in Planning of Vocational Services

During the next several decades, major changes will occur in the occupational framework of American society. A substantial decrease in entry-level skilled jobs will occur during the 1990s. Expansions will occur in the area of integrated employment opportunities for people with mental retardation. Training programs for transition to adulthood will expand, as mentioned. More linkages will be made between schools and business and industry. Training programs will develop for teachers to help them learn skills that will enable them to broker employment and service opportunities for people with mental retardation in community settings. Financing all these activities will still remain a problem.

Expansion of Technology

An increasing awareness of the importance of technology on the lives of people with mental retardation and other developmental disabilities will become more apparent during the 1990s. There are three major types of interaction between technology and the physical and mental lives of people with disabilities. These interactions include technology as it impacts on education and therapy, assistive technology, and finally, technologies as they are applied to the workplace, community, and home. In the 1990s and beyond, technology in the area of artificial intelligence will be explored and lead to techniques and interventions that will impact significantly on the lives of people with mental retardation. Major technological advances will clearly affect the life-styles and the quality of life of people with disabilities.

Expansion of Legal Protections for Persons With Special Needs

The involvement of the courts in issues related to developmental disabilities mushroomed during the 1980s. There is evidence that this trend will continue during the 1990s. A major activity of the courts will relate to the interpretation of many new statutes and laws related to legal protection concerns of people with disabilities. The new Americans With Disabilities Act of 1990, which is a major piece of civil rights legislation for people with disabilities, will have significant impact on much of the legal activities of the 1990s. Important legal concerns will relate to goals for saving the lives of infants with life-threatening conditions, improvement of access of educational services, implementation programs related to the right of habilitation, reform laws on guardianship, rights to community living arrangements, zoning and nondiscriminatory housing opportunities, protection from abuse and neglect, capital punishment concerns, and medical choices of people with mental disabilities.

Need for More Staff and Staff Training Programs

The 1990s will still see us concerned with a shortage of direct staff personnel in community programs for people with mental retardation. Turnover and low salaries will still be critical issues. Money for expansion of community programs will also be a problem. The staff shortages will include lack of professionally trained individuals as well as paraprofessionally trained individuals. Significant increases in volunteerism will occur. To promote more commitment to work in the mental retardation field, major efforts will be undertaken to develop training programs designed for individuals who will work in community settings.

Potential of Less Money With More Need

Because of budget deficits and shifting budget priorities, the mental retardation field will probably not be sufficiently funded over the next 10 years. Interstate variability in the commitment of money to community services will continue. States will be the primary source of funds for these programs throughout the 1990s. Major advocacy activities will need to be maintained throughout the 1990s to prevent any erosion of this state support. Federal funds will remain limited. The family will remain the largest provider of care. Proposed plans for Medicaid reform could change the funding patterns.

Increasing Need for Data

Despite the increasing need for data about people with mental retardation for planning purposes at the national level, there is little evidence that any form of uniform national data reporting system is on the horizon for the next decade (Rowitz, 1984). However, there is a partial attempt to remedy this concern in that the National Center for Health Statistics will be collecting some information on health-care use by people with mental retardation. During the 1990s, mental retardation data bases will primarily be state based. Any national data files that will be developed will be constructed out of data collected at the state and local level. Another change that will occur is that data collected will be tied to community-based systems and less to institution-based systems than in the past.

In this chapter, I have discussed many trends that will impact on the field of mental retardation during the 1990s and beyond. These trends are presented from information already at our disposal. Changing circumstances will change the trends and the directions in which they go. The trends will need to be modified as time goes by. In the following chapters, these trends will be discussed in greater detail. In the final chapter, a major listing of predictions will be presented for the 1990s and beyond. These predictions are a blueprint for action. Some will be implemented, and others will be modified as a result of our experiences.

References

Rowitz, L. (1984). The need for uniform data reporting in mental retardation. *Mental Retardation, 22,* 1–3.

Rowitz, L. (1988a). Caregiving—A lifetime concern. *Mental Retardation, 26,* iii–iv.

Rowitz, L. (1988b). The forgotten ones: Adolescence and mental retardation. *Mental Retardation, 26,* 115–117.

Rowitz, L. (1989). Trends in mental retardation in the 1990s. *Mental Retardation, 27,* iii–vi.

Part 1
Trends on Conceptual Issues

2
The Impact of Changing Paradigms of Disability on Mental Retardation in the Year 2000

Jane R. Mercer

Scientific thinking in the field of disabilities is moving from the functionalist–objectivist paradigm, which has dominated research and theorizing in the past, to multiparadigmatic thinking and varied conceptual models. This evolution has brought about changes in the definition of mental retardation, which in turn have influenced the characteristics of individuals who are being diagnosed as having this disability and the number and kinds of programs needed to serve them. Before we speculate about the changes that are likely to occur in the field of mental retardation by the year 2000, we must first understand the competing paradigms that have emerged during the past century.

The Nature of Scientific Paradigms

This analysis draws heavily on the seminal work of Kuhn (1970), who first defined scientific paradigms and described the nature of scientific revolutions. Kuhn argues that science is a social enterprise conducted by a community of scientists who create the paradigms that guide their activities as scientists. A scientific paradigm is the fundamental worldview that members of a given scientific community share. It tells them what entities exist in nature and how those entities behave. It includes the beliefs, values, and techniques shared by members of a given scientific community and systematically transmitted to new recruits through standard textbooks, case illustrations, and apprenticeships. In a fundamental sense, a scientific paradigm consists of the assumptions a scientific community makes about the nature of reality and the nature of society, assumptions that may not always be explicitly stated but are passed on as "tacit" knowledge to each new generation of scientists.

Emerging scientific communities tend to be "preparadigmatic," while more mature scientific communities coalesce around a single, dominant paradigm. As "normal science" is conducted within the dominant paradigm, anomalies may appear in the form of scientific findings that were not predicted and cannot be explained within the accepted worldview. When anomalies accumulate, the scientific community is thrown into crisis as scientists attempt to modify the dominant paradigm to account for unanticipated findings. "Extraordinary" science occurs when scientists go outside the traditional, accepted worldview of their scientific communities and create new paradigms in an attempt to better explain anomalous findings, to make better predictions, and to guide future research and practice. New paradigms then compete with the dominant paradigm and with each other for acceptance.

This sequence of events provides an accurate description of the past three decades in the field of disability. Before the 1960s, the scientific community concerned with disability was dominated by a single, functionalist–objectivist paradigm embodied in the medical model. Mental retardation was conceptualized within the psychomedical model, which is a derivative of the medical model. During the 1960s, major anomalies were uncovered when the dominant paradigm was used to diagnose mental retardation in racial and linguistic minorities (Heller, Holtzman, & Messick, 1982; Mercer, 1973). Alternative paradigms were proposed but, predictably, were rejected by the scientific community (Clarizio, 1979; Mercer, 1979b; Reschly, 1978). Nevertheless, anomalies continued to multiply as scientists continued to use the traditional paradigm to guide research and practice. The accumulation of anomalies led, in the 1980s, to more extraordinary science as individual scientists worked to create alternative paradigms that would better explain the natural and social world and would lead to more effective practice. Thus, the field has moved from a single dominant paradigm to multiple paradigms. The status of mental retardation in the year 2000 will depend on the nature of the paradigm or paradigms that become dominant in the field of disability during the decade of the 90s. Following are a brief description of the characteristics of the competing paradigms and an overview of their emergence and history.

Basic Paradigmatic Assumptions

Burrell and Morgan (1979) have proposed two dimensions that can be used to describe the fundamental assumptions of the four major scientific paradigms. Specific theoretical models used in the field of disabilities can be located within these four paradigms. Figure 2.1 presents a modification of Burrell and Morgan's typology (1979, p. 22).

The Nature of Reality: Objectivism Versus Subjectivism

The horizontal axis in Figure 2.1 describes the scientific community's view of the nature of reality, a view that can range from extreme "objectivity"

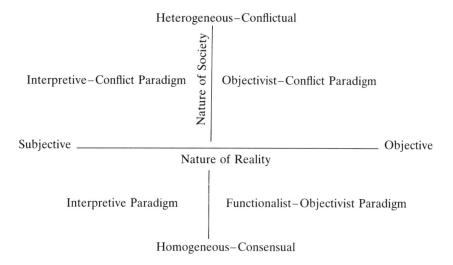

Heterogeneous–Conflictual

Interpretive–Conflict Paradigm   Nature of Society   Objectivist–Conflict Paradigm

Subjective ——————————————————————— Objective
Nature of Reality

Interpretive Paradigm   Functionalist–Objectivist Paradigm

Homogeneous–Consensual

FIGURE 2.1. Typology of four fundamental scientific paradigms. *Note.* From *Sociological Paradigms and Organisational Analysis* (p. 22) by G. Burrell and G. Morgan, 1979, Portsmouth, NH: Heinemann. Copyright 1979 by Heinemann. Adapted by permission.

on the right to extreme "subjectivity" on the left. The objective view sees reality as external to the individual, and as hard, measurable, predictable, and universalistic in meaning. Human nature is deterministic, shaped by heredity and environment, and predictable. Disability models located on the objective end of the horizontal axis assume the facticity of the social world and of disability; that is, they assume that ability and disability exist in the individual as entities that can be measured and diagnosed and that traits such as "intelligence" exist in the individual and can be assessed. For the objectivist, the only acceptable approach to creating knowledge about the world is through positivist, empirical research, and the only acceptable evidence comes through the human senses and must be verifiable and replicable. Experiments are the preferred methodology. Preferred practices are objective categorization, standardized assessment, and direct, standardized instruction.

The subjective view of reality emphasizes the fact that human cognition is the crucial screen through which all experience is interpreted. While it does not deny that there are objects and behaviors that are external to the individual, it insists that such objects and behavior have no intrinsic meaning. Meaning is created though social interaction in which human beings develop consensus about the meanings of various objects, behaviors, and events and develop common beliefs about the way in which individuals should act in regard to them. Human sense organs are capable of responding only to certain stimuli, and all incoming stimuli must be organized cognitively by the individual before they can be experienced as meaningful. Thus, the nature of reality is circumscribed not only by the limitations of human sensory equipment but by the cognitive structures that individuals have developed as part of their socialization to a particular cultural and linguistic system. Although individuals come to see these intersubjective realities as objective and factual, the subjective view takes the position that what individuals view as external reality is highly subjective.

Subjectivism, taken to its extreme, leads to solipsism, the denial of the possibility of any objective reality whatsoever. Subjective models of disability are not that extreme. Proponents of these models insist, however, that "disabilities" are social constructions and that the definition of what constitutes a "disability" not only will vary from society to society but will vary over time in the same society as individuals create and re-create their intersubjective realities. Such realities can be understood by outsiders only through the process of *verstehen*, in which the observer enters the subjective reality of those being studied, participates in their world of meanings, and is able to see the world as they see it. Ethnographies and participant observation are preferred scientific methodologies. Preferred instructional practices include meaning-oriented instruction, personalized learning acts, and individualized assessment.

The Nature of Society: Homogeneity Versus Heterogeneity

The vertical axis of Figure 2.1 deals with basic assumptions about the nature of society. Is society homogeneous or heterogeneous? Is it based on consensus, or is it filled with conflict? Is it basically integrated and stable or conflictual and unstable?

Scientific models that assume societal homogeneity, stability, integration, and functional coordination have been the most common. Proponents of these models assume societies are based on a broad value consensus that provides unity and cohesion. Some theorists use mechanistic analogies that visualize societies as huge machines with many interdependent parts. Each part has its function and contributes to the operation of the whole. When all parts fulfill their proper functions, society operates smoothly. Other theorists use organic analogies that visualize society as a living organism with many interdependent systems. When all systems function properly, there is homeostasis, and society, like a living organism, survives and thrives. When some systems do not function properly, the balance is disturbed, and society suffers.

Theories of disability based on assumptions of societal homogeneity and integration define behaviors that interfere with the smooth operation of society as dysfunctional and persons who behave dysfunctionally as deviant or "disabled." Hence, such theories emphasize the importance of programs and treatments that will make "disabled" persons more functional for society.

The top extreme of the vertical axis in Figure 2.1 sees society as heterogeneous, filled with conflict, unstable, and changing. It focuses on structural cleavages between social classes and ethnic groups and on differences between their social power, their cultural and linguistic backgrounds, and their norms and values. Society is characterized by the struggle for economic and political dominance. Inevitably, more powerful groups dominate less powerful groups and are able to enforce their norms, language, and culture on those who are subordinated. Part of the process of subordination consists of defining the language, behavior, values, and life-style of subordinated groups as unacceptable, thus "disabling" many members of subordinate groups by making them ineligible for full participation in the most desirable roles in society. Viewed as inadequate, they are then treated as surplus populations.

A Typology of Basic Paradigms

The two axes form four basic paradigms. The functionalist–objectivist paradigm, which assumes objective reality and societal homogeneity and integration, is the most widely employed in social science and in the field of disability. The objectivist–conflict paradigm, which assumes objective reality and societal heterogeneity and conflict, is widely used in social science but was first introduced into the field of disabilities during the civil rights era. Similarly, the interpretive paradigm, which assumes that reality is subjective but focuses primarily on mechanisms by which individuals create the consensus that holds society together, did not appear in the field of disabilities until the 1960s, although it has been a popular paradigm in social science since the 1920s, when George Herbert Mead first introduced symbolic interactionism. The interpretive-conflict paradigm with its emphasis on subjective reality and societal conflict has not been used in the field of disabilities and will not be discussed further.

Models of Disability Within the Typology of Paradigms

Figure 2.2 presents seven models of disability that have emerged in the scientific community and places them conceptually within the typology of paradigms. Space permits only a brief description of each of the models, an overview of their major elements, and summary of their impact on

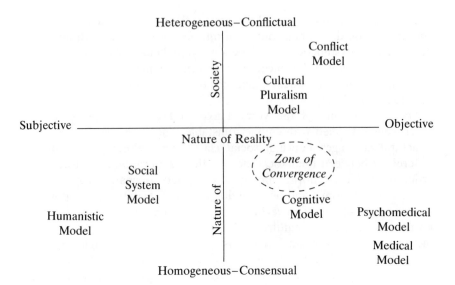

FIGURE 2.2. Seven models of mental retardation within the four fundamental scientific paradigms.

social policy. The models will be presented in historical order to clarify their relationships to each other and to identify the direction of change over the past century. By establishing intellectual trends, we will be in a better position to hypothesize about future developments.

The Medical Model

The earliest model of disability to emerge in the scientific community came from medicine. Initially, the scientific community classified as disabilities only conditions with clear biological components manifested in biological anomalies, such as blindness, deafness, and physical deformity. Only persons with severe behavioral and learning problems were regarded as "feebleminded." The "idiots" and "imbeciles" of the 19th century usually had physical anomalies as well as gross intellectual limitations that were evident even to untrained observers. Their treatment was in the hands of medical practitioners, who were also responsible for certifying placements in special institutions. This situation continued into the early decades of the 20th century.

The medical model occupies an extreme position on both axes in Figure 2.2. It assumes the objective reality of observed symptoms and the facticity of a disabling condition that exists in the individual. It assumes the disability exists, regardless of whether it has been diagnosed, and that it has been caused by factors that can be identified and studied, such as genetic flaws, disease processes, or trauma. Uncovering the cause of the disability through empirical research is essential. Once the cause is known, treatments can be developed, and appropriate preventive measures can be taken. Accurate diagnosis is central to practice because proper treatment depends on correct diagnosis. Different disabilities require different treatments.

The medical model assumes a very high level of societal consensus and homogeneity. Because the human organism is similar in all societies, the cultural setting is not relevant to diagnosis, nor is it a crucial element to prevention or treatment. Diagnoses and treatments are cross-cultural. Because many medical conditions become worse when untreated, there is a strong bias in the medical model toward type 2 errors (finding a disability when none exists) and avoiding type 1 errors (declaring the individual healthy when, in fact, there is unrecognized pathology).

Policy Impact of the Medical Model

As long as the medical model was dominant, the term "feebleminded" was used, and the number of persons diagnosed as feebleminded was small and prevalence rates were low. Medical diagnoses converged with lay diagnoses because most persons labeled as "idiots" or "imbeciles" had obvious physical and behavioral anomalies. Hence, there was no controversy about the diagnostic process and there were no racial or ethnic disproportions in prevalence rates. Viewed as having an incurable medical condition, the feebleminded were placed in custodial institutions initially called "training schools" or "colonies" but later renamed "hospitals." The latter were administered by medical directors.

The medical model has had a pervasive impact on practice in the field of mental retardation. Its emphasis on the centrality of diagnosis, its focus on categorization before treatment, its preference for segregated settings where treatment can be administered by experts, and its insistence on certification of eligibility through diagnosis by experts before treatment is made available are tacit knowledge in the field of mental retardation. From it flows the focus on cause, the assumption that there is a biological basis to all disability, the rejection of social and cultural factors as relevant to diagnosis, the bias toward type 2 errors, and the belief that treatment is benign.

The Psychomedical Model

The psychomedical model of disability also occupies the extreme lower right corner of the typology of paradigms in Figure 2.2. It is an extension of the medical model in which a statistical definition of "normal" is superimposed on the basic premises of the medical model. The psychomedical model emerged with the advent of "intelligence" testing in the first decade of the 20th century and continued to be refined for the following seven decades. Its ultimate contours were most clearly delineated by Jensen (1980).

The psychomedical model assumes that "IQ" tests measure "intelligence," a highly heritable trait that is relatively stable throughout an individual's lifetime because it is based on the biological substrate. Hence, a low score on an IQ test can be interpreted within a medical model as a symptom of mental subnormality, a hard, objective scientific fact. Indeed, soon after the introduction of IQ tests in the United States, Goddard identified and named a new class of feebleminded persons not formerly recognized because they did not have biological stigmata— "morons" who scored above "idiots and imbeciles" but below "normals" (mental age 12 and above) on IQ tests (cited in Doll, 1962). Soon, the existence of "morons" was accepted as an objective scientific fact.

When standardized tests of academic achievement were later introduced, it was assumed that they measure what the individual has learned, while IQ tests measure "intelligence," that is, what a person is capable of learning. In the psychomedical model, "intelligence" and "achievement" are treated as dimensions that can be separated both conceptually and operationally. It argues that IQ tests are valid measures of "intelligence" because they accurately predict performance on "achievement" tests. Correlations between them vary between .80 and .90 (Jensen, 1980, p. 323). Further proof of their validity is that IQ tests correlate highly with each other, having an overall mean correlation of about .67 (Jensen, 1980, p. 315).

When IQ testing was challenged for alleged "cultural bias," the scientific community of measurement psychologists argued that IQ tests are not culturally biased because they have similar predictive validity for persons of different cultural backgrounds, that is, the regression lines predicting academic achievement test scores from IQ test scores have similar slopes for different groups (Cleary, Humphreys, Kendrick, & Wesman, 1975). Subsequently, this argument was further elaborated with the claim that IQ tests are not culturally biased because they have comparable internal validity for different groups, that is, comparable reliability and stability, similar patterning of item difficulty levels, and similar factor structures (Jensen, 1980; Sandoval, 1979). The fact that some ethnic groups earn higher average scores on IQ tests than others is not regarded as an indication of bias in the tests. Such differences are interpreted as evidence that some groups have more "intelligence" than others. Finally, proponents of the psychomedical model specifically argue that society is culturally homogeneous and that a single set of norms is appropriate for all groups (Cleary et al., 1975; Jensen, 1980).

Policy Impact of the Psychomedical Model

The policy impact of the psychomedical model was immediate and profound. Mass testing of military recruits in World War I, which found millions of morons in the general population, led to widespread concern about the future of the nation and the deterioration of the national gene pool. The identification of thousands of "morons," especially among poor, migrant, non-English–speaking populations, led to the establishment of immigration quotas by national origin (Kamin, 1974; Mercer & Richardson, 1975). Large numbers of "morons" found in delinquent and prison populations created major concerns about the "menace of the feebleminded," which led to their widespread institutionalization and sterilization and fed the eugenics movement.

The social situation following World War II was auspicious for extending the psychomedical model into the public schools and medicalizing the educational problems of "backward" students. The terms *feebleminded* and *morons* had been replaced by the less pejorative *mental retardation*. Persons labeled as mentally retarded were no longer perceived as a social menace. A large influx of migrants from the rural South and from Mexico had created a burgeoning population of students who had difficulty mastering the standard public school curriculum. Large urban centers faced the problem of financing programs for such children. Special education for the physically handicapped, blind, deaf, and cerebral palsied was well established, and categorical funding based on the medical model was an accepted practice. Because many "backward" children were not only failing academically but also scored as "morons" on IQ tests, it was a simple matter to identify them as "mentally retarded" and to argue that they also needed special categorically funded programs to treat their disability.

During the 1950s and 1960s, the number of children diagnosed as "mentally retarded" and placed in special programs in the public schools increased exponentially and soon greatly outnumbered students with identifiable biological anomalies. One major consequence of applying the psychomedical model in the public schools was that disproportionately large numbers of children who had no biological stigmata but were from racial, ethnic, and linguistic minorities were diagnosed as "educable mentally retarded." These disproportions were accepted as objective facts by the psychometric community, although such disproportions appeared only among "morons" (now relabeled "educable mentally retarded") and did not appear among students with physical handicaps or among very low-functioning students with biological stigmata diagnosed as "trainable mentally retarded"—the "idiots" and "imbeciles" of yesteryear (Mercer, 1973).

The Social System Model of Disability

The interpretive paradigm was first used to conceptualize mental retardation in the 1960s when the social system model of mental retardation was introduced (Mercer, 1973). Rather than seeing mental retardation as a condition having universalistic meaning, the social system model sees it as a subjective cognition, a social construction emerging from social interactions in which social actors evaluate each other's behavior in relation to socially agreed on norms as to what constitutes "intelligent" behavior. Persons in society develop a consensus on what they consider to be "normal" or "intelligent" behavior, and that consensus becomes part of their intersubjective reality. The nature of the intersubjective reality that they create is not predetermined. From the perspective of the interpretive paradigm, mental retardation is a socially constructed category. At the level of the individual, it is an achieved social status, albeit a devalued, deviant one. Sociologists see the acquisition of any deviant social status as a social process involving at least two persons: the rule breaker, whose behavior or demeanor violates social norms, and the definer(s). The deviance process goes through two distinct stages. Primary deviance occurs when the actor behaves and the definer evaluates that behavior as violating some social norm and communicates that negative evaluation to the rule breaker and/or to others. At this juncture, the rule breaker may change his or her behavior to conform to the social norm, thus terminating the deviance process. If not, the definer and/or others may try to "normalize" the rule breaker's behavior informally by applying positive and/or negative sanctions. This failing, the rule breaker may be referred to agencies that have been given authority by society to determine whether the norms have been violated, the nature of the violation, and the appropriate societal response. Law enforcement and the courts, psychiatric clinics, and psychological assessment systems in the public schools are examples of such evaluating agencies. They have the power to alter the individual's life career by assignment to a deviant status (mental patient, criminal, delinquent, or "mental retardate"). Such assignments typically result in the person being perceived and treated as a deviant by others with whom they interact and being accorded the social stigma associated with their particular status. The final stage of the deviance process, secondary deviance, is reached when the individual accepts the deviant status as appropriate and incorporates the deviant role into the self-system. Of course, the deviance process may be aborted at any point, depending on various contingencies. The role of the social scientist is to study the deviance process and the various contingencies that result in some persons being defined as "disabled" while others are not.

Rather than accepting disproportionate rates of disability among minority populations as an objective, empirical fact, the interpretive paradigm sees it as a result of the manner in which the deviance process operates in society. Individuals and groups with the greatest social power have the greatest influence on the consensus formation, which creates the intersubjective reality that guides societal action. They are able to establish their view of "normal" behavior as the societal standard against which everyone will be judged. Inevitably, members of the dominant group will be advantaged because those standards will reflect their values, beliefs, language, and customs while nondominant groups will be disadvantaged. Because the scientists who devised IQ tests were members of the dominant English-speaking group in American society, they created tests that covered the linguistic and cognitive skills valued by their own group and normed them on populations consisting primarily of members of their own group. Inevitably, outsiders, such as racial and linguistic minorities, do less well on such tests than members of the dominant group and earn lower average scores because they do not share the same intersubjective reality. Consequently, they are more likely to be labeled as "mentally retarded."

The social system model of mental retardation differs profoundly from the psychomedical model. Where the psychomedical model sees "mental retardation" as an objective, empirical fact, the social system model sees it as a social construction. Because the definition of "mental retardation" is socially negotiated, it not only varies from society to society but changes over time. Where the psychomedical model sees "mental retardation" as a disability that one "has," the interpretive model sees it as a status that one holds as a result of a variety of social contingencies. A person can be "retarded" in one group and not in another. Retardation is a social enactment.

Policy Impact of the Social System Model

The social system model operating within the interpretive paradigm is value neutral. It takes no position for or against any particular set of tests, norms, or assessment procedures. It does not favor one intersubjective reality over another. It does not pass judgment on the "correctness" or "validity" of the outcomes of the deviance process it describes. To do so would be inconsistent with its own premises. Nevertheless, the very act of applying an interpretive analysis to professional practices conducted within the functionalist–objectivist paradigm was perceived by many of those operating from that paradigm as an attack on those practices. Furthermore, civil rights advocates were quick to use the interpretive perspective to build legal arguments on behalf of minority students placed in special education classes. If the meaning of mental retardation has been socially negotiated and has changed over time, then that meaning can be renegotiated. If diagnoses are social constructions rather than "facts," then they are open to dispute. Whose intersubjective reality shall prevail?

By emphasizing the deviance process and the stigmatization that accompanies placement in any kind of a devalued status, the interpretive paradigm directly challenged the assumption of the psychomedical model that type-2 errors are preferable to type-1 errors in making diagnoses. Overdiagnosis, formerly seen as benign because it provided special education services to children having educational difficulties, was redefined as malignant because it stigmatized persons who were not disabled by assigning them to a disesteemed social status and by triggering a deviant career. Hence, the social system model of mental retardation provided the rationale for challenging current diagnostic practices, especially in relation to racial and ethnic minorities, both in the academic community and in the courts.

The Cultural Pluralism Model of Mental Retardation

The cultural pluralism model is an objectivist view of mental retardation that takes into account societal heterogeneity and cleavages. Thus, it is located toward the heterogeneous–conflictual end of the vertical axis and the objectivist end of the horizontal axis in Figure 2.2. Like the psychomedical model, it assumes the facticity of mental retardation and operates on the assumption that some persons are "really" mentally retarded. Unlike the psychomedical model, it assumes that society is heterogeneous and contains racial, ethnic, and cultural cleavages. As a result of these social cleavages, it is impossible for the psychomedical model, which assumes social homogeneity, to accurately separate members of minority groups into those who are "really" retarded and those who are not. The solution to this dilemma is to modify the psychomedical model to take into account societal diversity.

The cultural pluralism model of mental retardation proposes two primary modifications in the psychomedical model. First, instead of relying exclusively on the IQ test, diagnosis includes a measure of the individual's social adaptation to their own social group. For children, this means securing information from the mother on the child's performance in a variety of social settings. If children are performing well in nonacademic environments, that is accepted as evidence that they are not mentally retarded, even though they may have academic difficulties in school and may score in the subnormal range on IQ tests.

The second method used to differentiate those who are "really" mentally retarded from those who only appear to be retarded among cultural minorities is to use multiple normative frameworks for interpreting the IQ test score. Each individual's performance is compared with that of others from similar linguistic, educational, and cultural backgrounds. Their "intelligence" is then inferred by comparing what they have learned about the language, information, and skills covered in the test with that learned by others who have had similar opportunities to learn those materials (Mercer, 1979a,b). The standard test norms currently used to infer "intelligence" are not to be used to infer the "intelligence" of children from minority sociocultural groups. Their performance relative to those standard norms is used to make first-level inferences about their current functioning level relative to the dominant society. Only sociocultural norms are used to make second-level inferences about their "intelligence."

The System of Multicultural Pluralistic Assessment (SOMPA), based on the pluralistic model, was developed for Anglo, Hispanic, and African American children 5 through 11 years of age (Mercer, 1979b). It measures each child's adaptive behavior based on an extensive, standardized interview with the child's mother. Significantly, the average adaptive behavior score of children from Anglo, Hispanic, and African American backgrounds is almost identical. There is no need for separate sociocultural norms for the three groups in making assessments of adaptive behavior. SOMPA also provides sensitive sociocultural norms for the Wechsler Intelligence Scale for Children—Revised (WISC—R) administered in English (Wechsler, 1974). Sociocultural norms are also available for the same test administered in Spanish and normed in Mexico (Gomez-Palacio, Padilla, & Roll, 1984). These norms are based on the linguistic, educational, and cultural characteristics of each child's family. Only the sociocultural norms are used to make inferences about the child's "intelligence."

Policy Impact of the Pluralistic Model

Sociocultural norms for the IQ test and the measurement of adaptive behavior eliminates ethnic disproportions when used to diagnose mental retardation (Mercer, 1979b). Inevitably, they also greatly reduce the total number of children diagnosed as mentally retarded because they are reducing type-2 errors—that is, reducing the number of children diagnosed as mentally retarded who are not, in fact, retarded. Those diagnosed as mentally retarded using the SOMPA are very similar to the very low-functioning persons who were labeled as "feebleminded" before the introduction of the psychomedical model.

Predictably, the pluralistic model was rejected by those committed to the psychomedical model (Clarizio, 1979) and by those concerned about possible shrinkage in the size of special education programs (Reschly, 1978). Some critics, misunderstanding the premises of the cultural pluralism model, argued that separate norms were demeaning to minority groups because they implied that minorities were not as "intelligent" as persons in culturally dominant groups. Others argued that multiple norms were not necessary because all social groups in American society have approximately equal access to the cultural mainstream (Jensen, 1980). Some contended sociocultural norms are not necessary because current tests are not culturally biased (Cleary et al., 1975; Jensen, 1980; Reschly, 1978; Sandoval, 1979). Others took the position that it is impossible to measure adaptive behavior reliably and that the multidimensional view should be abandoned (Cleary et al., 1975; Zigler, Balla, & Hodapp, 1984). One critic, operating from the interpretive paradigm, argued that "tissue is not the issue" and faulted the SOMPA for assuming that mental retardation is an objective reality that can be diagnosed, given culturally sensitive instruments (Goodman, 1979).

Although the SOMPA was adopted in some states and several thousand psychologists were trained to use the system, the cultural pluralism model of mental retardation has never been widely accepted. Although it is based on objectivist assumptions, it moves further into the conflict paradigm than the scientific community has been prepared to go.

The Conflict Model

The conflict paradigm was introduced into the field of mental retardation during the civil rights era at approximately the same time as the social system and cultural pluralism models were being proposed. It formed the basis for the complaints filed by advocates for minority groups in the legislative and judicial battles over the disproportionately large numbers of minority students, especially African American and Hispanic, who were being placed in classes for the mentally retarded.

As can be seen in Figure 2.2, the conflict model of mental retardation, like the psychomedical model, accepts the objective reality of mental retardation as a disability. However, it does not view society as homogeneous and consensual. Rather, it sees the social structure as filled with linguistic, racial, and social class cleavages and, instead of consensus, sees a continual struggle for dominance and power among various groups. The groups who prevail are able to make their language, values, beliefs, and cultural systems the standard for the entire society and the yardstick by which all members of the society are judged. Dominant groups determine the language of instruction and content of the curriculum of the schools, which exist as an instrument to preserve their social and economic dominance. They determine the language and content of the tests used in public education and the categories to which students will be assigned. Consequently, persons from nondominant groups are disadvantaged in gaining access to the educational and economic resources of the society. Through the standardized testing and sorting that takes place in the schools, they are systematically devalued, oppressed, and discriminated against (Bowles & Gintis, 1972–1973; Gould, 1981; Kamin, 1974; Karier, Violas, & Spring, 1973).

From this perspective, the categories of "moron," "educable mentally retarded," and "mildly mentally handicapped"—categories defined entirely by low test scores rather than biological symptoms—are used as mechanisms to control racial and cultural minorities and persons from the lower classes.

In short, IQ tests are culturally biased against racial and ethnic minorities and persons from lower social classes. Placing subordinate groups in special classes that stigmatize them as inferior and provide them with limited educational opportunities is simply discrimination legitimated by "scientific" testing. If tests are tools for discrimination and segregation, there is but one remedy—abolish the tests and the segregated classes.

Policy Impact of the Conflict Model

Needless to say, the conflict model of mental retardation has never been accepted by the scientific community of measurement psychology because it sees them as the intelligentsia providing scientific legitimacy to the administration of culturally biased tests that discriminate against social and cultural minorities. However, the conflict model of mental retardation formed the philosophic basis for the class action suits against the state of California filed on behalf of Hispanic and African American students who had been placed in classes for the mentally retarded using their scores on IQ tests as the main criterion (*Diana v. California Board of Education*, 1969; *Larry P. et al. v. Wilson Riles*, 1979). Consequently, the conflict model has had a profound influence on public policy. Civil rights lawyers argued that IQ tests are culturally biased against minority children, have not been validated for identifying mental retardation in minority children, and have been used to deprive minority children of an equal educational opportunity by segregating them into dead-end special education programs with a limited curriculum.

In *Larry P. et al. v. Wilson Riles* (1979), the scientific community responded to these complaints by presenting the major postulates of the psychomedical model. Early in the trial, the defense attorney rejected a compromise settlement that would have permitted the state to use sociocultural norms and adaptive behavior measures when assessing minority children, the approach proposed in the cultural pluralism model and operationalized in the SOMPA. Such an abrupt paradigm shift was unthinkable. Instead, she presented testimony from the most elite members of the measurement community, testimony that presented the psychomedical view of mental retardation. Operating from the assumptions of the functional–objectivist paradigm, she argued that the mental retardation diagnosed in the plaintiffs was an objective fact and that the treatments offered by the schools were beneficial and nonstigmatizing.

Nevertheless, the court found in favor of the plaintiffs in *Larry P.* (1979) and banned the use of IQ tests in the identification and placement of black students in classes for the mentally retarded in the state of California (Bersoff, 1980; Elliott, 1987). *Diana v. California Board of Education* (1969) was also settled, out of court, on terms acceptable to the plaintiffs. Subsequently, the prohibition was further expanded until, today, IQ testing is not permitted in the evaluation and placement of minority students in any type of special education programs in California. Some cities with large minority populations, such as New York and Chicago, have also prohibited IQ testing, and the ban appears to be spreading gradually to other cities and states.

The Cognitive Model

A cognitive model of learning difficulties has recently become popular in the scientific community (Feuerstein, 1979; Gelsheiser & Shepherd, 1986). Although there are various versions of this model, they are sufficiently similar to treat them as a single conceptual framework. They fall within the functional–objectivist paradigm, lying slightly to the left of the psychomedical model along the objective–subjective axis (see Figure 2.2). The cognitive model is not based on the medical model and is not closely tied to statistical definitions of normal. Like the psychomedical model, however, it takes an objectivist view of reality and a consensual view of society. Attributes such as learning problems, learning strategies, motivational attributions, and cognitive skills are perceived as objective realities. Thus, this model fits easily into traditional worldviews, and persons schooled in the psychomedical model can adopt the cognitive model without making a paradigmatic shift. Many have done so.

Persons operating from the cognitive model tend to attribute learning difficulties to inefficient learning strategies resulting from insufficient mediated learning rather than to some biologically based disability. They assume that learning will improve when the learner becomes actively involved in the learning process and uses effective learning strategies. The role of assessment is to identify the student's motivational status and to analyze the learning strategies that the student is currently using. The role of instruction is to modify the student's motivational status and to teach the student more efficient learning strategies.

Because standardized achievement and IQ tests provide only information on the end products of learning, they are not seen as very useful. Instead, assessment in the cognitive model generally involves an attempt to study how the student processes information in a learning situation and typically follows some type of test-mediate-observe-retest approach. By observing the learning process itself, the assessor can determine the extent to which a student profits from instruction, can question the student about strategies used in solving different types of problems, and can ascertain the extent to which the student's lack of confidence in the efficacy of employing various learning strategies may be a factor in failure to learn.

Cognitive psychologists have identified three major categories of cognitive processes that are important in efficient self-regulated learning. One category consists of metacognitive skills that make individuals aware of their own thinking processes. These skills include evaluating a novel problem to determine what kind of plan is reasonable, deciding what to do if the plan fails, checking one's own performance, being actively involved in identifying various learning options, modifying one's behavior when a strategy proves inefficient, and so forth. A second category consists of specific cognitive skills that are useful in particular learning tasks. For example, the following are some effective strategies to improve reading comprehension: rereading a passage; skimming a passage to study it; paraphrasing a main idea to summarize important points; identifying the topic sentence; writing a topic sentence for paragraphs that have no topic sentence; hypothesizing about what topic will be discussed next, asking oneself questions while reading, and so forth. Intervention involves directly teaching students the appropriate strategies for the learning task rather than expecting students to discover those strategies on their own.

Motivation is the third major category in the cognitive model. If the assessor finds motivational problems, then attributional retraining is initiated to convince the student that the lack of learning is the result of inefficient learning strategies and low effort rather than low ability.

Policy Impact of the Cognitive Model

The switch to a cognitive model from the psychomedical model has important implications, even though both are well within the functional–objectivist paradigm. Persons using a cognitive model see children who are having academic difficulties differently than those who use a psychomedical model. They do not see such children as disabled, in a medical sense, and reserve the term "mental retardation" to describe only very low-functioning children who usually have physical anomalies as well as learning problems. They assume most normal-bodied children can learn if they can be motivated to apply themselves and are taught effective learning strategies. The categories "educable mentally retarded," "borderline mentally retarded," and "mildly mentally retarded" atrophy. They disappear from the thoughts and vocabularies of persons using a cognitive model because they serve no purpose in that model.

Equally important, the cognitive model, unlike the psychomedical model, addresses the issue of motivation positively rather than negatively. Diagnostic labeling in the psychomedical model encourages negative self-attributions, undermines self-esteem, and fosters secondary deviance by convincing the student, teacher, and family that the child has low ability. Thus, IQ testing compounds children's learning difficulties by convincing them that it is useless to make an effort to learn. Children whose self-esteem is already low because of repeated academic failures are deprived of any motivation to make a vigorous effort to learn when they are told that their failures are the result of deficiencies that cannot be remedied. Cognitive models, on the other hand, see these very negative self-attributions as important elements causing academic failure, elements that must be reversed through attributional retraining before children can be motivated to make the strenuous effort required for successful learning. Children must believe they *can* learn before they will make the effort to use the cognitive strategies that make learning possible. This movement away from medical model thinking is a major break with the past.

The Humanistic Model

Recently, the functionalist–objectivist view of mental retardation has faced a new challenge from the interpretive paradigm. The humanistic model is even more subjective in its assumptions about reality than the social system model. It emphasizes the uniqueness of each individual child, the importance of getting inside the child's world and understanding the child's reality, and the necessity of tailoring instruction to the specific interests and needs of each child. It abhors standardized assessment, that compares children with each other. It focuses on their individualities rather than their similarities. It rejects objectivist thinking, which places children into categories and divides their wholeness into measurable traits, attributes, abilities, and disabilities. It sees reality as holistic and relationships as nonlinear. Organisms are open systems (Heshusius, 1988; Poplin, 1984).

The humanistic model opposes direct, standardized instruction that treats children as undifferentiated objects. It advocates highly individualized instruction based on sensitive, interpersonal interaction between student and teacher in a warm and caring environment.

Policy Impact of the Humanistic Model

It is too soon to know what the impact of the humanistic model will be on the field of mental retardation. Its power lies in its affirmation of the worth and individuality of each student and each teacher and its rejection of categorization, standardization, and mechanization. It goes well beyond the cognitive model in this respect and adds momentum to the movement away from the psychomedical model of disabilities and mental retardation, away from categorization and placement, and away from standardized testing and measurement. It has faith that good things will happen if teachers are given the autonomy necessary to accept real ownership in their tasks and the freedom to work with each individual child in an open-ended, naturalistic manner. It places responsibility for learning outcomes squarely on the teacher.

Mental Retardation in the Year 2000

Mental retardation, which once was a field based on a single paradigm, has become multiparadigmatic. There is little agreement on the nature of the phenomenon being studied and, consequently, little agreement on treatments. People talk past each other because they are operating from different assumptions. The field is in the midst of a scientific revolution.

While I hesitate to predict the outcome of that revolution, there are strong underlying intellectual currents that portend future directions.

During the early 20th century, the field of mental retardation moved from a medical model to a psychomedical model, which dominated the field for most of the century. Both are located in the most extreme corner of the functionalist–objectivist paradigm. After midcentury, the psychomedical model was challenged by the interpretive paradigm—the social system model and, more recently, the humanistic model. In the 1970s, challenges appeared from models based in the conflict paradigm—first, the cultural pluralism model and, soon after, the conflict model. The historic movement in the field has been toward the greater subjectivity of the interpretive paradigm and the greater recognition of societal heterogeneity of the conflict paradigm.

The recent popularity of the cognitive model is the response of "normal science" to these undercurrents. The cognitive model is slightly more subjective and somewhat more pluralistic than the psychomedical model but is still securely anchored in the functionalist–objectivist paradigm. Accepting a cognitive model does not require a paradigm shift, only a shift in models within the same paradigm. Nevertheless, the shift is in the general direction of greater subjectivity, less standardization and categorization, and more attention to individual differences.

Although the trend toward a more interpretive view of reality and toward more sensitivity to societal heterogeneity will be impeded by the fact that the psychomedical model is built into federal and state statutes, we can anticipate that the trend will continue through the coming decade. By the year 2000, the field will undoubtedly be multiparadigmatic and the center of intellectual gravity will have moved toward the location in Figure 2.2 where the two axes cross—a general location indicated by the circle. This movement will probably have an effect on assessment, categorization, prevalence, and educational programming for those children who have been classified as mentally retarded by the psychomedical model.

Changes in Assessment

Assessment will gradually become more truly multidimensional rather than pseudomultidimensional. Although there have been statutory requirements for multidimensional assessment since the 1970s, the measurement community has systematically resisted these mandates by conducting assessments in which multiple tests are given (several "achievement" tests and several IQ tests), but all tests are measuring the same dimension— cognitive skills in English. Assessments seldom measure cognitive skills in languages other than English. They have not included measures of social competence in a variety of social situations, measures of motivational status, measures of physical dexterity and coordination, or measures of health and physical well-being. Nor have they included measures of the environment, either at home or at school. Sociocultural factors have been totally ignored. By the year 2000, pseudo-multidimensional assessment will no longer be acceptable. Pressure from the interpretive paradigm will insist on more humanistic evaluations of children in their individual social environments. Pressure from the conflict paradigm will insist that socio-cultural and linguistic differences be taken into account when interpreting the meaning of particular performances.

A second important change in assessment will be a gradual decline in the belief that disabilities can be diagnosed by studying patterns of stan-dardized test scores. Even staunch defenders of the psychomedical model, such as Jensen, have now conceded that "achievement" and "intelligence" are indistinguishable and that "achievement" tests and "intelligence" tests are measuring the same dimensions of performance (Jensen, 1989). When the premise that "intelligence" and "achievement" can be measured separately is removed from the psychomedical model, the entire model collapses. "Intelligence" testing is no longer intellec-tually or operationally defensible.

Nevertheless, "intelligence" testing will undoubtedly persist to some extent throughout the next decade. There is always a lag between changes in scientific models and changes in practice. It takes time to change statutory requirements and training programs. It takes time for individ-uals to unlearn outmoded ways of thinking and to learn alternative approaches. Eventually, however, the notion that we can measure "intel-ligence" separately from achievement will die. It no longer has any major defenders in the scientific community. To the extent that they are used at all, psychometric assessments by the year 2000 will include only stan-dardized measures of achievement, and there will be no pretense of measuring "intelligence" as a separate dimension.

Changes in Categorization

If "intelligence" tests and "achievement" tests simply measure the same dimensions of performance, then it is not possible for the diagnostician to differentiate between "low achievers" and the "mentally retarded," between ignorance and stupidity. This is precisely the conclusion reached by Judge Peckham after hearing testimony in *Larry P.* (1979). Further-more, if IQ and achievement tests measure the same dimensions, diag-nosticians cannot differentiate between "low achievers" and the "learning disabled" simply by looking at the discrepancy between "intelligence" and "achievement" test scores. If disabilities can no longer be defined simply as patterns of standardized test scores, then categories of disability such as "moron," "educable mental retardation," "borderline mental retardation," and "mild mental retardation" are no longer useful. They will disappear.

Changes in Prevalence and the Reemergence of the Medical Model

The gradual demise of the psychomedical model, hastened by litigation, has already had an impact on prevalence rates for "mental retardation." In many educational jurisdictions, very few children are being diagnosed as "educable mentally retarded," and those who are being diagnosed generally have some type of clear biological involvement. The rates for "trainable mental retardation" (moderate, severe, and profound retardation) remain unaffected. They are the "feebleminded" (idiots and imbeciles), who have been recognized for centuries without benefit of "intelligence" testing. Those who are labeled are identified primarily with the medical model.

We can anticipate that this trend will continue. It will be accelerated as truly multidimensional assessments are used, because the more knowledge diagnosticians have about an individual the more likely they are to discover motivational, cultural, environmental, and educational factors that explain the individual's low performance and the less likely they are to place the person in that residual category of unknown cause, "educable mentally retarded." Such are the results when diagnosticians use the SOMPA. We would expect similar results when diagnosticians use any multidimensional assessment. Consequently, "mental retardation" will increasingly become a category consisting of persons whose low performance has clear biological origins, a category once again conceptualized within the medical model. The medical model will reemerge as the primary model in the field of mental retardation.

Changes in Treatment

What then happens to those formerly labeled "educable mentally retarded"—those whose only clinical symptom consisted of a low score on an IQ test?

During the past decade, some students formerly classified as educable mentally retarded have been reclassified as "learning disabled," using the psychomedical model. Others, who did not show a "significant discrepancy" between "intelligence" and "achievement," were returned to the regular classroom without additional services. An anomaly of the psychomedical model is that, under present definitions, those who score low only on one test, an "achievement" test, are eligible for extra assistance as "learning disabled," while those who score low on two tests ("achievement" and "intelligence") are not eligible for any special education services at all!

With the demise of the psychomedical model, we can anticipate that "learning disability" defined solely by psychometric discrepancies will also bifurcate. Only those few individuals who have clearly identified biological problems, such as dyslexia, will continue to be defined as "learning disabled." Like mental retardation, "learning disability" will also return to the medical model, where it first originated (Coles, 1987). The large majority of persons now diagnosed as "learning disabled" using the psychomedical model will no longer be so categorized, because their difficulties have no substantiated biological source. In addition, persons formerly diagnosed as "mentally retarded" with the psychomedical model will no longer be reclassified as "learning disabled." Thus, the prevalence rate for "learning disability" will shrink, just as the rate for mental retardation has already declined.

What will happen to those persons who are having learning difficulties in the regular classroom but are no longer perceived as "disabled" and no longer qualify for special education services as either "mentally retarded" or "learning disabled"? They are better conceptualized within the cognitive model of the functional–objectivist paradigm and/or the humanistic model of the interpretive paradigm. Multidimensional assessment can assist educators in locating the sources of their learning difficulties. Are their learning difficulties the result of cultural and linguistic differences? motivational problems? ineffective cognitive strategies? disadvantaged home environment? negative academic environment? lack of an interested, caring adult? poor social skills? With a full array of useful information, teachers will be better able to plan an appropriate program of intervention and personalized instruction.

We anticipate that by the year 2000 there will be two dominant paradigmatic clusters: the medical model in the most extreme corner of the functional–objectivist paradigm and some amalgam of the interpretive and conflict paradigms. With the psychomedical model gone, the medical model will reemerge as the basis for diagnosing and treating both mental retardation and learning disability. The functional–objectivist paradigm will continue to be dominant for this relatively small number of persons.

For the large majority of persons with learning difficulties, the paradigm will have shifted toward the intersection of the two axes in Figure 2.2. Although the details of this multiparadigmatic model are difficult to foresee, the new model will be located in the vicinity of the social system model and will include many elements of the cognitive, humanistic, and cultural pluralism models. The scientific community will become more comfortable with multiparadigmatic thinking and will use the model most appropriate for understanding the needs of each individual. Freed of the rigidities and blind spots of the psychomedical model, scientists and educators will find ways of conceptualizing the learning difficulties of children in our increasingly complex world that will lead to more effective educational programs.

References

Bersoff, D. N. (1980). Larry P. v. Riles: Legal perspective. *School Psychology Review, 9*(2), 112–122.

Bowles, S., & Gintis, H. (November/December, 1972–1973 January/February, 1973). I. Q. in the U. S. class structure. *Social Policy*, pp. 65–99.

Burrell, G., & Morgan G. (1979). *Sociological paradigms and organisational analysis*. Portsmouth, NH: Heinemann.

Clarizio, H. F. (1979). In defense of the IQ test. *School Psychology Digest, 8,* 79–88.

Cleary, T. A., Humphreys, L. G., Kendrick, S. A., & Wesman, A. G. (1975). Educational uses of tests with disadvantaged students. *American Psychologist, 30,* 15–41.

Coles, G. (1987). *The learning mystique: A critical look at "learning disabilities."* New York: Pantheon Books.

Diana v. California State Board of Education (1969). United States District Court, Northern District of California, C-70 37 RFP.

Doll, E. E. (1962). A historical survey of research and management of mental retardation in the United States. In E. P. Trapp & P. Himelstein (Eds.), *Readings on the exceptional child* (pp. 47–97). New York: Appleton-Century-Crofts.

Elliott, R. (1987). *Litigating intelligence*. Dover, MA: Auburn House.

Feuerstein, R. (1979). *The dynamic assessment of retarded performers*. Baltimore, MD: University Park Press.

Gelzheiser, L. M., & Shepherd, M. J. (Eds.). (1986). Competence and instruction: Contributions from cognitive psychology [Special issue]. *Exceptional Children, 53*(2).

Gomez-Palacio, M., Padilla, E. R., & Roll, S. (1984). *WISC-RM. Estandarizacion de la Bateria de Pruebas SOMPA en Mexico D.F.: Informe sobre teoria y resultados*. Mexico, DF: Direccion General de Educacion Especial.

Goodman, J. F. (1979). Is tissue the issue? A critique of SOMPA's models and tests. *The School Psychology Digest, 8*(1), 47–62.

Gould, S. J. (1981). *The mismeasure of man*. New York: W. W. Norton.

Heller, K. A., Holtzman, W. H., & Messick, S. (1982). *Placing children in special education: A strategy for equity*. Washington, DC: National Academy Press.

Heshusius, L. (1988). The arts, science, and the study of exceptionality. *Exceptional children, 55*(1), 60–65.

Jensen, A. R. (1980). *Bias in mental testing*. New York: The Free Press.

Jensen, A. R. (1989). *Psychometric "g" and manifest achievement*. Report for the National Commission on Testing and Public Policy funded by the Ford Foundation.

Kamin, L. J. (1974). *The science and politics of I. Q.* New York: John Wiley & Sons.

Karier, C. J., Violas, P. C., & Spring, J. (1973). *Roots of crisis: American education in the twentieth century*. Chicago: Rand McNally College.

Kuhn, T. S. (1970). *The structure of scientific revolutions* (2nd ed.). Chicago: University of Chicago Press.

Larry P. et al. v. Wilson Riles, Superintendent of Public Instruction for the State of California et al., C71 2270 REP (U.S. District Court for the Northern District of California, 1979).

Meyen, E. L., & Skrtic, T. M. (Eds.) (1988). *Exceptional children and youth* (3rd ed.). Denver, CO: Love Publishing.

Mercer, J. R. (1973). *Labeling the mentally retarded.* Berkeley, CA: University of California Press.

Mercer, J. R. (1979a). In defense of racially and culturally nondiscriminatory assessment. *The School Psychology Digest, 8*(1), 89–115.

Mercer, J. R. (1979b). *SOMPA: Technical and conceptual manual.* New York: Psychological Corporation.

Mercer, J. R., & Richardson, J. G. (1975). Mental retardation as a social problem. In N. Hobbs (Ed.), *Issues in the classification of children: Vol. 2. A sourcebook on categories, labels, and their consequences* (pp. 463–496). San Francisco: Jossey-Bass.

Poplin, M. (1984). Toward an holistic view of persons with learning disabilities. *Learning Disability Quarterly, 7*, 290–294.

Reschly, D. J. (1978). WISC-R factor structure among Anglos, blacks, Chicanos, and native American Papagos. *Journal of Consulting and Clinical Psychology, 46*, 417–422.

Sandoval, J. (1979). The WISC-R and internal evidence of test bias with minority groups. *Journal of Consulting and Clinical Psychology, 47*(5), 919–927.

Wechsler, D. (1974). *Manual for the Wechsler Intelligence Scale for Children— Revised.* New York: Psychological Corporation.

Zigler, E., Balla, D., & Hodapp, R. (1984). On the definition and classification of mental retardation. *American Journal of Mental Deficiency, 89*(3), 215–230.

3
Ethics and Mental Retardation: Steps Toward the Ethics of Community

Paul R. Dokecki

What kind of ethical community will we have in the year 2000? What will be the nature of the social interactions between persons with mental retardation and the rest of us? (Does it already prejudice the case to base ethical questions on the distinction between "them" and "us"?) What role will those of "us" in the professional community play in shaping this social world? Specifically, will mental retardation researchers, scholars, and professionals be willing and able to contribute significantly to ethical discourse in the community?

Initial insights concerning the future of ethics and mental retardation may be derived from two sources outside the field. First, it is impressive how many different people from diverse disciplines have cited *Habits of the Heart* (Bellah, Madsen, Sullivan, Swidler, & Tipton, 1985). In that work, Robert Bellah and colleagues probed the outlook of many seemingly successful Americans only to find a sense of alienation and lack of commitment. In effect, these people claimed to have worked hard, played the game ethically according to the established rules, and consequently, reaped many promised material rewards. But they are experiencing an unexpected sense of emptiness and incompleteness. America's prevailing individualism seems to be at the heart of this disappointment, especially what Bellah et al. called *ontological individualism*, "a belief that the individual has a primary reality whereas society is a second-order, derived or artificial construct" (p. 334). *Social realism* is the uncommon opposing belief "that society is as real as individuals" (p. 334). A sign of our times, then, is our individualism-based difficulty in articulating a meaningful vision of community and social reality. Whether or not and how we develop such a vision will be crucial in shaping the future ethical community and the nature of public choices affecting all of us, including persons with mental retardation.

In a second recent book, *The Cycles of American History*, Arthur Schlesinger (1986) viewed the Bellah et al. (1985) individualism-social realism issue in sweeping historical context. For Schlesinger, a fundamental contrast concerns the shifting throughout American history between national moods motivated by pursuit of either private interest or public purpose. Throughout much of the 1970s and 1980s, we have experienced the most recent manifestation of concern for private interest, and we have lived in an era of materialism, hedonism, privatization, and individualism. Sometime around 1990, however, argued Schlesinger, we will once again return to a more socially conscious concern for public purpose, having increasingly experienced "undercurrents of dissatisfaction, criticism, ferment, protest" (p. 28) in the recent individualistic years. This social tension is preparing us for a new period of social concern and innovation like those experienced under Theodore Roosevelt (early 1900s), Franklin Roosevelt (1930s), and John Kennedy (1960s). "The 1990s should be the turn in the generational succession for the young men and women who came of political age in the Kennedy years" (p. 47). And the Kennedy years, of course, saw a significant increase in public purpose concern for persons with mental retardation. Will this same level of concern characterize the ethical community of the year 2000? And beyond mere amount of concern, what will be the nature of this concern?

My purpose in this chapter is to describe emerging ethical trends that might, and should, come to characterize society's approach to mental retardation. The great advances we have made over recent decades—moving away from an often dehumanizing paternalistic approach to mental retardation to an emphasis on the individual civil rights and personal autonomy of persons with mental retardation—have left us with an ethical framework that is insufficient for confronting many of the ethical issues that will arise in the future. Mental retardation comprises a complex set of bioecological and socioecological conditions that confront society with difficult decisions at the levels of individual cases, the service system, and public policy. Should we diagnose as early as possible and perhaps engage in gene therapy? Should we abort, deliver, treat, or not treat? Should we engage in controversial treatments? What constitutes adequate community care? What research should we be conducting? What is informed consent really about? What constitutes a just level of expenditures to correct inequities? Unfortunately, these questions are typically understood in terms of the metaphor of the "divided community." People typically distinguish between "them"—persons with mental retardation and their families—and "us"—the rest of us. Such distinctions often lead to decisions to care for "them" in ways decidedly inferior to ones we would deem acceptable for "us."

I argue that we should work toward an ethical conception of community, which convincingly establishes that all persons are fundamentally equal as human beings. This ethical community of the future would require active redress of inequalities produced by genetic, environmental, or other conditions destructive of human development.

The Future as History

In the very first formal description by J. Langdon Down of the syndrome that eventually came to bear his name, we encounter language infused with the metaphor of the "divided community," the language of "otherness," of "them" and "us". Operating from a belief in the mental superiority of European Caucasians, Down described "the great Mongolian family . . . of congenital idiots." A child from this "family" is so different from us "that it is difficult to realize that he is the child of Europeans, but . . . there can be no doubt that these ethnic features are the result of degeneration" (cited in Rynders, 1987, p. 2). Further, Rynders cited subsequent allegations of the "otherness" of persons with Down syndrome, such as Crookshank in 1924 asserting that Down syndrome represents "regression to a nonhuman species (i.e., to an orangutan)" (p. 3) and Bard and Fletcher in 1968 asserting that someone with a developmental disability such as Down syndrome is not even a person.

Individuals who are beyond the Western racial-ethnic community and who are supposedly not even members of the same species as the rest of us would presumably not deserve to live among us. The late 19th- and early 20th-century move to build large congregate institutions for persons with mental retardation followed fairly logically from such a view. With the advice and consent of most professional people, "us" and "them" were separated by segregating them and their genes in colonies away from population centers. Paternalistic physicians and professional people—acting in the presumed best interests of a paternalistic society, of the public health, and of all concerned, including persons with mental retardation and their families—acted so as to divide the community, and they made even more unequal the lives of those born with any number of biological and social inequities. Ethical decisions were made according to a framework in which experts were presumed to know best and in which individual rights could be fairly easily compromised for the sake of the public good. In this regard, Brandt (1988) recounted the willingness of American society during the early 20th century to infringe individual rights, especially those of prostitutes, in order to safeguard the public health during sexually transmitted disease epidemics. This history has many disturbing parallels in aspects of society's current response to the acquired immune deficiency syndrome (AIDS) epidemic (Dokecki, Baumeister, & Kupstas, 1989), an issue with many implications for the mental retardation field (Klindworth, Dokecki, Baumeister, & Kupstas, 1989).

The paternalistic attitudes that informed the ethics of dealing with persons with mental retardation remained strong and dominant until about 1950, and they can be detected even today. After World War II, however, American social thinking began to shift somewhat. Public horror over Nazi atrocities and the Nuremberg war crimes trials raised consciousness about the abuse of human rights. In addition, long-standing concerns about civil rights for African Americans and other minorities grew in intensity throughout the late 1940s and the decade of the 1950s, culminating in a flurry of very visible national events and a spate of civil rights legislation in the mid-1960s.

Quietly at first, and then with growing visibility and intensity, the rights of persons with disabilities similarly came to be recognized. We have come to witness the deinstitutionalization movement; the enactment of the Education for All Handicapped Children Act (PL 94-142), its downward extension to the early childhood years (PL 99-457), and the Rehabilitation Act of 1973 (PL 93-112); and a spate of ethically oriented cases such as Baby Doe and Philip Becker.

This history warrants the conclusion that a concern for individual rights and personal autonomy has replaced an outmoded and problematic paternalism. Things are better, but all is not yet well. And Perske (1987) reminded us that "some individuals still cling to an older view based on misunderstanding, confusion, fear, and false assumptions. . . . And such persons who fight to exclude individuals with disabilities from their circle of acceptance can cause disastrous setbacks" (p. 286). Excluding persons with mental retardation from the "circle of acceptance" suggests the metaphor of the "divided community." Developing a convincing ethical framework to prevent social divisiveness and to help create a united community is a task that remains to be accomplished in the future. What initial conceptual steps might be taken in that direction?

Steps Toward the Ethics of Community[1]

So far, I have begun to suggest that ethical thinking grounded mainly in the notions of individual civil rights, personal autonomy, and the autonomous individual is not adequate for framing decisions regarding mental retardation. Colleagues and I (Dokecki et al., 1986) noted that the image of the autonomous individual is a vivid one in current ethical discourse. The early 1970s saw patients clamoring to be free from the "tyranny of technology" (Veatch, 1984, p. 38), a struggle embodied in the challenge posed by the principle of autonomy to the traditional principle of Hippocratic paternalism, which had physicians do whatever was believed to be in the best interests of patients. Great benefits ensue when autonomy has ethical priority over paternalism, including the pro- tection of "the rights of individuals and of their personal dignity; the execution of a powerful bulwark against moral and political despotism; a

---

[1] Parts of this section appear in Dokecki et al. (1986), Dokecki and Heflinger (1988), and Dokecki et al. (1989).

becoming humility about the sources of certainty of moral causes and demands; and a foundation for the protection of unpopular people and causes against majoritarian domination" (Callahan, 1984, p. 40). Veatch asserted that "the case is overwhelming that autonomy takes moral precedence over paternalism" (p. 38), but he added that this is "a temporary triumph of autonomy" (p. 40), since many of autonomy's implications are limited to the special situation where its competition is the principle of paternalism.

It is simply the case that autonomy has limited implications and has socially corrosive uses in everyday life, especially as we approach the year 2000. As identified by Callahan (1984), the community-threatening uses of autonomy include the prevailing beliefs that (a) each person is a moral agent walled off from others, (b) social relationships are exclusively contractual and voluntary, (c) respect for autonomy is all that I owe others and they me, and (d) morality is relativistic and subjective. As we have seen, the principle of individual autonomy produces many benefits, and Callahan cautioned that we meddle with it at our peril; therefore, we should not completely jettison it from our ethical framework.

Autonomy should be a moral good, not a moral obsession. It is *a* value, not *the* value. If, as too easily happens, it pushes other values aside, and if (all the worse) it rests on the conviction that there can be no common understanding of morality, only private likely stories, then it has lost the saving tension it competitively needs with other moral goods. Among them are piety toward tested and long-standing moral traditions, a search for morality in the company of others, community as an ideal and interdependence as perceived reality, and an embracing of autonomy as a necessary but not sufficient condition for a moral life. (Callahan, 1984, p. 41)

Consistent with Callahan, the person with mental retardation is a member of a community, an ethical community, and individual civil rights and personal autonomy must be understood in the context of that community. Only when ethical decision making is grounded in the ethical community will the individual rights and personal autonomy of persons with mental retardation be truly protected and advanced. But how are we to understand the nature of the ethical community?

In recent work on pediatric AIDS, my colleagues and I (Dokecki, Baumeister, & Kupstas, 1989) have found Beauchamp's (1986, 1988) ideas to be provocative. Beauchamp (1986) introduced the notions of the "tightly bounded" and "loosely bounded" community. A tightly bounded community is exclusive about granting membership and is quick to remove certain people from membership, presumably for the common good. Tightly bounded community thinking leads to institutionalizing persons with mental retardation, keeping them out of the educational mainstream, using restrictive services, and denying them treatment and life itself. Ross (1988) saw that this viewpoint is characterized by use of the metaphor of "otherness," a pervasive thought pattern about the divided community permitting speakers to put linguistic distance between themselves and the perceived threat posed by people with mental retardation.

A loosely bounded conception of community, I argue, is much to be preferred to a tightly bounded one as an ethical basis for structuring social life as lived together by people with mental retardation and the rest of us. Loosely bounded community thinking tends toward, among many things, community living, mainstreaming, least restrictive measures, and a view of the sanctity of human life (Dokecki, 1983). The social reality of the complex bioecological and socioecological conditions that constitute mental retardation requires the use of metaphors promoting not the divided community of otherness but the united community. This social reality involves the view that we are all in the reality of mental retardation together—persons with mental retardation, their families, their social networks, service providers, and the rest of us. We have a mutual responsibility for each other. How are we to understand this mutual responsibility that forms the basis of the ethical community?

Zaner's (1988) *Ethics and the Clinical Encounter* made a promising beginning in developing a mutual responsibility rationale. He identified the limitations of "the idea of the autonomous moral agent" (p. 288), and in the spirit of Callahan (1984), Dokecki et al. (1986), and Veatch (1984), challenged the ethical priority and centrality of individual rights and personal autonomy. Zaner argued that "to the contrary, moral life is essentially communal at its root, and it is mutuality (in all its complex forms), not autonomy, that is foundational" (p. 292).

Zaner elaborated the concept of mutuality by reliance on some of the little known ideas on ethics of the noted phenomenological philosopher Herbert Spiegelberg. Spiegelberg (1944, 1975) argued that a basic feature of being human, a feature that constitutes the basis of ethics, is that we are all subject to undeserved discriminations that produce inequalities of birth. An undeserved discrimination is an unequal lot in life, either privilege or handicap, which we inherit through no fault or dessert of our own, in effect, through moral chance.

We find ourselves simply born into quite different stations in life, different social environs and groups, and diverse families, nations, denominations, and classes, having neither chosen them nor been consulted about them. Awakening at some point in our lives to self-consciousness, we discover that we are already male or female, white or black, native or foreign, and that we have different physical abilities and biological endowments. None of these was chosen or deserved owing to some action or non-action of our own. (Zaner, 1988, p. 299)

The ethical import of these undeserved discrimination-produced inequalities of birth, which include many forms of mental retardation, is that they are ethically unwarranted and cry out for redress. Since we are all "fellows together" in sharing susceptibility to these inequalities, "fellowship, then, not autonomy, is basic in human life" (Zaner, 1988, pp. 300–301). Zaner argued that "there is something deeply wrong if people who share similar situations are subject to discrimination that favors the more 'fortunate' by the mere happenstance of good luck and disfavors the 'unfortunate' as mere victims of bad luck" (p. 303). Moreover, argued Zaner, "not only is something wrong about this, but in addition something ought to be done about it" (pp. 302–303), hence, the ethical imperative. In other words, when faced with the inequalities of birth produced by moral chance, we are ethically bound to redress those inequalities and move toward a community characterized by equality.

The notion of equality as the foundation of the ethical community has also been developed by Robert Veatch (1986) in *The Foundations of Justice: Why the Retarded and the Rest of Us Have Claims to Equality*. Veatch argued that the aforementioned dichotomy of "us" and "them" stands in the way of achieving equality for persons with disabilities. Just as the Spiegelberg (1944, 1975)–Zaner (1988) position asserts the fundamental equality of all persons in being subject to undeserved discriminations that result in inequalities of birth, Veatch argued that we are all equal by being finite and, therefore, are handicapped according to one or another societal standard. Some of us can't do statistics or are intimidated by computers, others can't read or write well, still others can't throw a football, serve an ace in tennis, or drive a car with skill. "We are all handicapped," argued Veatch, "and in some area or another we are likely to be seriously handicapped" (p. 200).

Although some of us may be generally more handicapped than most of the rest of us, as perhaps one might argue is the case with many persons with mental retardation, this specific set of handicapping conditions is different in degree not in kind from the condition of the rest of us, and we must continually remind ourselves that *we are all handicapped*. Moreover, inequalities and handicaps would entitle *all of us* to be compensated, "if only the resources were adequate" (Veatch, 1986, p. 200).

We must be careful not to trivialize the needs of persons with mental retardation by asserting that they are really no different from the rest of us in being handicapped. On Veatch's egalitarian view, however,

the goal is not simply to get the less well off up to a mythical average. The goal is to identify the worst off and bring them up to the next group then bring that (now larger) group up seriatim so that the floor continuously rises. That means that everyone (except perhaps the one hypothetical best-off person) is eventually on the agenda. That in no way dilutes the priority for those nearer the bottom. (Veatch, 1986, p. 201).

The last sentence of Veatch's provocative book lays out a political, economic, social agenda for the ethical community in the 21st century:

The welfare of the retarded and others with handicaps is served in the long run by acknowledging that we are all in some sense equal in our finitude, that resources are available to meet needs as they arise in order to give people a chance to live out that equality, and that as a community we all share a responsibility for bringing about that restoration. (Veatch, 1986, p. 202)

What ought we be working for in the ethical community that would improve the lot of persons with mental retardation and their families in the 21st century?

To exemplify some of the specifics of a community-based ethical position, I turn to the value and ethical issues encountered in developing programs and policies for persons with mental retardation and their families. In this regard, I have recourse to a community-oriented value analytic framework my colleagues and I recently developed (Dokecki, 1983), which served to focus policy research on the family's role in child development (Hobbs et al., 1984) and which has been used in analyzing several public issues concerning developmental disabilities (Dokecki & Heflinger, 1988, 1989; Dunst, Trivette, & Deal, 1988; Kaiser & Hemmeter, 1988).

To emphasize the ethics of community in mental retardation is to promote interrelated community and human development values, expressed as two sides of the same ethical coin:

1. The aim of intervention should be to *enhance community* . . . so that individuals and their families may develop to their potential. Individuals and families have a legitimate claim on community resources and support in the performance of their developmental tasks.
2. The aim of intervention should be to *enhance human development* so that individuals and their families might be effective participants in the community. The community can legitimately expect individuals and families to master their developmental tasks. (Dokecki, 1983, pp. 115–116)

The pursuit of these values relative to persons with mental retardation suggests four general questions about possible programs and policies. Does a given program or policy (1) enhance the community of persons with mental retardation and their families, (2) strengthen the families of persons with mental retardation, (3) enable the parents of persons with mental retardation to do their jobs well, and (4) enhance the individual development and protect the rights of individual members of the families of persons with mental retardation? Brief elaboration is in order.

An ethical analysis of a program's or a policy's capacity to *enhance the community of persons with mental retardation and their families* requires additional specific questions. Is the program or policy demeaning by devaluing and stigmatizing these people and their families, causing them to lose self-esteem? Is it divisive by separating persons with mental retardation from their community and allowing, even encouraging, invidious social comparison? On the positive side, does it increase shared heritage, mutual aid, and community building by bringing persons with mental retardation and their families together with other people and families, highlighting commonalties and shared values? In a related vein, Seymour Sarason (1984) has asked in the title of a recent controversial article: "If It Can Be Studied or Developed, Should It Be?" He is willing to say yes only if such study or development contributes to our sense of community. I agree with Sarason that this concern with community must be kept clearly in view when we consider whether or not to pursue certain lines of work in genetics and other biomedical, psychoeducational, and psychosocial intervention.

A program's or a policy's capacity to *strengthen the families of persons with mental retardation* can be assessed, first, by asking about its ability to improve the capacity of families to master a broad range of development tasks through services that enhance parental knowledge, skill, and ability to make decisions. Does the program or policy improve the liaison or linkage functions that mobilize social resources and supports needed by these families? Families should be helped both to identify and to make use of formal human service agency networks and to look toward primary social supports, such as family members, kinship groups, neighbors, and voluntary associations. Finally, does it protect these families from unwarranted intrusion and allow parents choice by providing a variety of service options and adequate information about these options?

Ethical assessment of a program's or a policy's capacity to *enable the parents of persons with mental retardation to do their jobs well* suggests these questions. Does it minimize stress by making available to these parents time and energy, knowledge, and resources to carry out their parental functions? Does the program or policy promote shared responsibility among parents and service providers; in other words, does it operate according to empowerment principles? Parents are strengthened when they are treated as capable adults and helped by professionals to become even more capable. Empowerment also occurs when parents are provided with resources and legal rights so they may negotiate effectively with societal institutions.

The final value element of the community-oriented ethical framework, *enhancing the individual development and protecting the rights of all the members of families with persons with mental retardation*, suggests several questions. Does the program or policy enhance all individual family member's opportunities for the development of competence and self-realization? Does it protect individual members of the family from abuse and severe neglect?

Conclusion

This chapter began with the evocative and hopeful ethically relevant observations of Bellah et al. (1985), who suggested the need for social realism to mitigate society's rampant ontological individualism, and of Schlesinger (1986), who suggested that the 1990s will witness the turning to an emphasis on public purpose to mitigate the recent emphasis on private interest characteristic of the Reagan years. What followed was an attempt to outline some of the dimensions of a community ethics for mental retardation that might issue from these newly emerging social and public societal visions.

Although I believe that there is reason for optimism in the further development of society's ethical consciousness about mental retardation, one must be realistic. In that regard, it is helpful to recall Rowitz's (1989) prediction about ethics in his article, "Trends in Mental Retardation in the 1990s." In a section entitled "Ethics Without Power," he wrote:

During the 1990s, there will continue to be much concern about the ethical issues associated with service delivery or the rationing of that service, scientific misconduct, and philosophical concerns related to euthanasia, aversive treatments, denial of rights due to determination that no improvement in physical or mental status is possible, setting priorities for program development based on the effectiveness of lobbying organizations rather than on a humanity basis, and so on. There will continue to be all sorts of position papers on ethics. Most of these papers will lead to a short-term flurry of activity in the media and then will tend to be forgotten. Although I am presenting a rather pessimistic scenario, I hope that efforts in the 1990s will lead to the development of effective strategies for the implementation of ethical principles throughout society. (Rowitz, 1989, p. iv)

Rowitz's "pessimistic scenario" seems to derive from an analysis in which power is the basis for ethical decision making in society. Might makes right, and persons with mental retardation and their families do not have much might, except through the lobbying process. It is hard to argue against the proposition that societal decisions, with or without ethical import, are strongly influenced by power relations. It was ever so, is now, and probably ever will be. It certainly seems that power relations have been central to modernity. But many philosophers, historians, and social analysts have argued that we have been moving out of modernity into a postmodern era and that power issues are changing.

A particularly insightful prophet of the postmodern age has been the noted historian and philosopher of science, Stephen Toulmin. Having been among the first to see the breakdown of the modern view of science grounded in Newtonian thinking and logical positivism (Toulmin, 1953), he has recently been exploring the broader societal implications of the movement from modernism to postmodernism (Toulmin, 1982, 1990). To oversimplify greatly his complex analysis, Toulmin (1990) sees moral argument as beginning to hinge less on power and force and more on moral influence. Toulmin observed that "we have seen power and force run up against their limits," and in the emerging postmodern age, "the name of the game will be *influence*, not force" (p. 208). In that regard, today the only institutions whose moral opinions command general respect and are generally heard as stating "the decent opinion of Humankind" are Amnesty International, the World Psychiatric Association, and similar organizations, which are devoid of physical power or "armed force." . . . Institutions with bigger and bigger guns have, in practice, less and less claim to speak on moral issues with the small voice that carries conviction. (Toulmin, 1990, p. 197)

A provocative metaphor capturing the shift from power to influence is the juxtaposition of Stalin's cynical question, "How many divisions has the Pope?" and Gorbachev eagerly seeking to establish warm relations with the Pope. Toulmin's prophetic view of the 21st century echoes Bellah et al. (1985), Schlesinger (1986), and the argument I have been developing.

This chapter's identification of value-laden programmatic and policy issues, as well as the general argument for needed future ethical development, should not be construed as an outright dismissal of the importance of power relations, individual rights, and personal autonomy. The gist of the argument, however, is that an individual rights position will not stand on its own in giving a convincing rationale for the ethics of dealing with persons with mental retardation in the future. As we approach the year 2000, the society in general and the field of mental retardation in particular must reconceptualize the nature of our social interventions and decision making involving persons with mental retardation. We must attempt to move toward a more caring and competent society (Hobbs et al., 1984), in which the values of human development and community are paramount in our ethical thinking and in which moral influence comes to be based in the ethical community.

References

Beauchamp, D. E. (1986). Morality and the health of the body politic. *Hastings Center Report, 12*, 30–36.

Beauchamp, D. E. (1988, March). *Testimony of Dan E. Beauchamp before the Presidential Commission on the Human Immunodeficiency Virus Epidemic*, Nashville, TN.

Bellah, R. N., Madsen, R., Sullivan, W. M., Swidler, A., & Tipton, S. M. (1985). *Habits of the heart: Individualism and commitment in American life*. New York: Harper & Row.

Brandt, A. M. (1988). AIDS in historical perspective: Four lessons from the history of sexually transmitted diseases. *American Journal of Public Health, 78*, 367–371.

Callahan, D. (1984). Autonomy: A moral good, not a moral obsession. *Hastings Center Report, 14*(5), 40–42.

Dokecki, P. R. (1983). The place of values in the world of psychology and public policy. *Peabody Journal of Education, 60*(3), 108–125.

Dokecki, P. R., Able, H., Allred, K., Beck, B., Donovan, W., Jr., Heflinger, C. A., Lowitzer, A., & Smith, S. (1986). Scholars and ethics: Toward an ethically relevant agenda for scholarly inquiry in mental retardation. In P. R. Dokecki & R. M. Zaner (Eds.), *Ethics of dealing with persons with severe handicaps: Toward a research agenda* (pp. 17–37). Baltimore, MD: Paul H. Brookes.

Dokecki, P. R., Baumeister, A. A., & Kupstas, F. D. (1989). Biomedical and social aspects of pediatric AIDS. *Journal of Early Intervention, 13,* 99–113.

Dokecki, P. R., & Heflinger, C. A. (1988). Families and the developmental needs of dually diagnosed children. In J. A. Stark, F. I. Menolascino, M. N. Albarelli, & V. C. Gray (Eds.), *Mental retardation and mental health: Classification, diagnosis, treatment, services* (pp. 435–444). New York, Springer-Verlag.

Dokecki, P. R., & Heflinger, C. A. (1989). Strengthening families of young children with handicapping conditions: Mapping backward from the street level. In J. Gallagher, P. Trohanis, & R. M. Clifford (Eds.), *Policy implementation for children with special needs* (pp. 59–84). Baltimore, MD: Paul H, Brookes.

Dunst, C., Trivette, C., & Deal, A. (1988). *Enabling and empowering families: Principles and guidelines for practice.* Cambridge, MA: Brookline Books.

Hobbs, N., Dokecki, P. R., Hoover-Dempsey, K., Moroney, R. M., Shayne, M., & Weeks, K. (1984). *Strengthening families.* San Francisco, CA: Jossey-Bass.

Kaiser, A. P., & Hemmeter, M. L. (1988). Value-based approaches to family intervention. *Topics in Early Childhood Special Education, 8*(4), 72–86.

Klindworth, L. M., Dokecki, P. R., Baumeister, A. A., & Kupstas, F. D. (1989). Pediatric AIDS, developmental disabilities, and education: A review. *AIDS Education and Prevention, 1,* 291–302.

Perske, R. (1987). Attitudes, acceptance, and awareness: The changing view toward persons with Down syndrome. In S. M. Pueschel, C. Tingey, J. E. Rynders, A. C. Crocker, & D. M. Crutcher (Eds.), *New perspectives on Down syndrome* (pp. 273–287). Baltimore, MD: Paul H. Brookes.

Ross, J. W. (1988). Ethics and the language of AIDS. In C. Pierce & D. Vanderveer (Eds.), *AIDS: Ethics and public policy* (pp. 39–48). Belmont, CA: Wadsworth.

Rowitz, L. (1989). Trends in mental retardation in the 1990s. *Mental Retardation, 27,* iii–vi.

Rynders, J. E. (1987). History of Down syndrome: The need for a new perspective. In S. M. Pueschel, C. Tingey, J. E. Rynders, A. C. Crocker, & D. M. Crutcher (Eds.), *New perspectives on Down syndrome* (pp. 1–17). Baltimore, MD: Paul H. Brookes.

Sarason, S. B. (1984). If it can be studied or developed, should it be? *American Psychologist, 39,* 447–485.

Schlesinger, A. M. (1986). *The cycles of American history.* Boston: Houghton Mifflin.

Spiegelberg. H. (1944). A defense of human equality. *Philosophical Review, 53,* 101–124.

Spiegelberg, H. (1975). Good fortune obligates: Albert Schweitzer's second ethical principle. *Ethics, 85,* 227–234.

Toulmin, S. (1953). *The philosophy of science: An introduction.* New York: Harper & Row.

Toulmin, S. (1982). *The return to cosmology: Postmodern science and the theology of nature.* Berkeley CA: University of California Press.

Toulmin, S. (1990). *Cosmopolis: The hidden agenda of modernity.* New York: The Free Press.

Veatch, R. M. (1984). Autonomy's temporary triumph. *Hastings Center Report, 14*(5), 39–40.

Veatch, R. M. (1986). *The foundations of justice: Why the retarded and the rest of us have claims to equality.* New York: Oxford University Press.

Zaner, R. M. (1988). *Ethics and the clinical encounter.* Englewood Cliffs, NJ: Prentice-Hall.

4
Quality of Life and Quality of Care in Mental Retardation

SHARON A. BORTHWICK-DUFFY

Landesman (1986) identified quality of life as one of the new buzz words among professionals in the field of mental retardation. Frequently, a buzz word denotes a term that is trendy, lacks substance, and in the long run, affects neither policy nor practice. In 1986, quality of life had not been adequately defined and was not being reliably measured, thus limiting its credibility in the scientific community. Professionals in the past 4 years have responded to Dr. Landesman's challenge to make quality of life a meaningful variable in the evaluation of decisions about the lives of individuals and groups of people with mental retardation. Although notable progress has been made, many of the important issues are still being debated. In this chapter, I will review the early work in this area, summarize the current state of knowledge, and suggest issues that are likely to be the focus of study in the 21st century.

Historical Overview

The 1960s were characterized in the United States by the recognition of the civil rights of individuals with mental retardation and other disabilities. The Scandinavian principle of normalization was embraced in this country and was operationalized by numerous changes in service-delivery systems. Many residential and educational settings were transformed to reflect a new respect for the dignity of all individuals, including those individuals with severe disabilities. The widespread belief that small residential settings were preferable to large congregate facilities resulted in the transfer of thousands of people from state institutions to other kinds of community placement. To evaluate changes in the life conditions of these individuals, the first follow-up studies focused on either a dichotomous outcome of success (remaining in the smaller setting) or failure (return to the institution), or on the length of time an individual remained in the new placement. Quality of life, per se, was not addressed. It was assumed, for philosophical reasons, that people would experience an improved quality of life in the smaller setting because it was likely to be more normalized and be geographically closer to the heart of community life. A monograph of the American Association on Mental Deficiency (Meyers, 1978) titled *Quality of Life in Severely and Profoundly Mentally Retarded People: Research Foundations for Improvement* did not contain any references to quality of life and focused on a variety of topics from reducing problem behaviors to teaching children to read, write, and speak.

Deinstitutionalization and the development of a wide range of community residential alternatives continued throughout the 1970s. Concomitantly, the concept of placement success was broadened to include evaluations that extended beyond mere tenure, including such variables as the actual degree of community involvement, friendship patterns, and the degree of normalization in the home. These outcomes were generally referred to as aspects of "community adjustment," and although the term *quality of life* had not yet emerged in the mental retardation literature, the same factors thought to be important at the time are currently placed within quality of life frameworks.

Whereas earlier studies on the effects of deinstitutionalization (and other residential moves) had often examined single outcomes, it was during the 1980s that a more holistic approach was taken, and investigators acknowledged the multidimensional aspects of "success." The term *quality of life* became popular and referred to an overall evaluation of an individual's life circumstances, preferably from the viewpoint of the person.

The American Association on Mental Retardation recently published another monograph called *Quality of Life: Perspectives and Issues* (Schalock, 1990b, see Note 1). In contrast to the earlier monograph, each of the 22 chapters focuses directly on the concept of quality of life and covers issues of definition, measurement, and application. As Landesman (1986) predicted, there are differences of opinion on each of the issues. Nevertheless, the road has been paved for a healthy discussion, and hopefully, a better understanding of how people are affected by mental retardation and the services they are provided.

Definition

What is quality of life? The concept has an abstract meaning that is difficult to put into words. Nevertheless, it is generally understood in the scientific community as it is used in daily discourse. Examples of descriptions in the mental retardation literature include one's satisfaction with one's lot in life, an inner sense of contentment, fulfillment with one's experience in the world (Taylor & Bogdan, 1990), general well-being, life satisfaction, happiness, contentment, or success (Stark & Goldsbury,

1990), empowerment, autonomy, independence, personal satisfaction (Keith, 1990), and opportunities to pursue and achieve meaningful goals (Goode, 1990).

Common to most discussions is the notion that the evaluation of a person's quality of life takes into account his or her individual characteristics and natural endowment (Borthwick-Duffy, 1990; Stark & Goldsbury, 1990; Taylor & Bogdan, 1990). Does this imply that quality of life has a similar or a different meaning for persons with and without disabilities? In Goode's (1990) opinion, quality of life for persons with disabilities comprises the same factors and relationships that are important to persons without disabilities. Schalock, Keith, and Hoffman (1990) also contend that the construct of quality of life is essentially the same for persons with and without disabilities and that every person has the same wants and needs for affiliation, sense of worthiness, decision making, and choices. Flanagan (1982) has suggested, though, that some adjustments may have to be made to the dimensional structure of quality of life after conducting an empirical investigation of the opinions of people with various disabilities. Flanagan further asserts that the specific questions used to measure the dimensions might have to be modified to take into account the limits imposed by the disabilities. It has also been suggested that for people with mental retardation, comparisons of life quality must be made only within homogeneous groups of people, that is, taking into account such variables as age, level of cognitive ability, and health condition (Borthwick-Duffy, 1990). Significant correlations of quality of life scores with IQ in the standardization sample of Schalock et al. lend support to this position. Age was uncorrelated with quality of life scores, but this could have been due to the restricted age range of the sample of adults.

Definitional Issues

The descriptors of quality of life given here raise important questions. For example, is quality of life the same as personal satisfaction? Are such factors as opportunities offered, physical comforts, and control over one's life synonymous with quality of life, or do they instead impart a causal influence on a person's quality of life?

The multidimensionality of quality of life has been noted repeatedly in the literature, with empirical roots in the work of Flanagan (1978, 1982). Table 4.1 presents a summary of the various life domains that have been mentioned in the recent quality of life literature, focusing primarily on work in the area of mental retardation. The domains are grouped according to the same broad dimensions that were reported in an earlier summary of the variables associated with community adjustment: interpersonal relationships, community involvement, residential environment, and stability–security (Borthwick-Duffy, 1986). A fifth new category,

TABLE 4.1. Quality of life domains.

	Campbell (1981)	Keith (1990)	Keith, Schalock, & Hoffman (1986)	Blunden (1988)	Schalock (1990a)	Bellamy et al. (1990)	Borthwick-Duffy (1990)	Stark & Goldsbury (1990)
Personal Development								
Physical well-being				X				
Health	X	X			X			X
Self	X	X			X			
Education	X	X			X			
Independence						X		
Independent survival skills		X						
Cognitive well-being				X				
Variety						X		
Interpersonal Relationships								
Marriage	X	X						
Family life	X	X						X
Interpersonal/social relation.		X	X					
Friendships	X	X			X			
Social well-being				X				
Social welfare					X			
Community Involvement								
Community involvement			X				X	
Leisure activity					X			X
Physical integration						X		
Social integration						X		
Residential Environment								
Residential environment							X	X
Housing	X	X			X			
Neighborhood	X	X			X			
City or town	X	X						
Nation	X	X						
Environmental control			X					
Safety					X			
Security–Stability								
Security–stability						X	X	
Employment		X						
Work	X	X						X
Standard of living	X	X			X			
Material well-being				X				

personal development, is taken from Flanagan (1978) and may overlap with individual characteristics (e.g. health, education, adaptive behavior). Thus, personal development might be viewed as containing influences on quality of life, rather than dimensions of it. The purposes of Table 4.1 are (a) to illustrate how different people conceptualize the dimensions of quality of life, (b) to show how similar terminology is used differently by various investigators, and (c) to show how the dimensions can be placed into broader categories.

Social and Psychological Indicators

Schalock (1990a) distinguished between social indicators of quality of life, which are external, environmentally based conditions such as education, social welfare, friendships, housing, leisure, and so on, and psychological indicators, which focus on a person's subjective reactions to life experiences. Considerable overlap is evident in the dimensions, suggesting that most life domains can be identified as both types of indicators (e.g., Schalock, Keith, & Hoffman, 1990). Thus, for each dimension shown in Table 4.1, one should be able to evaluate the condition or experience itself (social indicator) as well as the individual's feelings about the condition (psychological indicator).

Quality of Life: Is It Life Conditions, Satisfaction With Conditions, or a Combination of the Two?

Reading the quality of life literature can be a frustrating experience as one encounters three different perspectives on what defines quality of life. Figure 4.1 is intended to untangle the overlapping terminology and discrepant viewpoints in the work on quality of life. It should be noted that the authors cited as exemplars have not presented their views in the form of the models shown, and the assignment to a particular view is based only on my interpretation of what they have written. Moreover, this is a rather crude breakdown of a definitional issue, and authors who are classified as having the same viewpoint may differ with regard to other ideas about quality of life.

Landesman (1986) and Edgerton (1990) represent one view that distinguishes between quality of life and personal life satisfaction (Figure 4.1a). Quality of life is defined by objective, social factors (e.g., housing, family, leisure, etc.) or life conditions, some of which can be modified by communities, service systems, and significant others. According to this view, quality of life has an impact on an individual's well-being or personal satisfaction; however, personal satisfaction is seen as a separate construct that can be influenced by factors other than quality of life. In his thought-provoking essay, Edgerton (1990) suggested that even if we can identify system or otherwise imposed changes that would appear to improve quality of life, it is ultimately the choice of the individual to

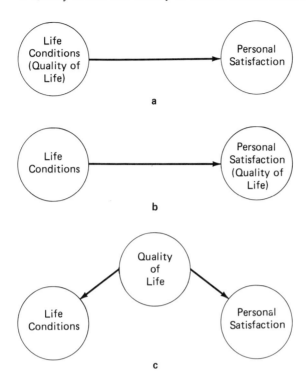

FIGURE 4.1 Perceptions of quality of life. (a) Quality of life is defined by objective measures of life conditions. (b) Quality of life is defined by an individual's satisfaction with life conditions. (c) Quality of life comprises both life conditions and personal satisfaction.

accept or reject those changes, regardless of the anticipated impact on his or her level of personal satisfaction.

A second viewpoint (depicted in Figure 4.1b) equates quality of life with personal satisfaction. Taylor and Bogdan (1990) and Stark and Goldsbury (1990), for example, see quality of life as synonymous with satisfaction with one's life experiences. Objective or social indicators (life conditions) are not part of quality of life but have *an impact* on quality of life, which is simply the person's response to external factors and his or her feelings about them (psychological indicators).

The third viewpoint asserts that quality of life is a combination of social and psychological indicators (see Figure 4.1c). Schalock et al. (1990), for example, describe four quality of life dimensions that include both social indicators (competence–productivity, empowerment–independence, social belonging–community integration) and psychological indicators (satisfaction). Whether satisfaction is a separate dimension of quality of life or a descriptor of each social indicator is an empirical question that is still unresolved.

In all three views, social indicators and individual characteristics are thought to have a causal influence on an individual's subjective well-being, but the distinction of which component(s) of the model are considered to define quality of life is important to an understanding of the literature. In other words, when one hears or reads the term *quality of life*, it could refer to life conditions, life satisfaction, or both.

Quality of Care and Quality of Life

A discussion of the definition of quality of life must address the relationship between quality of life and quality of care. There is a general consensus that quality of care is a necessary but not sufficient aspect of quality of life. This is particularly true in the cases of individuals with severe and profound mental retardation who require more intense levels of care and are more likely to live outside their natural homes. Accountability of care provided, or quality assurance, has been an important component of delivery systems that serve people with mental retardation for several decades. Turnbull and Brunk (1990) assert that standards for residential care, educational, or vocational rehabilitation programs are intended to ensure a certain quality of life. It has been argued, though, that sometimes a focus on documentation and other requirements for certification can detract from the care and attention given to the people served (Riddle & Riddle, 1983). Bradley (1990) suggested that another problem with evaluating care in terms of standards is that the emphasis tends to be on meeting *minimum* requirements of care, rather than on challenging service providers to provide exemplary care that would truly impact an individual's quality of life. Conroy and Feinstein (1990) distinguish between an outcome orientation and a process approach to quality assurance. Whereas the process orientation focuses on licensing, standards, and accreditation, an outcome orientation examines the quality of the service in terms of measurable, desirable, outcomes. Incorporating more of an outcome orientation to the evaluation of care and services provided would be a positive response to some of the criticisms of the process approach.

Measurement

Until the phenomena of any branch of knowledge have been submitted to measurement and number it cannot assume the status and dignity of a science (F. Galton, cited in Cowles, 1989).

Galton's view might not be shared by everyone in the field of mental retardation, but it does explain why efforts to measure quality of life followed closely on the heels of the popularization of the term. Both scientific and practical needs have motivated the development of quality of life measures. Program evaluation, the evaluation of decisions regarding the lives of individuals, and the study of influences on life conditions and personal satisfaction require some kind of yardstick that can, at the very least, say something about "more" or "less," or "better" or "worse." Although more sophisticated methods of measurement will provide refined answers to the questions we have, definitional issues will need to be resolved before more effective measures can be developed. Moreover, the characteristics of people with mental retardation pose unique challenges to the measurement of quality of life. A number of concerns and recommendations for measurement have been suggested in the literature (see especially Borthwick-Duffy, 1990; Heal & Sigelman, 1990; Taylor & Bogdan, 1990):

1. Include both objective and subjective measures of life quality.
2. Do not assume a hierarchy of quality conditions, that is, theater and opera may not be "higher" quality than sports or television—it depends on the preference of the individual (Taylor & Bogdan, 1990).
3. Be careful of personal bias when asking a third party to respond regarding the feelings of the person with mental retardation.
4. Do not assume all changes in life conditions will have the same effect on all people—what enhances one person's quality of life may detract from another's.
5. Do not rely on a single measurement instrument to evaluate quality of life. Use multiple methods and multiple sources of information. Evaluate the relative contributions of method and substantive variance.
6. Examine quality of life within the different settings in which an individual spends his or her time.
7. Improve ways of estimating subjective well-being for individuals who are unable to communicate or may not understand the questions asked.
8. Empirically test the construct validity of instruments that are based on a dimensional structure of quality of life.
9. Examine the psychometric properties of both subjective and objective measures.
10. Do not assume subjective measures are stable. Individuals may vary their responses according to mood, recent events, or motivation to provide socially desirable responses. Obtain test–retest reliability and conduct longitudinal studies that will examine the stability of objective and subjective information.
11. Be aware that variations in wording, method of inquiry, format, and the like may influence responses.
12. To the extent possible, obtain open-ended, unstructured information through interview or observation to supplement quantitative data.
13. Be aware that people with mental retardation may have a greater tendency to acquiesce in their responses.

14. Recognize the heterogeneity of people with mental retardation and consider that they may hold very different views with regard to what makes a good quality of life.

The recommendations listed here pose a nearly impossible challenge to those who would dare to quantify the quality of life construct. In addition, the recommendations assume that there is a general consensus regarding the definition and interpretation of quality of life, which there is not. The process must begin so that it can be refined over time. However, we must be careful not to rush too quickly to arrive at a "score" that can become equated with the construct it purports to measure and assumed that it captures the full essence of it. Heal and Sigelman (1990) warn against "slapping together" a measure that may not be valid or reliable. Schalock and his colleagues (Keith, Schalock, & Hoffman, 1986; Schalock et al., 1990) in the United States and Cragg and Harrison (1986) in Britain have pursued this task in the face of predictable criticism, especially from those who reject the notion of quantification altogether. No doubt there are dangers associated with assigning quality of life scores to the subjective well-being of an individual, but a valid and reliable measure used properly can contribute to a fuller understanding of the lives of people with developmental disabilities (Heal & Sigelman, 1990).

Concerns About Measuring Quality of Life

There is little argument that quality of life is an important consideration in the evaluation of mental retardation policy and decisions regarding lives of individuals. For example, two recent class action suits, *Homeward Bound, Inc. et al.* v. *Hissom Memorial Center* (1988) and *Walter Stephen Jackson* v. *Fort Stanton State Hospital and Training School* (1990), addressed issues of residential placement and considered quality of life in their arguments. In the latter case, measured quality of life was presented as evidence by the plaintiffs. Quality of life has also been used to determine personhood or humanness, for purposes of justifying euthanasia of people with severe impairments (Lusthaus, 1985). The phrase is gaining a power of its own, and used irresponsibly, could become a dangerous weapon. Luckasson (1990) feels so strongly about this that she urges the disability community to reject the use of the phrase altogether. In her view, the potential denial of human rights on the basis of "pseudo-scientific predictions" of an individual's quality of life outweighs its usefulness. Taylor and Bogdan (1990) also suggest that people with mental retardation might be singled out by the very consideration of quality of life because we do not ordinarily measure quality of life for people without disabilities.

Some of the concerns over measuring quality of life echo those associated with the use of IQ scores for decision making in special education. When the IQ score is perceived as synonymous with intelligence or potential, it can be overused and misinterpreted. Likewise, if a quality of life summary score is equated with all that the construct is intended to represent, the term can take on a narrow meaning and be misused. Edgerton (1990) cautions that a quality of life quotient should not be used as a "template for action" (p. 150). These concerns should be taken seriously; however, in my opinion and in others' (e.g., Schalock et al., 1990; Stark & Goldsbury, 1990), when the limitations of quality of life data are taken into account, this information can be a useful tool in the decision-making process.

Recommendations for Future Study

Cross-Cultural Comparisons

The current interest in quality of life extends beyond the United States to Europe and other parts of the world. Goode (1990) reported that studies conducted independently in several countries have made similar discoveries on topics related to quality of life, and he suggested that a comprehensive analysis of international work should be undertaken. Given the subjective nature of the quality of life construct, cross-cultural studies, even within the United States, would provide useful comparisons related to the definition and dimensional structure of quality of life, as well as differences in measured life conditions and levels of satisfaction across cultures.

Validate the Quality of Life Construct

Landesman (1986) challenged us to better define the construct of quality of life. Schalock et al. (1990) likewise noted that the conceptualization of quality of life is still in its infancy. It is therefore important to examine the *construct* validity of the various dimensional structures of quality of life presented in the literature (such as those cited in Table 4.1). A multitrait-multimethod approach (Campbell & Fiske, 1959) would be useful with multiple sources and methods of input. It would address the potential problems of common method variance, identified by Heal and Sigelman (1990), that can overshadow substantive or trait variance. Scores on social and/or psychological indicators would be used to evaluate relationships among the measured variables and to determine whether the data gathered lead to meaningful and valid constructs. In addition, these analyses would contribute a great deal to understanding the theoretical construct of quality of life.

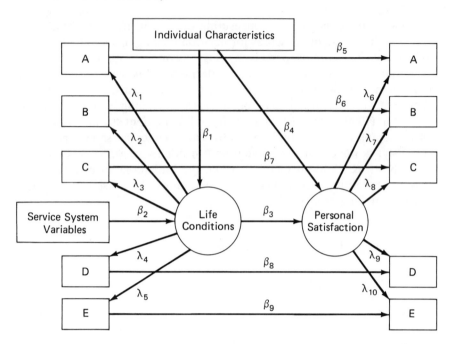

FIGURE 4.2 A testable quality of life model describing influences on life conditions and personal satisfaction.

Validate Implied Causal Effects

At the risk of adding yet another conceptual model to the many that have been reported in recent years, Figure 4.2 depicts a potentially *testable* model that incorporates the relationships commonly described in the quality of life literature. A person's individual characteristics (e.g., age, level of intelligence, abilities, health) and service-system variables (e.g., availability and cost of services) are hypothesized to impact life conditions, represented by causal paths (β_1 and β_2). Dimensions of life conditions and personal satisfaction (letters A to E), would be represented by factors (e.g., community involvement and interpersonal relationships) that would emerge from a study of the construct validity of quality of life (described previously). Paths from the latent variables, life conditions and personal satisfaction, are represented by the paths $\lambda_1-\lambda_{10}$ and suggest that these general factors determine conditions and satisfaction levels of each of the life domains. Other examples of the domains might include any of those listed in Table 4.1. The general construct of life conditions is expected to have an effect on the personal life satisfaction construct (path β_3). The possibility exists, and should be tested, that life conditions in a specific domain might impact personal satisfaction in the same domain, over and above the general influence of life conditions (paths $\beta_5-\beta_9$). Finally, we should test the possibility that characteristics of the individual (e.g., cognitive ability, personality, past experience) will influence personal satisfaction over and above the impact that is mediated through life conditions (path β_4). Testing this model and variations of it with structural equation modeling would shed light on the hypothesized relationships between social and psychological indicators of well-being, regardless of which component is identified as representing quality of life. Longitudinal studies allowing cross-lagged analyses would also examine the impact of change in circumstance or experience on the individual's own reaction to that change. As Stark and Goldsbury (1990) remind us, "despite the billions of dollars that have been allocated in implementing policies such as deinstitutionalization, mainstreaming, early intervention, and community integration, we have not yet answered the critical question: 'Has it really made a difference in improving the *quality* of life for persons with mental retardation?'" (p. 71). A shift from conceptual models to testable models represents an attempt to provide at least part of the answer we are seeking.

Conclusion

This chapter has outlined several issues related to the study of quality of life of people with mental retardation. Quality of life remains a subjectively defined construct. To presume that we can generate group-derived criteria for evaluating a person's personal values, experiences, and feelings is almost an invasion of privacy. The only justification for engaging in this kind of study is to do so with the objective of improving quality of life as it is viewed by the individual. Landesman (1986) challenged professionals in this field to confront the process of defining and measuring quality of life and personal life satisfaction:

Once we define *quality of life* and propose measurable standards (both subjective and objective), service providers and families will be better able to pursue innovative programs to achieve these outcomes; social scientists can focus on developing strategies to measure specific, sensitive outcomes; and administrators and policymakers can adopt more reasonable and effective means for monitoring their programs on a regular basis. (Landesman, 1986, p. 142)

For over two decades professionals in the field of mental retardation have recognized that quality of life extends well beyond the simple success–failure dichotomy that once guided evaluation procedures. The principles of normalization and least restrictive environment as well as the legislated guarantee of an appropriate education have each contributed significantly to improving quality of life among people with mental retardation. As we look forward to the 21st century, a direct but sensitive treatment of quality of life evaluation should continue to enrich the lives of this vulnerable group of people.

Acknowledgments. The author gratefully acknowledges work of the editor, Robert L. Schalock, and the contributors of the recently published Monograph of the American Association on Mental Retardation, *Quality of life: Perspectives and issues* (Schalock, 1990b). The monograph presents a wide range of backgrounds and current perspectives on issues related to quality of life. This chapter draws extensively from the research and ideas presented in the monograph. The work on this chapter was supported in part by Grants HD-21056 and HD-22953 from the National Institute for Child Health and Human Development.

References

Bellamy, G. T., Newton, J. S., Le Baron, N. M., & Horner, R. H. (1990). Quality of life and lifestyle outcomes: A challenge for residential programs. In R. L. Schalock (Ed.), *Quality of life: Perspectives and issues* (pp. 127–137). Washington, DC: American Association on Mental Retardation.

Blunden, R. (1988). Programmatic feature of quality settings. In M. P. Janicki, M. W. Krauss, & M. M. Seltzer (Eds.), *Community residences for persons with developmental disabilities: Here to stay* (pp. 117–122). Baltimore, MD: Paul H. Brookes.

Borthwick-Duffy, S. A. (1987). Quality of life of mentally retarded people: Development of a model (Doctoral dissertation, University of California, Riverside 1986). *Dissertation Abstracts International, 47,* 4322-A.

Borthwick-Duffy, S. A. (1990). Quality of life of persons with severe or profound mental retardation. In R. L. Schalock (Ed.), *Quality of life: Perspectives and issues* (pp. 177–189). Washington, DC: American Association on Mental Retardation.

Bradley, V. J. (1990). Quality assurance: Challenges in a decentralized system. In R. L. Schalock (Ed.), *Quality of life: Perspectives and issues* (pp. 215–225). Washington, DC: American Association on Mental Retardation.

Campbell, A. (1981). *The sense of well-being in America.* New York: McGraw-Hill.

Campbell, D. T., & Fiske, D. W. (1959). Convergent and discriminant validation by the multitrait-multimethod matrix. *Psychological Bulletin, 56,* 81–105.

Conroy, J. W., & Feinstein, C. S. (1990). Measuring quality of life: Where have we been, where are we going? In R. L. Schalock (Ed.), *Quality of life: Perspectives and issues* (pp. 227–233). Washington, DC: American Association on Mental Retardation.

Cowles, M. (1989). *Statistics in psychology: An historical perspective.* Hillsdale, NJ: Lawrence Erlbaum.

Cragg, R., & Harrison, J. (1986). *A questionnaire of quality of life* (pilot version). Wolverley, Kidderminster, Worcester, England: West Midlands Campaign for People with a Mental Handicap.

Edgerton, R. B. (1990). Quality of life from a longitudinal research perspective.

In R. L. Schalock (Ed.), *Quality of life: Perspectives and issues* (pp. 149–160). Washington, DC: American Association on Mental Retardation.

Flanagan, J. C. (1978). A research approach in improving our quality of life. *American Psychologist, 33*, 138–147.

Flanagan, J. C. (1982). Measurement of quality of life: Current state of the art. *Archives of Physical Medicine and Rehabilitation, 63*, 56–59.

Goode, D. A. (1990). Thinking about and discussing quality of life. In R. L. Schalock (Ed.), *Quality of life: Perspectives and issues* (pp. 41–57). Washington, DC: American Association on Mental Retardation.

Heal, L. W., & Sigelman, C. K. (1990). Methodological issues in measuring the quality of life of individuals with mental retardation. In R. L. Schalock (Ed.), *Quality of life: Perspectives and issues* (pp. 161–176). Washington, DC: American Association on Mental Retardation.

Homeward Bound, Inc. et al. v. Hissom Memorial Center, No. 85-C-437-E (N. D. Okla., 1988).

Keith, K. D. (1990). Quality of life: Issues in community integration. In R. L. Schalock (Ed.), *Quality of life: Perspectives and issues* (pp. 93–100). Washington, DC: American Association on Mental Retardation.

Keith, K. D., Schalock, R. L., & Hoffman, K. (1986). *Quality of life: Measurement and programmatic implications.* Lincoln, NE: Region V Mental Retardation Services.

Landesman, S. (1986). Quality of life and personal life satisfaction: Definition and measurement issues. *Mental Retardation, 24*, 141–143.

Luckasson, R. (1990). A lawyer's perspective on quality of life. In R. L. Schalock (Ed.), *Quality of life: Perspectives and issues* (pp. 211–214). Washington, DC: American Association on Mental Retardation.

Lusthaus, E. W. (1985). Involuntary euthanasia and current attempts to define persons with mental retardation as less than human. *Mental Retardation, 23*, 148–154.

Meyers, C. E. (Ed.). (1978). *Quality of life in severely and profoundly mentally retarded people: Research foundations for improvement.* Washington, DC: American Association on Mental Deficiency.

Riddle, J. I., & Riddle, H. C. (1983, January). The "joy quotient": Observations on our need to prioritize pleasure in the lives of the severely handicapped. *An occasional paper of the National Association of Superintendents of Public Institutions for the Mentally Retarded*, No. 20.

Schalock, R. L. (1990a). Attempts to conceptualize and measure quality of life. In R. L. Schalock (Ed.), *Quality of life: Perspectives and issues* (pp. 141–148). Washington, DC: American Association on Menal Retardation.

Schalock, R. L. (Ed.). (1990b). *Quality of life: Perspectives and issues.* Washington, DC: American Association on Mental Retardation.

Schalock, R. L., Keith, K. D., & Hoffman, K. (1990). *1990 Quality of life questionnaire: Standardization manual.* Hastings, NE: Mid-Nebraska Mental Retardation Services.

Stark, J. A., & Goldsbury, T. (1990). Quality of life from childhood to adulthood. In R. L. Schalock (Ed.), *Quality of life: Perspectives and issues* (pp. 71–83). Washington, DC: American Association on Mental Retardation.

Taylor, S. J., & Bogdan, R. (1990). Quality of life and the individual's perspective. In R. L. Schalock (Ed.), *Quality of life: Perspectives and issues* (pp. 27–40). Washington, DC: American Association on Mental Retardation.

Turnbull, H. R., & Brunk, G. L. (1990). Quality of life and public philosophy. In R. L. Schalock (Ed.), *Quality of life: Perspectives and issues* (pp. 193–209). Washington, DC: American Association on Mental Retardation.

Walter Stephen Jackson v. Fort Stanton State Hospital and Training School, Civ. No. 87–839 JP (New Mexico, 1990).

Part 2
Trends on Family and Life Course

5
Increasing Knowledge on Family Issues: A Research Agenda for 2000

BERNARD FARBER and IONE DEOLLOS

Since midcentury, changes have taken place in American society that have had a profound impact on both the family and the lives of mentally retarded persons. To yield highly relevant findings, future research on families with mentally retarded members will have to take these changes into account. This chapter suggests yet another perspective for future research in this area. In the discussion that follows, the terms *mentally retarded* (MR) and *severely developmentally disabled* (DD) are used interchangeably.

A review of research on families with mentally retarded offspring indicates that each historical era presents its own unique concerns about the role of the family in relation to mental retardation (Farber, 1986). As the American settlement moved from colonial status and then the early years of independence to the Jacksonian period and later through the Victorian era and on to the emergence of the welfare state and to the contemporary era, the social and cultural demands on the family have shifted. As these demands have changed, so have ideas about the primary tasks that the family is supposed to perform. In the past 200 years, writers on the American family have continually shifted in their perspective of the family: (a) In the Colonial era and early independence from England, the family was regarded mainly as a little government, focusing on control over deviant and dependent members (Demos, 1979; Morgan, 1966). (b) Afterward, during the Jacksonian and Victorian eras, the family was identified as resembling a business concern, with an emphasis both on producing individuals who are "useful" and "productive" and on isolating deviants residentially, often in asylums or "colonies," to avoid diverting the family from its main task (Degler, 1959; Howe, 1857; May, 1978; St. John, 1848). (c) Beginning with the Progressive era, at the beginning of the 20th century and continuing into the 1960s with the flowering of the welfare state, the family was perceived as a cohesive unit (the so-called companionship family), with a strong concern over the social and emotional functioning for its members and the delivery of supportive services in the case of individual or group deficits (Burgess, 1926; Burgess &

Locke, 1945; Burgess & Wallin, 1953; Folsom, 1943). (d) With the rise of
the civil rights movement of the 1960s and the personal rights movement
of the 1970s, the companionship model was severely criticized, and
another cultural paradigm shift occurred. A pluralistic family model
emerged, wherein it is assumed that *each* family member has the *right* to
develop to maximum potential (as opposed to the collective emphasis of
the companionship family). This paradigmatic shift subtly replaced the
emphasis in the companionship model on personal satisfactions in stable
family ties with a focus on personal rights, regardless of the stability of
family ties (Kobrin, 1978; Morse, 1979, p. 321; Orr, 1979). For severely
DD persons, the pluralistic family model implies a goal of "normalization," often involving "mainstreaming" in schools. (See Clignet, 1979, on
cultural paradigms.)

As the historical perspective on the American family indicates, the
character of the family has changed markedly over the years. The nature
of the family structure at the beginning of the 21st century will in turn
define the social problems of concern (and thereby the kinds of family
research needed) for formulating social policy and alleviating hardships.
Indications are that trends in divorce rates, nonmarital cohabitation, low
fertility, dual-earner families, and so on begun a generation ago, are
abating to some extent. However, it is unlikely that they will be reversed
in the near future. As a result, households in which a DD child is reared
during the first decade of the new century will be faced with a different
set of circumstances than those of a generation ago.

Developmental Disability and Social Context

How does having a child with a severe developmental disability affect
the lives of family members in ways that distinguish them from the
"ordinary?" In early research, particular emphasis was given to the issue
of residential institutionalization as a way of counteracting or anticipat-
ing family problems (e.g., Farber, 1959; Saenger, 1960; Fotheringham,
Skelton, & Hoddinott, 1972). After a surge of family studies during the
1950s and early 1960s, there was a lull in research in this area. However,
during the 1980s (perhaps because of the deinstitutionalization movement), there was a revival in concern about families with disabled children. This renewal in interest has stimulated the application of different
models to permit systematic investigation of the relationship between
family context and the presence of a developmentally disabled individual.
These models differ in their definition of what is problematic and in type
of utility. Three types of models discussed in this chapter are described as
the functional impact model, the family crisis model, and the variant
family organization model.

Functional Impact Model

Some models search for effects of the family context on the quality of the social and cognitive functioning of the developmentally disabled individual. One example of functional impact models is presented by Mink, Nihira, and Meyers (1983) and Mink (1986). This model is concerned with distinguishing between families that are "growth promoting" from those that are "growth defeating." The Mink model consists of variables in three areas: (a) environmental process of reinforcement aspects in the home, (b) the psychosocial climate of the home, and (c) child-rearing attitudes and practices. In families with trainable MR children, Mink et al. (1983, pp. 489–491) found five family types based on their model: cluster 1 (cohesive and harmonious), in which the DD children have effective adaptive behavior, high self-esteem, and good peer acceptance; cluster 2 (control-oriented and somewhat unharmonious), in which the children showed poor adaptive behavior, some maladjustment, and low self-esteem; cluster 3 (low-disclosure and unharmonious), in which the children had the highest adaptive behavior and high self-esteem; cluster 4 (child-oriented and expressive), whose DD children were self-sufficient but had low self-concepts; and cluster 5 (disadvantaged with low morale), with children low in adaptive behavior and low in self-esteem.

Another version of the functional impact model of the family is the systems model described by Turnbull, Summers, and Brotherson (1986). According to the Turnbull et al. model, "the elements of cohesion, adaptability, and communication are key determinants of successful family interaction" (p. 62) and the task of research is to identify the structural characteristics of families that exhibit these elements. These structural characteristics would include (a) family composition and "the nature of the extrafamilial system;" (b) cultural style (such as race and ethnicity, religion, socioeconomic status, and geographic location); and (c) ideological style, which would involve beliefs and values and coping styles. Such findings could then be applied to assisting parents to collaborate in and to adapt to developmental transitions associated with the family life cycle and particularly to the special needs of MR children in making these transitions.

The focus on the effects of the family on the disabled child seems to be a useful tool in educational and psychological therapy dealing with problems in the development of exceptional children. But in focusing on a single family member, the impact model ignores the consequences of both the problem and therapy for the other family members not only within the family but also in their lives outside the family—work, school, friendships, and so on. For example, the family may be "growth promoting" for the disabled child but "growth defeating" for the nondisabled siblings and parents (or vice versa). Likely, family members are affected differentially by the drain on the time and resources available for home care (Moroney, 1983, pp. 202–203; Perlman & Giele, 1983). Too often, parents report that the child's normal siblings do not lack attention and do not resent the care required, while the siblings themselves contradict their parents. Superficially, the family gives evidence of strong cohesion, open communication, and high cooperation—marks of high adaptation—whereas a probing analysis might reveal costs of which the parents are unaware.

Family Crisis Models

Another type of model deals with effects of the presence of a developmentally disabled individual on the quality of the functioning of the family. The family crisis model emerged during the mid-20th century, an era when the companionship family model predominated in the general population—when the family was seen as a haven from the harshness of the society-at-large, with its competitive-market mentality, and family cohesiveness was highly valued as a necessary basis for personal growth and achievement.

This model generally derives from the pragmatist perspective—the symbolic interactionist approach—whereby families proceed in habitual ways until a disruptive event occurs. At that point, it gains in self-awareness and seeks to resolve the crisis that has emerged so that it can again continue habitually. Perhaps the most popular exemplar of this model is the Hill (1949, 1958) ABCX scheme. (See also H. I. McCubbin & Patterson, 1983; Wikler, 1986.) According to the ABCX model, the degree to which a family experiences stress is a function of A (the stressor event) interacting with B (the family's crisis-meeting resources) interacting with C (the definition that the family applies to the stressor event) to produce X (the family crisis). M. A. McCubbin and McCubbin (1989) focus on the efforts made by the family to resolve the crisis, and they emphasize the family's problem-solving and coping abilities and the family's capability in resolving a demands–resources imbalance. For Wikler (1986), a crucial element in the crisis resolution is element B, family resources available (e.g., social support, finances, religiosity, the quality of the marriage). Among other family crisis models is the stress-adaptation model proposed by Farran, Metzger, & Sparling (1986), which plays off a description of changes associated with the stressful event against the adaptive capacity of the family members.

Implicit in the preceding two types of models—the functional impact as well as the family crisis models—is the assumption that, as an organic social entity, the family strives to regain (or attain) an equilibrium and thereby seeks to restore its previous state of affairs. Such a perspective is consistent with a concern in previous historical eras that divergence from norms was a sign of familial disequilibrium and therefore personally and socially pathogenic. For example, divorce was considered as the result of degeneracy or neuroticism, and explanations of religious or racial inter-marriage involved such concepts as self-hatred, opportunism in self-advancement, or revenge against parental or social authority. That was before the pluralistic family model, with its tenets regarding personal autonomy as a value. The pluralistic family model established "no-fault" divorce as a solution to the breakdown of relationships and explained intermarriage as a consequence of the decline of the significance of traditional racial, ethnic, and religious constraints. This change in attitudes toward pluralism is apparently relevant for families with disabled children as well.

Variant Family Organization Model

Still another series of models concerns the range in kinds of adaptation that families make to accommodate the presence of a developmentally disabled individual. This type of model derives from the tendency of families to avoid stigmatization and to be identified as "normal" (see Voysey, 1972), despite their departing from normative conduct. Derived from the pluralistic family paradigm, this perspective is perhaps the familial counterpart of the movement in mental retardation circles to promote the "normalization" of the lives of disabled persons as much as possible.

The "normalization" perspective is consistent with the successive minimal adaptations model of Farber (1975), which depicts a hypothetical series of increasingly more profound modifications in family life in response to continuing stress. The minimal adaptations model assumes that at any given time, family relations are organized to afford the personal growth and autonomy of each member as far as possible. Consequently, when a problem emerges, families will initially make the least amount of change in response to the problematic situation. When the least-modification solution fails, the family members go on to the next minimal change, and so on. Although these successive adaptations may take place without influence from outside the family, likely consultation with outsiders, knowledge of experiences of other parents, and observations of variant family-role patterns in the society influence decisions. This model is particularly sensitive to the influence of social networks on parents (e.g., kin, friends, and in particular, subcommunities based on interest in or concern with the developmentally disabled in one way or another). Consequently, the successive minimal adaptations model is the most responsive model to general changes and trends in family life that are occurring in the society.

Consistent with the variant family organization model, Wikler (1981) depicts a series of 10 stresses over transitions that families with pro-foundly retarded children must face over the years. Each of these stresses reminds the parents of their plight and the modifications in their lives that require decisions. As a series of events, these stresses represent a chronic state of grief and frustration over what might have been, and they stimulate a continual awareness of the nature of family organization as an accumulation of compromises. These familial stresses occur in two ways: first, the timing of ordinary role and status transitions, and second, making necessary troublesome arrangements with regard to the retarded offspring. The stressful times occurring in conjunction with ordinary role and status transitions include (a) from infanthood to toddler (associated with walking), (b) social intercourse through talking, (c) from preschool activities to school activities, (d) from childhood to adolescence (with the onset of puberty), and (e) from adolescence to adulthood (associated with the legal age of adulthood). Each transition reinforces the sorrow and pain of the circumstances; (f) the diagnosis of retardation as mental invalidism; (g) the prospect of residential placement of the child outside the home; (h) the changing rank ordering of the children, whereby socially, the retarded child moves to "youngest child" status (Farber, 1959); (i) the continual intervention of behavioral and medical treatments associated with the child's physical and mental conditions; and (j) the decisions with respect to the relinquishing of guardianship of the offspring. However, the family members' adaptations to these demands are considered to be the most "normal" under the circumstances. In the variant family organization model, departure from norms is seen as a coordinated response to divergent circumstances rather than as a sign of family disequilibrium and pathology.

The Normality of Families With Developmentally Disabled Children

The functional impact model and the family crisis model both focus on those elements in family life that are "abnormal." The functional impact model sees families with developmentally disabled children as requiring special techniques for "coping"—which some families are incapable of doing effectively. Similarly, the family crisis model deals with the presence of the child as a "stressor" and the attempts by family members to "cope" with this stressor. By way of contrast, the variant family organization model is concerned not so much with focusing on the child per se; rather it asks: Given the presence of a developmentally disabled child, how does the family deal with the tasks that all families are concerned with—facing the future, keeping peace in the household, making a living, interacting with friends and relatives, making consumer decisions, taking part in recreational activities, having additional children, helping the children and disciplining them, and so on? To a considerable extent, the factors that determine the handling of these family tasks in "ordinary" families would operate in a similar fashion in families with developmentally disabled children. Consequently, problems that are identified as peculiar to families with a developmentally disabled child in the functional impact or family crisis models are seen in the variant family organization model as possible analogs for other kinds of problems prevalent in other families. The question then becomes: To what extent do the same factors that explain the functioning of other families also explain the functioning of families with developmentally disabled children? Or asked in another way: When is it necessary to introduce the disabled child as a factor in explaining family functioning?

For example, in their review of family-research literature dealing with parents of disabled children, Sherman and Cocozza conclude that "the rate of divorce among families of the developmentally disabled, controlling for socioeconomic status, does not differ significantly from families with normal children" (1984, p. 98). Moreover, although "marital satisfaction may decrease over time in families with retarded children" (Crnic, Friedrich, & Greenberg, 1983, p. 129), the longitudinal study initiated by Burgess and Wallin (1953) (and continued at the University of Chicago under Foote) indicates that a similar decline also tends to occur in "ordinary" families (see Litwak, Count, & Haydon, 1960). These findings suggest that perhaps the same predictive factors that portend marital problems and divorce in "ordinary" families operate as well in families with disabled children.

Similarly, Farber's 1959 study of 240 families with severely retarded children found a tendency toward low marital integration among parents who scored low on a series of premarital items found in Burgess's research to be effective predictors of marital success generally (Burgess, Locke, & Thomes, 1963). In particular, the parents' reports of their own parents' marriage were enlightening.

A major hypothesis guiding the numerous marital prediction investigations under Burgess's direction was that people tend to reproduce the family ideologies and role enactments they had learned in their parents' marriage (often without awareness). In a series of marital prediction studies by Burgess and his associates, the best single predictor in a large battery of items was the respondent's report of the degree of parental marital happiness during the time that the respondent was "growing up" (Burgess & Wallin, 1953, p. 514).

As an indirect test of the Burgess family reenactment hypothesis, a reanalysis has been undertaken of Farber's Illinois data gathered in 1958 on about 400 families with severely retarded children (as yet unpublished). The reanalysis indicates the following: When the wife reported that her parents' marriage was of "less than average happiness," as compared with women from happier homes, her own marriage gave evidence of (a) a relatively high degree of role tension, (b) a greater display of anger and irritability, (c) a marked difference between husband

and wife on the relative importance to them of producing healthy and happy children and of regarding the home as a haven. The extent of initial emotional impact at the time of diagnosis of retardation was comparable to that found in the other families; however, at the time of the study, those parents whose own parents had been unhappily married were having more difficulty in handling their retarded offspring. In addition, other indications of enduring marital stress among these parents were found (e.g., a 1985 follow-up study showed a relatively low age at widowhood (or widowerhood) in families of women reporting in 1958 that their parents had been unhappily married.)

Given the ubiquitous potentiality for stress in families with DD offspring, the preceding results on parents' premarital background suggest that the marital prediction findings (and the parental–family reenactment hypothesis) may be particularly relevant for families with severely disabled children. During the 1990s, similar prediction devices and hypotheses might be tested with families in clinics engaged in diagnosing developmental disabilities to anticipate which families will require special attention as the disabled child matures. Such research may be particularly enlightening since many women and men entering adulthood during the 1990s may react against traditional ideas held by their parents about family roles and values. Moreover, in the 1950s, couples tended to stay together despite the presence of severe marital problems; however, in the coming decades, many such marriages will likely end in divorce.

The Changing Social Context

Sociologists of the family have depicted various trends in family life that will probably continue into the 21st century. (See Norton, 1983; Rowitz, 1985; Vietze & Coates, 1986; Thornton, 1989.) The following discussion deals with various issues relating to families with DD children in relation to these changes.

1. Changing patterns of household formation and childbearing.
2. High likelihood of dual employment of parents.
3. High prevalence of single-parent families.
4. Of particular reference to families with developmentally disabled children is the emergence of a special-interest DD community, and
5. Changing long-term versus short-term consequences for parents and siblings.

Changing Patterns of Household Formation and Childbearing

Historically, the correlation between age at household formation (or marriage) of couples, age at beginning childbearing, and number of children eventually born to a couple has been high. However, recent trends have affected this intercorrelation markedly. Whereas a generation ago, couples formed their households at the time of marriage, now more and more household formation precedes marriage (and may often continue without marriage), and the age at first marriage continues to rise. The birth of the first child may be delayed for several years while the members of the couple establish their individual careers, and other social and economic obstacles will result in fewer subsequent children.

The pluralistic family model (described briefly in the introduction to this chapter) places much emphasis on personal autonomy, growth, and gratification for each member, and in particular on an ability to control one's destiny. Each step in the family life course is considered as a separate matter of choice and compromise: marriage, child rearing, continuing a pregnancy, counseling, occupational priorities, remaining together, and so on—rather than a taken-for-granted element of marriage. Given the preceding characteristics, the pluralistic family model evokes an additional burden of self-blame over the long run, particularly in cases where amniocentesis has indicated the presence of a severe DD (e.g., Down's syndrome). The parents must decide whether to risk an abortion or to continue the pregnancy (Seals, Ekwo, Williamson, & Hanson, 1985; Sells, Roghmann, & Doherty, 1978). Regardless of their decision, there may be a lingering sorrow and consequent stress.

High Likelihood of Dual Employment of Married Parents

Changing labor-force participation of women has important implications for their role in the family. Especially in the middle classes, married women have tended to see their roles as wife and mother as a "greedy" demand, dwarfing the importance of their out-of-home activities. Rather, they believe that a balance should exist between their domestic roles and the development of a business or professional career. Often, marriage and childbearing are delayed for the sake of career establishment or advancement.

For mothers of disabled children, labor-force activity is associated with racial characteristics, socioeconomic variables, and marital status. First, married mothers who are African American have a lower degree of labor-force participation than whites. Second, there is a reduction in "the probabilities of maternal labor force participation [among married women] in families with income below the median" (Breslau, Salkever, & Staruch, 1982, pp. 179–180).

The findings thus indicate that race, socioeconomic status, and marital status have a differential effect on the extent to which the lives of women who might ordinarily work, are modified by the presence of a disabled child. Since Breslau et al. (1982) found a "modest" but statistically significant influence of the severity of the child's disability on maternal employment, presumably, the differential effect results from the need for full-time maternal involvement at home. Apparently, the married mothers whose income is above the median are able to arrange for the special care needs of their disabled children. But for low-income families, likely "the cost of acceptable substitute child care often outweighs the potential contribution to family income from the mother's paid work" (Breslau et al., 1982, p. 169). Inasmuch as the Breslau et al. findings refer to a single area (Cleveland) and to children with diverse disabilities and ages, more refined analyses are needed to determine effects of particular areas, populations, disabilities, and ages of disabled children.

High Prevalence of Single-Parent Families

According to social-demographic predictions, breakdown of marital relationships is expected to continue at high levels into the 21st century. As a result of this trend, large percentages of children will grow up (for at least a part of their childhood) in one-parent families. Findings on divorce indicate that, whereas the financial state of the divorced men generally improves after the breakup, the standard of living for divorced women and their children is usually reduced considerably (Weitzman, 1985).

The enhanced economic demands of having a disabled child place divorced (or otherwise unmarried) mothers in a particularly stressful situation. In the case of single mothers (i.e., widows, divorcees, separated or never-married women), regardless of the mother's race or income, the presence of a disabled child does not significantly affect her labor-force participation (Breslau et al., 1982, pp. 179–180). Probably the most stressed are the single mothers who must work to survive (see Beckman, 1983, p. 150). One direction for future research is to determine the care arrangements made by these women (as well as by those low-income married women who do work) for their disabled children. Since such care arrangements likely involve siblings more than in other families, the question is evoked: To what extent are the disabled child's siblings faced with additional stresses in a single-parent family?

The Emergence of a Special-Interest Community Built Around DD

Since World War II, the number and types of special-interest communities have expanded considerably. (A special-interest community consists of families, professionals, and associated groups and institutions with a particular concern for the welfare of a needy group—e.g., the elderly, alcoholics, drug-abusers, Alzheimer's patients, minority ethnic groups, etc.) Of concern here is the interrelated set of institutions and groups with a common interest in MR (or DD). This community consists of (a) the developmentally disabled and their families; (b) medical, educational, legal, and social supporting professionals and their respective institutions; (c) the family's kith and kin as interested parties; (d) co-workers and employers, particularly in sheltered workshops; (e) university research and educational personnel; (f) advocacy and professional organized movements, and so on (e.g., Birenbaum, 1970; Rowitz, 1981; Voysey, 1975). When a child is labeled as MR or DD, the family becomes incorporated into the DD community to a greater or lesser degree. Such a community creates (and transmits) both revisions of interpretations of DD and new ways of dealing with people labeled as DD and with their families. However, little systematic research has been undertaken on the role of the mental-retardation community in making the life of families with retarded members more "ordinary."

Before the latter half of the 20th century, one could not speak literally of a DD or MR special-interest community. There were professionals who formed associations and special interest groups focusing on the MR population. Yet the families whose lives were often transformed by the presence of a retarded child tended to be isolated from one another. However, shortly after World War II, families with retarded children organized into parent's groups, and government agencies undertook the development of educational, medical, and social programs dealing specifically with mental retardation. With the increased interaction among people interested in the destiny of families with retarded members, the traditional prevalent views regarding mental retardation have been questioned, and new ways of handling family predicaments deriving from the moment a child is assigned a DD or MR status have been sought.

Long-Term and Short-Term Consequences: Discontinuous or Stable?

Both the functional impact and family crisis models are oriented toward the implementation of early interventions in problematic families, because presumably, the greater the family disequilibrium, the more deleterious the impact on the disabled child as well as the other family members. Hence, for the family's general welfare, intervention should take place as soon as possible.

Yet various difficulties are implicit in such an approach: (a) What is "growth conducive" (or beneficial) for some family members may be "growth defeating" (destructive) for others; (b) what appears to be beneficial at one period in the family's life course may yield later problems for various family members (or vice versa); (c) what appears to be inconsequential at one time may eventually have profound significance (or vice versa); and/or (d) beneficial or harmful effects may vary with historical era. As a result, interventions based on family-disequilibrium findings should be undertaken with caution.

The need for caution in acting on family-disequilibrium findings is suggested by the 1986 follow-up of the earlier Farber (1960a; Farber, Jenné, & Toigo, 1960) sample. According to the functional impact and family crisis models, one of the signs of a cohesive family is the participation of all family members in the upbringing and care of the DD child. Many parents with a DD child in the home report that the family collaboration tightens family ties and gives the siblings a deeper understanding and acceptance of the disabled child (e.g., Grossman, 1972; unpublished interviews in 1958 with parents in the Farber sample). However, the 1986 follow-up indicates that those siblings who interacted (usually as caretaker-playmate) frequently with their disabled sibling in the 1958 survey had more problems a quarter century later than did those whose childhood interaction was infrequent (Rowitz & Farber, unpublished).

Another area of caution is the short-run versus long-run effects on the profoundly DD child's mother as compared with the father. Invariably, research findings indicate that mothers suffer a greater stress both emotionally and through the burden of care than do the fathers. In addition, "a prolonged period of denying the reality of the handicap appears to be common among minimally involved fathers who do not interact with the children often enough to be forced to recognize the severity of the problem" (Bristol & Gallagher, 1986, p. 88). Because much evidence in epidemiological research indicates that stress is associated with high mortality rates, one would anticipate that the life span of the mothers would be more affected than that of the fathers. Yet, when one surveys the mortality experience of a sample of parents with severely retarded children (as was the case in the 1986 follow-up), the findings do not conform to expectations: It is the fathers rather than the mothers whose lives appear to be shortened by the presence of the disabled child.

In 1958, the mothers in the Farber studies (e.g., 1960a, 1960b)—as in other investigations—showed greater signs of stress than their husbands. They reported more difficulty in adapting to the child's disability, more difficulty in handling the child, and more chronically poor health. Yet, in 1986, the women survived to a far greater extent than did the men: The statistical analysis indicated that for women early stress did not affect survival. In contrast to the women, based on expected survival rates from 1958 to 1986 by age, men's nonsurvival in 1986 was associated with the following elements in the 1958 data: (a) placement of the retarded child in an institution before 1958; (b) men whose lives revolved around the retarded child and/or who felt worn out in 1958 from caring for the child; (c) attributing the child's disability to an explicit biological cause; (d) chronic poor health in 1958; and (e) withdrawal in 1958 from friends and kin (Farber, Rowitz, & DeOllos, 1987).

To attribute the gender difference to "genetics" begs the question. As behavioral scientists, we ask: What is it that women do and men do not (or vice versa) that accounts for the differential effect of stress on the life spans of fathers and mothers of DD children? From a historical perspective, one question that presents itself is: To what extent might the emergence of a special-interest community focusing on DD (as well as the pluralistic cultural model of the family) influence the future mortality rates of fathers of such children? The seriousness of the impact of having a DD child on the father's life span demands systematic longitudinal investigation by the year 2000.

Conclusion

Each historical era seems to have stimulated its own cultural paradigm regarding the nature of significant family relations and the solutions sought for remedying deviations (Farber, 1986). Stimulated by these historical paradigms, family researchers have produced conceptual models appropriate to studying the family problems and their solutions within the framework of these paradigms (Farber & Rowitz, 1986; see also Gallagher & Vietze, 1986). The historical paradigm that will be prevalent at the beginning of the 21st century emphasizes the values of personal rights, self-expression, and autonomy embodied in a pluralist family cultural paradigm. Consistent with the pluralist family model, the variant family organization research model suggests that presence of the DD child be viewed as a potential *obstacle* to normal social existence of other family members rather than as a chronic *stressor* in evoking family crisis. The research problem is then to determine those areas in which the DD child is an obstacle to normality so that ways of getting around this obstacle can be devised.

References

Beckman, P. J. (1983). Influence of selected child characteristics on stress in families of handicapped infants. *American Journal of Mental Deficiency, 88,* 150–156.

Birenbaum, A. (1970). On managing courtesy stigma. *Journal of Health and Social Behavior, 11,* 196–206.

Breslau, N., Salkever, D., & Staruch, K. S. (1982). Women's labor force activity and responsibilities for disabled dependents: A study of families with disabled children. *Journal of Health and Social Behavior, 23,* 169–183.

Bristol, M. M., & Gallagher, J. J. (1986). Research on fathers of young handicapped children. In J. J. Gallagher & P. M. Vietze (Eds.), *Families of handicapped persons: Research, programs, and policy issues* (pp. 81–100). Baltimore, MD: Brookes.

Burgess, E. W. (1926). The family as a unity of interacting personalities. *The Family, 7,* 3–9.

Burgess, E. W., & Locke, H. J. (1945). *The family: From institution to companionship.* Cincinnati. American Book.

Burgess, E. W., Locke, H. J., & Thomes, M. M. (1963). *The family: From institution to companionship.* (Third edition). New York: American Book Company.

Burgess, E. W. & Wallin, P. (1953). *Engagement and marriage.* Philadelphia: Lippincott.

Clignet, R. (1979). The variability of paradigms in the construction of culture. *American Sociological Review, 44,* 392–409.

Crnic, K. A., Friedrich, W. N., & Greenberg, M. T. (1983). Adaptation of families with mentally retarded children: A model of stress, coping, and family ecology. *American Journal of Mental Deficiency, 88,* 125–138.

Degler, C. N. (1959). *Out of our past.* New York: Harper & Row.

Demos, J. (1979). Images of the American family, then and now. In V. Tufte & B. Myerhoff (Eds.), *Changing images of the family* (pp. 43–60). New Haven: Yale University Press.

Farber, B. (1958). Unpublished interviews with parents of DD children.

Farber, B. (1959). Effects of a severely mentally retarded child on family integration. *Monographs of the Society for Research in Child Development* (Serial No. 71). Vol. 24.

Farber, B. (1960a). Family organization and crisis: Maintenance of integration in families with a severely mentally retarded child. *Monographs of the Society for Research in Child Development* (Serial No. 75). Vol. 25.

Farber, B. (1960b). Perceptions of crisis and related variables in the impact of a retarded child on the mother. *Journal of Health and Human Behavior, 1,* 108–118.

Farber, B. (1975). Family adaptations to severely mentally retarded children. In M. J. Begab & S. A. Richardson (Eds.), *The mentally retarded and society* (pp. 247–266). Baltimore, MD: University Park Press.

Farber, B. (1986). Historical contexts of research on families with mentally retarded members. In J. J. Gallagher & P. M. Vietze (Eds.), *Families of handicapped persons: Research, programs, and policy issues* (pp. 3–23). Baltimore, MD: Brookes.

Farber, B., Jenné, W. C., & Toigo, R. (1960). Family crisis and the decision to institutionalize the retarded child. *Council of Exceptional Children, NEA, Research Monograph Series* (Series No. A-1).

Farber, B. & Rowitz, L. (1986). Families with a mentally retarded child. In N. R. Ellis & N. W. Bray (Eds.), *International review of research in mental retardation, Volume 14* (pp. 201–224). Baltimore, MD: Brookes.

Farber, B., Rowitz, L., & DeOllos, I. (1987). Thrivers and nonsurvivors: Elderly parents of retarded offspring. Paper presented at the 1987 annual meeting of the American Association of Mental Deficiency, Detroit.

Farran, D. C., Metzger, J., & Sparling, J. (1986). Immediate and continuing adaptations in parents of handicapped children. In J. J. Gallagher & P. M. Vietze (Eds.) *Families of handicapped persons: Research, programs, and policy issues* (pp. 143–163). Baltimore, MD: Brookes.

Folsom, J. K. (1943). *The family in a democratic society.* New York: John Wiley & Sons.

Fotheringham, J. B., Skelton, M., & Hoddinott, B. A. (1972). *The retarded child and his family.* Toronto: Ontario Institute for Studies in Education.

Gallagher, J. J. & Vietze, P. M. (Eds.), (1986). *Families of handicapped persons: Research, programs, and policy issues*. Baltimore, MD: Brookes.

Grossman, F. K. (1972). *Brothers and sisters of retarded children*. Syracuse, NY: Syracuse University Press.

Hill, R. (1949). *Families under stress*. New York: Harper & Row.

Hill, R. (1958). Generic features of families under stress. *Social Casework*, *49*, 139–150.

Howe, S. G. (1857). *A letter to the governor of Massachusetts, upon his veto of a bill providing for an increase of state benefits at the School for Idiotic Children*. New Haven, CT: Ticknor & Fields.

Kobrin, F. E. (1978). The fall in household size and the rise of the primary individual in the United States. In M. Gordon (Ed.), *The American family in social-historical perspective* (2nd ed., pp. 100–112). New York: St. Martin's Press.

Litwak, E., Count, G., & Haydon, E. M. (1960). Group structure and interpersonal creativity as factors which reduce errors in prediction of marital adjustment. *Social Forces*, *23*(March), 217–223.

May, E. T. (1978). The pressure to provide: Class, consumerism, and divorce in urban America, 1880–1920. *Journal of Social History*, *12*, 524–527.

McCubbin, H. I., & Patterson, J. M. (1983). The family stress process: The double ABCX model of adjustment and adaptation. In H. McCubbin, M. Sussman, & J. Patterson (Eds.), *Advances and developments in family stress theory and research* (pp. 7–37). New York: Haworth Press.

McCubbin, M. A., & McCubbin, H. I. (1989). Theoretical orientations to family stress and coping. In Charles R. Figley (Ed.), *Treating stress in families* (pp. 3–43). New York: Brunner/Mazel.

Mink, I. T. (1986). Classification of families with mentally retarded children. In J. J. Gallagher & P. M. Vietze (Eds.), *Families of handicapped persons: Research, programs, and policy issues* (pp. 25–43). Baltimore, MD: Brookes.

Mink, I. T., Nihira, K., & Meyers, C. E. (1983). Taxonomy of family life styles: I. Homes with TMR children. *American Journal of Mental Deficiency*, *87*, 484–497.

Morgan, E. S. (1966). *The Puritan family*. New York: Harper & Row.

Moroney, R. M. (1983). Families, care of the handicapped, and public policy. In R. Perlman (Ed.), *Family home care: Critical issues for services and policies* (pp. 188–212). New York: The Haworth Press.

Morse, S. J. (1979). Family law in transition from traditional families to individual liberty. In V. Tufte & B. Myerhoff (Eds.), *Changing images of the family* (pp. 319–360). New Haven, CT: Yale University Press.

Norton, A. (1983). Demography of the family. *Journal of Marriage and the Family*, *45*, 267–275.

Orr, J. B. (1979). The changing family: A social ethical perspective. In V. Tufte & B. Myerhoff (Eds.), *Changing images of the family* (pp. 377–388). New Haven: Yale University Press.

Perlman, R. & Giele, J. Z. (1983). An unstable triad: Dependents' demands, family resources, community supports. In R. Perlman (Ed.), *Family home care: Critical issues for services and policies* (pp. 12–44). New York: The Haworth Press.

Rowitz, L. (1981). A sociological perspective on labeling in mental retardation.

Mental Retardation, 19, 47–51.

Rowitz, L. (1985). Proposal for information networks in mental retardation. *Mental Retardation, 23*, 1–2.

Rowitz, L. & Farber, B. (1986). Longitudinal study of families with mentally retarded adults. Paper presented at the annual meeting of the American Association of Mental Deficiency, Denver, CO.

Rowitz, L. & Farber, B. (unpublished). Growing up with a mentally retarded sibling.

Saenger, G. (1960). *Factors influencing the institutionalization of mentally retarded individuals in New York City.* New York: State Interdepartmental Health Resources Board.

Schilling, R. F., Gilchrist, L. D., & Schinke, S. P. (1984). Coping and social support in families of developmentally disabled children. *Family Relations, 33*, 47–54.

Seals, B. F., Ekwo, E., Williamson, R., & Hanson, J. (1985). Moral and religious influences on the amniocentesis decision. *Social Biology, 32*, 13–30.

Sells, R. R., Roghmann, K., & Doherty, R. (1978). Attitudes toward abortion and prenatal diagnosis of fetal abnormalities: Implications for educational programs. *Social Biology, 25*, 288–301.

Sherman, B. R., & Cocozza, J. J. (1984). Stress in families of the developmentally disabled: A literature review of factors affecting the decision to seek out-of-home placements. *Family Relations, 33*, 95–103.

St. John, J. A. (1848). Introduction to "Doctrine and Discipline of Divorce". In J. A. St. John (Ed.), *Collected prose works of John Milton* (Vol. 3, pp. 168–171). London: Henry G. Bohn.

Thornton, A. (1989). Changing attitudes toward family issues in the United States. *Journal of Marriage and the Family, 51*, 873–893.

Turnbull. A. P., Summers, J. A., & Brotherson, M. J. (1986). Family life cycle: Theoretical and empirical implications and future directions for families with mentally retarded members. In J. J. Gallagher & P. M. Vietze (Eds.), *Families of handicapped persons: Research, programs, and policy issues* (pp. 45–65). Baltimore, MD: Brookes.

Vietze, P. M., & Coates, D. L. (1986). Research with families of handicapped persons: Lessons from the past, plans for the future. In J. J. Gallagher & P. M. Vietze (Eds.), *Families of handicapped persons: Research, programs, and policy issues* (pp. 291–301). Baltimore, MD: Brookes.

Voysey, M. (1972). Impression management by parents with disabled children. *Journal of Health and Social Behavior, 13*, 80–89.

Voysey, M. (1975). *A constant burden: The reconstitution of family life.* Boston: Routledge & Kegan Paul.

Weitzman, L. J. (1985). *The divorce revolution.* New York: Free Press.

Wikler, L. (1981). Chronic stresses of families of mentally retarded children. *Family Relations, 30*, 281–288.

Wikler, L. (1986). Family stress theory and research on families of children with mental retardation. In J. J. Gallagher & P. M. Vietze (Eds.), *Families of handicapped persons: Research, programs, and policy issues* (pp. 167–195). Baltimore, MD: Brookes.

6
Family Caregiving Across the Full Life Span

MARSHA MAILICK SELTZER

Family care is and always has been the dominant residential arrangement for persons with mental retardation. The vast majority of persons with mental retardation live with their families, many for their entire lives. According to national estimates, fewer than 20% of the U.S. population with mental retardation live in any form of out-of-home placement, institutional or community-based (Fujiura, Garza, & Braddock, 1989; Lakin, 1985). While the risk of out-of-home placement increases with advancing age (Meyers, Borthwick, & Eyman, 1985), the rate of placement even in adulthood is not high. However, public policy initiatives and public resources have been directed primarily toward those who live away from their family home, which has reduced the visibility of family-based care. Although the desirability of family-based care for adults with retardation is not a matter about which all policy makers and advocates have agreed, it remains the single most common residential arrangement and, therefore, warrants our attention as we project ahead to the year 2000.

Until very recently, examination of family care for a person with mental retardation has focused on young children and their parents. This focus was a reflection of the orientation of the field of mental retardation, which has emphasized childhood and child development. Also until recently, the life expectancy of most persons with mental retardation was shorter than that of the general population, and it was uncommon for these persons to outlive their parents. At the present time, however, their life expectancy more closely approximates that of the general population. Further, many middle-aged adults with retardation continue to reside with their elderly parents, and often live for several decades after the parents are no longer able to provide care (Janicki & Wisniewski, 1985). However, the impact of long-term caregiving on parents and on other family members is not well understood because past research has focused primarily on the effects of relatively short periods of family care for young children with retardation.

This chapter will apply a life-span perspective to the phenomenon of family caregiving for persons with mental retardation. This perspective on family life recognizes that parenting is a life-long commitment (Lancaster, Altmann, Rossi, & Sherrod, 1987), that the roles of parent and child continue even after the child has become an adult, and that there are expectable changes across the life span in family functions, composition, stability, and other family life dimensions. As a result of these changes, patterns of individual and family adaptation, such as levels of cohesion, intimacy, and stress, that are observed during the first decade of a child's life may not be characteristic of how a family functions when the "child" is in his or her 30s or 40s and the parents are in their 60s or 70s. Little is known about the course of intraindividual and intrafamilial change and development over the full life span for families with a child with a disability or, for that matter, for families in general. There is thus a need to extend the focus of research on the family impact of a child with retardation through the old age of both the parents and the child.

In the discussion that follows, family caregiving across the full life span will be examined from several different perspectives. First, consideration will be given to the changing age structure of American society and the implications of these changes for lifelong family care for an individual with retardation. Second, an overview of the life-span perspective on family caregiving will be presented, followed by a description of two alternative explanations for observed differences between caregiving families at successive stages of the life span: age versus cohort effects. The chapter then presents a discussion of the family impacts of caregiving for a child with retardation at different stages of the family's and child's life span and an examination of the extent to which older siblings carry on the caregiving role once the parents are no longer able to do so. The chapter concludes with a summary section and an articulation of the most significant trends affecting family caregiving across the life span.

The research reviewed in this chapter examines life-span changes at both the family level and at the individual level. This dual focus is necessary because some changes are experienced by the family as a whole (such as changes in family cohesion) while other changes are manifested separately by the individuals in the family unit (e.g., changes in stress and coping). The impact of lifelong family care for a person with mental retardation is manifested at both the individual and the family level, with each locus of change having an effect on the other.

Changing Societal Age Structure

Projections about the nature of family caregiving in the year 2000 must be tempered by an understanding of trends affecting families with a child with retardation. Many social trends are expected to affect these families during the next decade, including changes in the ethnic and racial mix of the U.S. population and the developmental impact of congenital acquired immune deficiency syndrome (AIDS) and drug dependence. One trend in particular that is expected to alter the nature of family caregiving is the changing age structure of American society. This trend is manifested by a marked increase in the proportion of older persons in our society relative to younger persons. In the year 1900, about 44% of Americans were young (0–19 years) and only 4% were elderly (age 65 or older). By 1980, the younger group had decreased to 32% and the elderly group had increased to 11%. The younger group and the elderly group are expected to be about equal in size (23% and 22%, respectively) by the year 2050 (U.S. Senate Special Committee on Aging, 1985–1986). This shift is primarily the result of a decrease in fertility rates and an increase in the years of life expectancy. In fact, by the middle of the next century, the number of deaths per year in the United States is expected to exceed the number of births (Rossi, 1987).

These age-related trends have far-reaching implications for families with a child with retardation. First, as noted, whereas in the past, persons with retardation had a considerably shorter than average length of life, advances in medical care have extended their expected life span almost to that of the nonretarded population. As a result, the period of family responsibility for a relative with retardation is now prolonged and may include the involvement of siblings once the parents are deceased or no longer able to provide care.

Second, the ratio of older to younger caregiving families has increased and will continue to increase. In a society in which younger families predominate, the greatest family support needs are related to the education and socialization of children. However, in societies in which older families outnumber younger families, health maintenance and long-term care become increasingly important for family support. The trend toward increasing proportions of older families will put pressure on family support services to emphasize programs needed by older families in particular, such as respite care, health-care services, and residential placements. While few would argue against the merits of investing in services designed to prevent disabilities, such as early intervention, an age-driven shift in the emphasis of family support services may well be implemented at the expense of some services currently targeted for younger families.

Third, the dependency ratio (i.e., the proportion of caregivers to care recipients) is becoming less favorable. In American society, there are now considerably fewer members of the younger generation available to care for members of the older generation than there were in the past. Thus, a mother of a child with retardation probably has more substantial caregiving responsibilities for her own parents than did her counterpart 30 or 40 years ago because her parents live longer and because she has fewer siblings with whom to share the burden of parent care. Contemporary mothers probably experience greater role strain than did mothers in the past and may be under considerably greater physical and emotional pressures. In fact, Seltzer and Krauss reported that almost 20% of the Wisconsin mothers in their sample, all of whom were between the ages of 55 to 85 and provided in-home care for a son or daughter with retardation, also cared for another family member (Seltzer & Krauss, 1989b).

Fourth, U.S. society currently includes a larger proportion of single-parent, primarily female-headed families than in the past (Masnick & Bane, 1980). The trend toward increased proportions of single-parent families is due to two factors: (a) the increasing divorce rate and (b) the widening gender gap in longevity, with women outliving men by almost 10 years (Rossi, 1987). As a result of these large-scale social trends, fewer children, including those with a disability, currently live in two-parent households than was the case in the past. Given the special demands and stresses facing single-parent families, the potential for long-term family care in such families may be reduced.

In summary, it is now common for caregiving family members to have lifelong rather than time-limited responsibility for a relative with retardation, for caregivers to have more than one family member dependent on them at the same time, and for caregivers to have less marital support. The impacts of these demographic changes in U.S. society on families with a child with a retardation are not fully understood. However, it is possible that these changes may signal an increase in the fragility of families and may make it more difficult for them to provide life-long care to a relative with retardation. Any projection about the nature of family caregiving in the year 2000 must be tempered by the impact of these larger population trends.

A Life-Span Perspective on Families

Life-span research on parent–child relations—in families with or without a child with retardation—represents a departure from the traditional focus of family research, which has tended to emphasize either the beginning or the end of life. Hagestad (1987) noted that even though it is now the norm for an individual to be a child (i.e., to have a living parent) for fully 50 years, research on parents and children has focused either on the first decade of the *child's* life (child development research) or on the last decade of the *parent's* life (gerontological research), leaving a 30-year gap in our understanding of the parent–child relationship. Recently, however, there has been increasing interest in human behavior across the full life span, and, in this context, researchers have begun to examine the continuing impact of early life experiences on adult development (e.g., Ainsworth, 1989; Richardson, Koller, & Katz, 1985) and the earlier life antecedents of adaptation to old age (e.g., Ryff, 1989a, 1989b; Labouvie-Vief, DeVoe, & Bulka, 1989).

In a parallel fashion, a life-span perspective has influenced research on how families develop and on age-related changes in family functions and tasks. During the past 30 years, many researchers have conceptualized the discrete stages of the family life span (e.g., Duvall, 1957; Olson, McCubbin, & Associates, 1983), and although the number and names of the stages differ from study to study, they generally begin with young married couples without children and end with aging families in retirement. While there is acknowledgment of substantial individual variation in the rate at which families move from stage to stage, especially as a result of the impact of divorce and remarriage, family life-course theory is based on the assumptions that there are fairly predictable changes that families experience across the life span and that these changes have an impact on family functioning.

According to most family-stage theories, the primary family functions during a family's early years are establishing a household and childbearing. However, as the children age, socialization and education take over as primary family functions. Another family function, which increases in importance as the family matures, is the enhancement of the parents' social roles, including their careers, social networks, and community relationships. In old age, family functions include maintaining the extended family and providing support and care to members who have limitations in their independent functioning.

The extent to which these functions are performed differently by families with a child with a disability—or the extent to which they experience a different set of stages—has been the subject of very little research, especially with respect to the later stages of the family life span (Krauss & Giele, 1987; Turnbull, Summers, & Brotherson, 1986). Rather, the limited number of applications of stage theory to a family with a child with retardation has focused on stages of parental adjustment to the birth of the child (Blacher, 1984a).

A few studies have examined how families with a child with retardation at different stages of the life span differ from one another. For example, several studies have examined the relation between the age of a child with retardation and the risk of out-of-home placement. Tausig (1985) reported age-related differences in families' reasons for seeking out-of-home placement for their child with retardation. For children under the age of 21, placement was sought primarily when there were multiple problems in the family, while for those age 21 or older, placement was sought specifically when there were family health problems. Suelzle and Keenan (1981) also examined age-related placement patterns and found that the risk of out-of-home placement is highest when the child is between 6 and 12 years of age and again between 19 and 21 years of age. The authors relate these findings to the higher level of family stress during transition points in the child's life, particularly when beginning and completing school. Olson et al. (1983), in a study of families without a child with a disability, found that family satisfaction was highest for young couples without children and for couples whose grown children no longer live at home, while stressful life events were experienced most frequently by families "launching" adolescent children into independent living. The findings of these cross-sectional studies, which highlight the existence and magnitude of between-stage differences, underscore that it is unwarranted to generalize from the results of research conducted on young families to older families, as families at different stages are very different from one another.

Age Versus Cohort Effects

While the existence of between-stage differences in family adaptation and functioning is now well-accepted, it is much more difficult to pinpoint the specific causes of such differences. There are two primary explanations that have been discussed in the literature to account for the between-stage differences that have been observed at various points of the life span for individuals and for families (Schaie, 1988). They are (a) age or maturational effects and (b) cohort effects.

Age or Maturational Effects

Age or maturational effects are the patterns of individual and family functioning that are associated with chronological age and that result in intraindividual and intrafamilial change over the life span. As Frey, Fewell, and Vadasy (1989) note, change is possibly the most important feature of family functioning, inevitably caused by factors such as the aging of family members, changes in the composition of the family, and the continuing influence of each family member on the others. Maturational changes include the transition from nonparenthood to parenthood, from parenting adolescent children to parenting adult children, from employment to retirement, etc. Such maturational changes can only be detected by studying the same families longitudinally, and identifying the changes in family and individual functioning that emerge over the course of time.

One longitudinal investigation of family functioning is the research reported by Friedrich, Wilturner, and Cohen (1985) on mothers of children with retardation (mean age = 10.5, range = 3 to 19 years). They found that over time, as the severity of parent and family problems increased, there was a concomitant increase in maternal depression. Other individual and family characteristics—such as family relations and locus of control—remained stable between the two assessments. This study illustrated that both stability and change are characteristic of individual and family development, and that the specific patterns of maturational influences can only be detected through longitudinal research.

Cohort Effects

Cohort effects are the second source of differences between stages that have been conceptualized. A cohort is a group of persons born in the same time interval, who share a common social and demographic history, and who age together (Ryder, 1965). The experiences and life histories of one cohort may differ substantially from those of earlier and later birth cohorts (Hogan, 1987). Because persons born at different times—and because families formed at different times—are the products of different personal and societal circumstances, they cannot be expected to move through the life course in identical trajectories. For example, two families with a son or daughter with retardation of different ages—say, 45 and 15 years of age in 1990—might be quite different in their patterns of individual and family adaptation for reasons *other than the age of the child.* In addition to the age differences between these two families, there may be large cohort differences. While the older "child" is a member of the baby-boom generation, the younger child is a member of a much smaller birth cohort. The number of age peers competing for resources is much greater for the 45-year-old than for the 15-year-old. Further, the 45-year-old was reared and educated in the era of post-World War II prosperity, a politically conservative time, while the 15-year old's childhood was a period of economic recession and political liberalism. As a result of these cohort differences, the younger family *never will be just like* the older family, and the older family *never was just like* the younger family, in spite of powerful maturational influences.

In another example of cohort effects, Krauss and Seltzer (1986) compared two age groups of adults with retardation who resided in both institutional and community-based settings, with respect to cognitive, medical, and functional impairments: those age 22 to 54 and those age 55 and over. While Krauss and Seltzer hypothesized, based on expected aging effects, that the older group would be more impaired cognitively, medically, and functionally than the younger group, it was found that the younger cohort was actually significantly more impaired. The explanation for these unexpected findings was that the older and younger cohorts were composed of a different mix of persons. These differences were the result of differences in diagnostic practices, placement patterns, and mortality that have occurred during the last century. Thus, the members of the younger cohort included a higher proportion of persons with severe and profound retardation, who in the past were less likely to survive past childhood, while the older cohort included a higher proportion of persons labelled "borderline" mental retardation, who were not included in the younger group as a result of contemporary diagnostic practices. This example illustrates the distinction between true aging influences and cohort effects, and cautions us to carefully separate the two.

Whereas age effects are relatively stable, cohort effects are dynamic, and they modify age effects. Featherman (1985) and Riley (1988) have clarified how the interaction of age and cohort effects produces unique changes in the life course experienced by any given individual or family. Persons grow old in a different society from the one in which they were born as a result of social change. Macrolevel influences, such as demographic changes, the introduction of new technology, and changing policies regarding services for persons with disabilities, to name just a few, have a lasting effect on the social context in which individuals and families function. Individuals and families reach each stage in the life span at a unique point in historical time. According to Riley (1988), "because society changes, people in different cohorts age in different ways" (p. 29).

To understand family caregiving for a member with retardation, one must examine the influences of the maturational or aging process on both the family as a whole and on each individual and also must be cognizant of how cohort effects change the course of development. Thus, our expectations regarding family caregiving for persons with mental retardation in the year 2000 are a function of the passage of historical time—namely, the social, demographic, and political developments that will occur during the next 10 years—and the passage of personal time—the aging of individuals and families during the next 10 years. It is only at the intersect of historical and personal time that the impact of family caregiving across the full life span can be adequately studied and fully understood.

The Impact of Life-Span Considerations on Family Caregiving

For decades, researchers have investigated the impact of a child with retardation on the members of his or her family (Blacher, 1984b; Farber, 1959; J. J. Gallagher & Vietze, 1986). Among the outcomes that have been examined are the well-being of the parents as individuals, the quality of their marital relationship, and the adjustment of the other children in the family. It is increasingly recognized that overall family adaptation in families with a child with retardation is quite varied, with some families coping well and others manifesting more serious problems. Furthermore, specific risk factors and protective mechanisms have been identified that account for variation in family adaptation. The risk factors include having a child with more severe retardation, poorer health, maladaptive behavior, and older age (Crnic, Friedrich, & Greenberg, 1983; Seltzer & Krauss, 1984). The protective mechanisms include strong and satisfying parental social support networks (Tausig, 1985), effective personal coping skills (Friedrich, et al., 1985), and the quality and strength of the parental relationship with the child (Blacher, 1984b). However, the durability of these risk and protective mechanisms across the life course is presently unknown.

Family caregiving for a child with retardation has both stressful and gratifying aspects (Bristol & Schopler, 1984). While families at all stages of the family life span experience both stresses and gratifications, the balance of the negative and positive aspects of caregiving is not uniform across the life span. Caregiving is said to be most stressful at expected times of family transitions, such as when the child completes school, and it is least stressful during periods of continuity and stability in family roles (Wikler, 1986).

One source of life-span variation in the frustrations and gratifications of caregiving derives from the extent to which having a dependent child is a normative versus an "off-cycle" role. Past research on the impact of life events has demonstrated that the timing of events plays a large role in determining their subjective impact (Brim & Ryff, 1980; Riley, 1986). When a child with mental retardation is an infant or a preschooler, the provision of care by a parent is a normative role, as the parents' peers are also performing this caregiving function for their young (non-handicapped) children. However, once the "child" has reached adulthood and the parents are in middle or old age, the continuation of caregiving by parents is not normative and represents an off-cycle role. Farber (1959) and Birenbaum (1971) noted that families with a child with mental retardation may experience an "arrest" in the family life cycle because their children are never fully launched to independent adulthood. This perspective would hypothesize that caregiving becomes more stressful for a family with a child with a disability as the family ages.

A related perspective on the long-term impact of family caregiving is that the cumulative stressful effects of caregiving affect the family negatively. As the child ages, he or she often presents a more formidable physical and emotional challenge just at the time that the parent's energy level has begun to diminish. The "wear and tear" hypothesis of family caregiving suggests that over time, the impact on the family is progressively more negative (Bristol & Schopler, 1984; Seltzer & Krauss, 1984). For example, in a study of families with a child with autism, Holroyd, Brown, Wikler, and Simmons (1975) found family stress to be higher in families of older as compared with younger children.

Other research evidence suggests that the "wear and tear hypothesis" may not describe life-span variation in family caregiving impact. For example, Townsend, Noelker, Deimling, and Bass (1989), in research on caregiving by adult (nonretarded) children for their aged parents, unexpectedly found that over time adult children adapted to the caregiving role and some improved in psychological functioning, rather than manifesting the deterioration that the researchers had originally expected. This adaptational hypothesis regarding the impact of long-term family caregiving suggests that stressful events and roles can be opportunities for personal and psychological growth. Some preliminary support for this hypothesis is suggested by research conducted by Seltzer and Krauss (1989a) on older mothers who provided long-term care for their adult sons and daughters with retardation. Comparison of these mothers with other groups of older women and with caregivers for the elderly suggests that adaptational processes might have occurred. Specifically, a higher proportion of the women in the Seltzer and Krauss (1989a) sample viewed their physical health as good or excellent (78%) than did women in a national probability sample of older women (60%; Bumpass & Sweet, 1987). Similarly, the sample of older mothers with adult children with retardation reported substantially higher life satisfaction than did a sample of caregivers for the elderly and slightly less caregiving stress and feelings of burden than other samples of caregivers (Friedrich, Greenberg, & Crnic, 1983; D. Gallagher et al., 1985; Zarit, Reever, & Bach-Peterson, 1980).

Qualitative data from the Seltzer and Krauss (1989a) study also support the adaptational hypothesis. The mothers' responses to open-ended questions suggest that they did not view long-term family caregiving in primarily negative terms. In fact, the majority described the gratifications as well as the frustrations associated with the process of rearing a child with retardation to adulthood. The following examples are illustrative.

"Being an 'older mother' with aching bones, etc., I sometimes want to just throw in the towel. I know that this negative attitude would spread like a disease and affect my whole life. A positive attitude is a happy one, full of surprises. It bounces off each member of the family and our son gets the benefit from it all."

"This child has taught me an appreciation for the little things in life that we all take for granted. My other children learned about love and caring for others from Cindy. I don't ask, 'Why, me?' I ask, 'Why not me?' "

"It took me five years to accept Bob's limitations and come to value who he is. Our other seven children are better people because of Bob's presence in our lives. I had to grow, too. My advice to other parents is to value who he is, not who he isn't. Forgive yourself. Keep special time for yourself, and the other members of the family. Martyrs are hard to live with."

These quantitative and qualitative data provide only tentative support for the adaptational hypothesis, as they have several methodological limitations. First, they are based on an analysis of the later years of the life span only. Second, no comparisons can be made between present levels of functioning and the patterns manifested by these families when they were younger. Third, only those mothers who continued as caregivers were studied. It is likely that when stresses outweigh gratifications, mothers make efforts to place their child out of the home, while those who perceived a more favorable ratio of positive and negative outcomes of caregiving have maintained their role as caregiver. Future research should sample families from all stages of the life span and should attempt to determine which families are affected more negatively over time by caregiving (as predicted by the "wear and tear" hypothesis) and which manifest positive as well as negative outcomes (as predicted by the adaptation hypothesis). Such investigations will also clarify the extent to which parenting a child with retardation has unique effects at different stages of the life span and will help to identify sources of gratification and positive effects as well as the sources of frustration and negative effects.

Siblings as Caregivers

While in most families, parents function as the primary caregivers for persons with mental retardation throughout their lives, in some families siblings assume this responsibility after the parents are no longer able to provide care. Research on siblings of persons with mental retardation, like research on families in general, has tended to emphasize relationships among siblings in childhood (Farber, 1963; Gath, 1974; Simeonsson & Bailey, 1986; Seltzer, 1985; Simeonsson & McHale, 1981). While most of this body of research describes the negative impacts on siblings of a brother or sister with retardation, some research has provided evidence of positive adaptation. However, few studies have used comparison groups to provide normative data on the expected range of affection and conflict in sibling relationships.

It is only recently that sibling relationships across the full life span have received attention, despite the long-lasting duration of these relationships. In one of the few studies that included a wide age range (12 to 69 years of age), Begun (1989) reported numerous age-related and birth-order differences in the relationships between siblings. For example, siblings who were several years older than the sibling with retardation were more satisfied with the sibling relationship than those several years younger than the sibling with retardation. Similarly, Zetlin (1986) described the heterogeneity of sibling relationships between adults with mild mental retardation and their brothers and sisters. She noted that these relationships differed at various points in the family life span, with middle-aged siblings perceived by their sisters and brothers with retardation to be the closest and most supportive, while young adult siblings were perceived as being less dependable.

Even when parents remain the primary caregivers, siblings tend to assume more responsibility for their brother or sister with retardation as the parents age. Seltzer, Begun, Seltzer, and Krauss (1991) found that mothers between the ages of 55 and 85 reported feeling less stressed and less burdened by care giving when there was more social interaction between the nonhandicapped sibling and those with retardation. Further, the majority of mothers (62%) expected a sibling to assume the responsibility for their son or daughter with retardation after they are no longer able to provide care or supervision. Indeed, mothers who had made explicit plans for a sibling to assume caregiving responsibility reported significantly less stress than mothers who had not made long-term care arrangements.

Conclusions

This chapter has presented several compelling theoretical reasons for embracing a life-span perspective on family caregiving. This perspective is increasingly supported by the results of empirical research, as well. While a life-span perspective is increasingly accepted by researchers, theoreticians, and service providers, a great deal remains to be learned about the specific course of intraindividual and intrafamilial change and stability. Much more research is necessary to fill the many gaps in our understanding of the adaptability and well-being of families of children with mental retardation across the life span. This research will be strengthened by attending to several methodological issues. First, a multi-disciplinary perspective will clearly be more productive than a single-discipline approach, because the well-being of caregiving families across the life span has biological, psychological, and social dimensions. Second, both normative and non-normative life events and social roles warrant careful description to promote understanding of how families of children with retardation differ from, and are similar to, their counterparts who have nonhandicapped children, as well as families who care for a dependent member other than a child. Third, future studies should include investigation of both the individual development of family members and the development of the family as a whole. The disaggregation of individual-level change from family-level change and the mapping of the mutual influences of these loci of development provide both a formidable challenge and a unique opportunity for future researchers. Finally, there is a need to relate knowledge gained about one age group or one stage in the family life span to similar knowledge about other age groups or other stages, in order to develop an understanding of the processes of change and stability over the full family life span.

References

Ainsworth, M. D. S. (1989). Attachments beyond infancy. *American Psychologist, 44*, 709–716.
Begun, A. L. (1989). Sibling relationships involving developmentally disabled people. *American Journal of Mental Retardation, 93*, 566–574.

Birenbaum, A. (1971). The mentally retarded child in the home and the family life cycle. *Journal of Health and Social Behavior, 12*, 55–65.

Blacher, J. (1984a). Sequential stages of parental adjustment to the birth of a child with handicaps: Fact or artifact. *Mental Retardation, 22*, 55–68.

Blacher, J. (Ed.) (1984b). *Severely handicapped children and their families: Research in review.* New York: Academic Press.

Brim, O. G., & Ryff, C. D. (1980). On the properties of life events. In P. B. Baltes & O. G. Brim (Eds.), *Life-span development and behavior: Vol. 3* (pp. 368–388). New York: Academic Press.

Bristol, M. M., & Schopler, E. (1984). A developmental perspective on stress and coping in families of autistic children. In J. Blacher (Ed.), *Severely handicapped children and their families: Research in review* (pp. 91–141). New York: Academic Press.

Bumpass, L., & Sweet, J. (1987). *A national survey of families and households.* Madison, WI: Center for Demography and Ecology, University of Wisconsin-Madison.

Crnic, K., Friedrich, W. N., & Greenberg, M. T. (1983). Adaptation of families with mentally retarded children: A model of stress, coping, and family ecology. *American Journal of Mental Deficiency, 88*, 345–351.

Duvall, E. (1957). *Family development.* Philadelphia: Lippincott.

Farber, B. (1959). Effects of a severely mentally retarded child on family integration. *Monographs of the Society for Research in Child Development, 24*(2, Serial No. 71).

Farber, B. (1963). Interaction with retarded siblings and life goals of children. *Marriage and Family Living, 25*, 96–98.

Featherman, D. L. (1985). Individual development and aging as a population process. In J. R. Nesselroade & A. von Eye (Eds.), *Individual development and social change* (pp. 213–241). New York: Academic Press.

Frey, K. S., Fewell, R. R., & Valdasy, P. F. (1989). Parental adjustment and changes in child outcome among families of young handicapped children. *Topics in Early Childhood Special Education, 8*, 38–57.

Friedrich, W. N., Greenberg, M. T., & Crnic, K. (1983). A short form of the Questionnaire on Resources and Stress. *American Journal of Mental Deficiency, 88*, 41–48.

Friedrich, W. N., Wilturner, L. T., & Cohen, D. S. (1985). Coping resources and parenting mentally retarded children. *American Journal of Mental Deficiency, 90*, 130–139.

Fujiura, G. T., Garza, J., & Braddock, D. (1989). *National survey of family support services in developmental disabilities.* Mimeo: University of Illinois-Chicago.

Gallagher, D., Rappaport, M., Benedict, A., Lovett, S., Silven, D., & Kramer, H. (1985). *Reliability of selected interview and self-report measures with family caregivers.* Paper presented at the 38th Annual Meeting of the Gerontological Society of America, New Orleans, LA.

Gallagher, J. J., & Vietze, P. M. (Eds.) (1986). *Families of handicapped persons: Research, programs, and policy issues.* Baltimore, MD: Brookes.

Gath, A. (1974). Sibling reactions to mental handicap: A comparison of the brothers and sisters of mongol children. *Children of Child Psychology and Psychiatry and Allied Disciplines, 15*, 838–843.

Hagestad, G. O. (1987). Parent–child relations in later life: Trends and gaps in past research. In J. B. Lancaster, J. Altmann, A. S. Rossi, & L. R. Sherrod (Eds.), *Parenting across the life span: Biosocial dimensions* (pp. 405–433). New York: Aldine de Gruyter.

Hogan, D. P. (1987). Demographic trends in human fertility, and parenting across the life span. In J. B. Lancaster, J. Altmann, A. S. Rossi, & L. R. Sherrod (Eds.), *Parenting across the life span: Biosocial dimensions* (pp. 315–349). New York: Aldine de Gruyter.

Holyroyd, J., Brown, N., Wikler, L., & Simmons, J. Q. (1975). Stress in families of institutionalized and non-institutionalized autistic children. *Journal of Community Psychology, 3*, 26–31.

Janicki, M. P., & Wisniewski, H. M. (Eds.). (1985). *Aging and developmental disabilities: Issues and approaches.* Baltimore, MD: Brookes.

Krauss, M. W., & Giele, J. Z. (1987). Services to families during three stages of a handicapped person's life. In M. Ferrri & M. B. Sussman (Eds.), *Childhood disability and family systems* (pp. 213–230). New York: Haworth Press.

Krauss, M. W., & Seltzer, M. M. (1986). Comparison of elderly and adult mentally retarded persons in institutional and community settings. *American Journal of Mental Deficiency, 91*, 237–243.

Labouvie-Vief, G., DeVoe, M., & Bulka, D. (1989). Speaking about feelings: Conceptions of emotion across the life span. *Psychology and Aging, 4*, 425–437.

Lakin, K. C. (1985). Service system and settings for mentally retarded people. In K. C. Lakin, B. Hill, & R. Bruininks (Eds.), *An analysis of Medicaid's intermediate care facility for the mentally retarded (ICF-MR) program.* Minneapolis: University of Minnesota.

Lancaster, J. B., Altmann, J., Rossi, A. S., & Sherrod, L. T. (Eds.). (1987). *Parenting across the life span: Biosocial dimensions.* New York: Aldine de Gruyter.

Masnick, G., & Bane, M. J. (1980). *The nation's families: 1960 to 1990.* Cambridge, MA: Joint Center for Urban Studies.

Meyers, C. E., Borthwick, S. A., & Eyman, R. (1985). Place of residence by age, ethnicity, and level of retardation of the mentally retarded/developmentally disabled population of California. *American Journal of Mental Deficiency, 90*, 266–270.

Olson, D. H., McCubbin, H. I., & Associates (1983). *Families: What makes them work.* Beverly Hills: Sage.

Richardson, S. A., Koller, H., & Katz, M. (1985). Relationship of upbringing to later behavior disturbance of mildly retarded young people. *American Journal of Mental Deficiency, 90*, 1–8.

Riley, M. W. (1986). Overview and highlights of a sociological perspective. In A. B. Sorensen, F. E. Weinert, & L. R. Sherrod (Eds.), *Human development and life course* (pp. 153–175). Hillsdale, NJ: Princeton University Press.

Riley, M. W. (1988). On the significance of age in sociology. In M. W. Riley (Ed.), *Social structures and human lives* (pp. 24–45). Beverly Hills: Sage.

Rossi, A. S. (1987). Parenthood in transition: From lineage to child to self-orientation. In J. B. Lancaster, J. Altmann, A. S. Rossi, & L. R. Sherrod (Eds.), *Parenting across the life span: Biosocial dimensions* (pp. 31–81). New York: Aldine de Gruyter.

Ryder, N. B. (1965). The cohort as a concept in the study of social change. *American Sociological Review*, *30*, 843–861.

Ryff, C. D. (1989a). *Getting better, getting worse with time: Beliefs about personal change from young adulthood through old age*. Paper presented at the Meeting of the International Society for the Study of Behavioral Development, Finland.

Ryff, C. D. (1989b). In the eye of the beholder: Views of psychological well-being among middle-aged and older adults. *Psychology and Aging*, *4*, 195–210.

Schaie, K. W. (1988). The impact of research methodology on theory building in the developmental sciences. In J. E. Birren & V. L. Bengston (Eds.), *Emergent theories of aging* (pp. 41–57). New York: Springer.

Seltzer, G. B., Begun, A. L., Seltzer, M. M., & Krauss, M. W. (1991). Adults with mental retardation and their aging mothers: Impacts of Siblings *Family Relations*, *40*, 310–317.

Seltzer, M. M. (1985). Informal supports for aging mentally retarded persons. *American Journal of Mental Deficiency*, *90*, 259–265.

Seltzer, M. M., & Krauss, M. W. (1984). Placement alternatives for mentally retarded children and their families. In J. Blacher (Ed.), *Severely handicapped children and their families: Research in review* (pp. 143–175). New York: Academic Press.

Seltzer, M. M., & Krauss, M. W. (1989a). Aging parents with mentally retarded children: Family risk factors and sources of support. *American Journal on Mental Retardation*, *94*, 303–312.

Seltzer, M. M., & Krauss, M. W. (1989b). *Preliminary report on long-range planning*. Unpublished manuscript, University of Wisconsin, Madison.

Simeonsson, R. J., & Bailey, D. B. (1986). Siblings of handicapped children. In J. J. Gallagher & P. M. Vietze (Eds.), *Families of handicapped persons: Research, programs, and policy issues* (pp. 67–77). Baltimore, MD: Brookes.

Simeonsson, R. J., & McHale, S. M. (1981). Review: Research on handicapped children: Sibling relationships. *Child: Care, health, and development*, *7*, 153–171.

Suelze, M., & Keenan, V. (1981). Changes in family support networks over the life cycle of mentally retarded persons. *American Journal of Mental Deficiency*, *86*, 267–274.

Tausig, M. (1985). Factors in family decision-making about placement for developmentally disabled individuals. *American Journal of Mental Deficiency*, *89*, 352–361.

Townsend, A., Noelker, L., Deimling, G., & Bass, D. (1989). Longitudinal impact of interhousehold caregiving on adult children's mental health. *Psychology and Aging*, *4*, 393–401.

Turnbull, A. P., Summers, J. A., & Brotherson, M. J. (1986). Family life cycle: Theoretical and empirical implications and future directions for families with mentally retarded members. In J. J. Gallagher & P. M. Vietze (Eds.), *Families of handicapped persons: Research, programs, and policy issues*. Baltimore, MD: Brookes.

U.S. Senate Special Committee on Aging (1985–1986). *Aging America: Trends and projections*. Washington, DC: US Government Printing Office.

Wikler, L. (1986). Family stress theory and research on families of children with mental retardation. In J. J. Gallagher & P. M. Vietze (Eds.), *Families of handicapped persons: Research, programs and policy issues* (pp. 167–195). Baltimore, MD: Brookes.

Zarit, S., Reever, K., & Bach-Peterson, J. (1980). Relatives of the impaired elderly: Correlates of feelings of burden. *The Gerontologist, 20,* 649–655.

Zetlin, A. (1986). Mentally retarded adults and their siblings. *American Journal of Mental Deficiency, 91,* 217–225.

7
Adolescence and Community Adjustment

Laraine Masters Glidden and Andrea G. Zetlin

Adolescence is frequently conceptualized as a transitional stage, as a bridge between the emotional and economic dependency of childhood and the autonomy and independence orientation of adulthood. Although this notion of transition is reasonable, it should not lead to the mistaken belief that what occurs during adolescence is unimportant, or no different in kind from what occurs during other developmental periods of the life span. In Western industrialized societies especially, adolescence is a rather lengthy period of preparation wherein the man or woman child is given the opportunity to try on and train for the various roles of adulthood (Hopkins, 1983, p. 9).

These roles and the experiences that are crucial for their successful performance are not equally relevant for all adolescents. For example, whether voluntarily or not, some adults will not take on the role of parent, and others may not be wage earners. Determinants of role ascription and attainment include societal and cultural features as well as individual characteristics. Some cultures, for instance, might forbid the role of religious adherent, whereas others will either sanction or even mandate it. Sometimes, societies assign roles on the basis of individual characteristics. Many cultures and subcultures, for example, differentiate adolescent and adult roles on the basis of gender.

In contemporary American society, one important determinant of role assignment is intellectual ability. For persons with mental retardation, adult roles and the preparation in adolescence for those roles may be substantially different from those for individuals without mental retardation. Furthermore, differences often depend on the degree of mental retardation. The person with mild or borderline mental retardation, like the one without mental retardation, may expect and be expected to be economically independent, to marry and to parent, and to be generally a fully functioning citizen of the society. In contrast, the profoundly retarded individual is not expected to perform any of these roles.

Nonetheless, the focus of this chapter, that of adolescence and community adjustment, is relevant for all individuals with retardation, regardless of level of functioning. However, the emphasis is different, depending on functional level. Many adolescents with mild or borderline levels of mental retardation will blend into the anonymity of unlabeled and unserved adults once they leave the school system. For them, the emphasis is on how they will adjust to the community (Edgerton, 1984). The demands that the community may make on them in the year 2000 are critical. In contrast, for the lowest functioning retarded persons, the issue is more how the community will adjust to them as they move from childhood into adulthood, and lifelong dependence becomes a reality rather than a prognosis.

For prediction to the year 2000, a number of general trends are relevant. First, the demographics of the adolescent population for that year are already largely determined by the birth rate and the numbers of children born in the 1980s. The birth rates, or number of children born per 1,000 individuals in the population, were at historic lows throughout most of the 1980s. For example, during the 1984 to 1988 period, the rate averaged 15.7, in comparison to 19.6 in 1965, about two decades earlier (U.S. Bureau of the Census, 1990). Nonetheless, despite the low birth rate, cohort group size, or the number of children born, actually increased each year during the 1980s. For example, in 1988, 3.91 million children were born, in contrast to 3.61 million in 1980. This 3.91 million was larger than the 1965 cohort group of 3.76 million despite a birth rate of 19.4 per 1,000 women in 1965 in comparison with 15.9 in 1988. The birth of more children, despite declining birth rate, is a function, in part, of the large number of women, the baby boomers, having children in the 1980s. It is also the result of high birth rates among selected segments of the population, that is, African American and Hispanic women. These children will, of course, be in adolescence in the year 2000.

Thus, for all adolescents, community adjustment will be affected by the sheer size of the cohort group. An important consequence for adolescents with mental retardation concerns service provision. Because these children have been raised during an era of extensive service provision (e.g., educational, health, and social-vocational programs), community agencies will need to expand to continue to offer the level of service that has come to be expected.

These larger numbers may also collide with societal problems, which may produce adolescents with mental retardation. For example, economic analyses show that the 1980s was a decade in which the rich got richer and the poor got poorer. The top 20% of income earners increased their share of the American wealth, whereas the bottom 80% got less. Although its overall effect has been limited, immigration, particularly of poor Hispanics, has contributed to this trend. For example, there were 50% more Hispanic households in 1989 than there were in 1980, representing 20% of the increase of all households (Samuelson, 1989).

Poverty is a risk factor and one of the defining criteria for mental retardation that is due to psychosocial disadvantage (Grossman, 1983). Thus, just on the basis of birth and poverty indices alone, we should expect a higher prevalence of mentally retarded adolescents by the year 2000. Of course, poverty is often linked with additional risk factors such as young and single parenthood, low educational level, and drug abuse. Some of these risk factors, such as maternal crack cocaine use, increased dramatically during the 1980s and led to vulnerable babies who may well be mentally retarded adolescents by the year 2000.

Furthermore, it is likely that the 1980s' trend toward delabeling and mainstreaming those individuals with IQ scores in the 55 to 70 range will reverse. Although mainstreaming, especially combined with individualized instruction, does seem to benefit children whose IQs are above 70, results are more equivocal for those with lower IQs (Madden & Slavin, 1983). Furthermore, influential scientists and educators have begun to emphasize the negative aspects of mainstreaming and delabeling (e.g., MacMillan, 1989; Pollaway, 1985; Siperstein, Bak, & O'Keefe, 1988). In addition, an increasingly complex society will demand ever higher functioning individuals (Glidden, 1988).

Another aspect of this predicted reversal is the trend toward early classification and service provision exemplified by PL 99–457 and infant and toddler identification initiatives. As intended, early identification and intervention may lead to some prevention. The prevention may be primary, as in removing children from a high-risk to a low-risk environment; secondary, as in infant-stimulation programs for children exhibiting developmental delays; or tertiary, as in teaching manual language to children unable to use oral language. Regardless of the nature of the intervention, however, in addition to prevention, current efforts may lead to even more lifelong labeling and intervention.

The prediction of more adolescents with mental retardation by the year 2000 and the recognition of the importance of adolescence as a life stage combine to make the issue of adolescence and community adjustment a critical one. Equally critical, however, is that adolescence has not generally been given much attention in the mental retardation literature (Rowitz, 1988; Shapiro & Friedman, 1987). Nor have specialists in adolescence much concerned themselves with mental retardation. Indeed, textbooks and reviews of the literature on the subject tend to ignore the issue (Fuhrman, 1986; Manaster, 1989; Petersen, 1988).

This neglect is unfortunate because the developmental tasks of adolescence are conceptually important for understanding the experiences and adjustment of the adolescent with mental retardation. Havighurst (1953) describes 10 different tasks that are the "stagework" of the adolescent. These tasks focus on the development of self; on relationships with agemates, parents and other adults; and on preparing for the future in terms of occupation, marriage and the family, and citizenship. Most adolescents with mental retardation will need to tackle at least some of these developmental tasks because they are functioning at a level where they will be expected to become independent or semi-independent as adults.

In the next section, we discuss these relatively high-functioning adolescents, focusing on four major aspects of their lives: personal characteristics, the home environment and relations with parents, peer relations, and the school environment. Within each of these domains, all critical to the issue of community adjustment, we will address the difficulties that adolescents with mental retardation may have in successfully completing the relevant developmental tasks.

High-Functioning Adolescents With Mental Retardation

Personal Characteristics

Although "Sturm und Drang" versions of the adolescent experience are now perceived as more myth than reality, there does appear to be a higher incidence of behavioral disturbance among adolescents with mild retardation than among adolescents without retardation (Chess, 1977; Koller, Richardson, Katz, & McLaren, 1982, 1983; MacMillan, 1982; Syzmanski, 1977). Brier (1986) reported that some 20% to 35% of adolescents with mental retardation experience behavioral disorders compared to 14% to 18% in the nonretarded population. Furthermore, Zetlin (1985) found that at least 61% of her sample had exhibited some form of problem behavior during their teen years. Community-based adults with mild retardation and their parents described instances of drug or alcohol abuse, temper tantrums, destructive behavior, and withdrawal. The nature of the adolescents' concerns were similar to those felt by many adolescents but were intensified by retardation (Zetlin & Turner, 1985). Parent–child relations were a central area of tension, but issues of independence were more complex because of parental concerns about the adolescent's competence and judgment. Similarly, efforts to establish a sense of identity were complicated by (a) the need to acknowledge their "differentness" and the effect it was having on their lives and (b) having to deal with overt rejection and discrepancies between their achievements and those of their siblings and age-mates.

The stereotypes and perceptions that others have of people with mental retardation play a vital role in the identity that the adolescent with retardation must develop. One of Havighurst's adolescent tasks is the development of an appropriate masculine or feminine social role. The adoption of such a role may be particularly difficult when the perceptions and expectations of others conflict with that role. The story of Colette as told by her mother is an especially poignant example of these difficulties (Kaufman, 1986). Colette wanted independence, love, marriage, a family, a job that she enjoyed, a car, and many of the other accoutrements that are part of the American ideal. Her mother, however, had considerably lower expectations for her, and only gradually came to understant the "normalness" of Colette's identification with her feminine social role.

Despite their expectations of a normal life, even the highest functioning adolescents with mental retardation may not possess many of the competencies that allow them to achieve what they want. For example, comparison of the coping responses of adolescents with and without mild retardation revealed that adolescents with mild retardation were less apt to take control of problem situations or attempt to actively resolve conflict (Wayment & Zetlin, 1989). Adolescents with mild retardation tended to invoke less-developed negotiative styles and more passive emotional responses, whereas nonhandicapped adolescents showed a greater willingness to confront conflict, especially when placed in the position of hypothetical victim, when seeking increased autonomy, or when faced with a stressful problem. The authors argued that socialization practices that fostered dependence in adolescents with mild retardation, as well as repeated exposure to failure, may have resulted in these young people having had less opportunity to understand and assert personal power.

Despite their adjustment difficulties with establishing an identity and coping with daily problems, adolescents with mental retardation do not appear to be at risk for many of the chronic problems and pathologies that begin to make their appearance during this stage. For example, the extent of alcohol and substance abuse among adolescents with mild retardation still needs to be explored. Even those individuals who were involved with drugs and alcohol as adolescents in Zetlin's (1985) sample did not continue their substance abuse into their adulthood. Furthermore, studies conducted on various adult populations with mild retardation suggest that neither drug nor alcohol use pose significant problems for individuals with retardation (Edgerton, 1986). A small percentage of heavy users was identified in Zetlin's (1987) study of high school students with mild retardation, but only among those who were most integrated into a nonhandicapped peer group. As mainstreaming encourages closer associations between adolescents with and without retardation, this relatively "drug-free" population may be at risk for substance abuse much like their nonhandicapped counterparts.

Home and Family Environment

Many writers have addressed the issue of parental protection and overprotection (e.g., Paulson & Stone, 1973; Tingey, 1988). Because parents of adolescents with retardation are unclear or in conflict as to what their child's adult role will be, it may not be easy for them to withdraw protective supervision. As their child with retardation matures, they may inadvertently encourage dependency, obedience, and child-like behavior rather than independence, self-direction, assumption of responsibility, and sexual awareness. Murtaugh and Zetlin (1988) compared the process of increasing autonomy in adolescents, with and without mild retardation, and found adolescents with retardation slow to shed close supervision by parents. Adolescents with retardation were more likely to stay in close proximity to home during free time (i.e., weekends, after school, holidays/vacation periods) and were less inclined to challenge parental restrictions. Patterns of parental control established during the childhood period seemed to be the same patterns in effect even as these individuals approached high school graduation. The pressures faced by parents of nonhandicapped adolescents to break patterns of protective care were, for the most part, absent in the families of adolescents with mild retardation. The authors felt that the passive acceptance of low levels of autonomy by these teenagers with mild retardation prolonged conditions of dependency.

In a related study, Morrison and Zetlin (1988) found that when questioned about parental control adolescents with and without retardation similarly indicated an increasing desire to disengage or emotionally separate from families. Responses by parents of the nonhandicapped adolescents seemed to acknowledge the need for developmental change, but responses by parents of adolescents with retardation emphasized the need for continued structure and supervision at home. A collision course appeared likely unless the parents of adolescents with retardation began to recognize the need for increased autonomy and began revising their overcontrolling practices. There seems to be a need for a gradual decrease of parental restrictions beginning in early adolescence to encourage less-dependent behavior and more active coping responses so young people with retardation can assume increasing control of their lives.

Of course, parents are frequently provided with a double message regarding supervision of their children, adolescents, and adults with mental retardation. On the one hand, increasingly, we expect parents to be decision makers, advocates, case managers, and teachers (Allen & Hudd, 1987). On the other hand, we expect them to disengage as their children grow up. The latter expectation may be especially difficult for parents to fulfill as adolescents become young adults, and the many services that they were guaranteed by educational law and policy become unavailable or inaccessible as soon as they reach their 21st birthdays.

Peer Relations

For most persons, whether with or without mental retardation, adolescence is a time of increasingly frequent and psychologically important peer relationships. Even adolescents with moderate mental retardation are quite similar in their classroom social relationships to nonretarded peers. Siperstein and Bak (1989), in a study of seven different classrooms reported that friendship choices were both selective and reciprocal, and some classmates were popular and others were rejected. Nonetheless, there are also differences that are relevant to community adjustment. Zetlin and Murtaugh (1988), in a comparison of the friendship patterns of adolescents with and without retardation, found differences in both the nature and structure of the peer group. Adolescents with retardation had fewer friendships than their nonhandicapped counterparts, and these friendships tended to be with same-sex peers, some of whom were close relatives. For at least half, peer contact occurred during school hours only with some evening or weekend phone conversations. These friendships were also less stable and more discordant than those of nonhandicapped teenagers, and there was less evidence of intimacy and empathy among associates.

Examination of why peer relations between adolescents with retardation were conflictive and short-lived revealed the use of less-effective interaction strategies as compared to those employed by nonhandicapped peers (Zetlin, 1989). Adolescents with retardation invoked egoistic strategies that were provocative and increased the probability of continued conflict. These strategies were characteristic of younger children. Nonhandicapped teens, on the other hand, were more likely to acquiesce or negotiate confrontations that lessened the likelihood of future conflict. Cognitive factors and changing emotional needs were believed to account for only a small portion of the differences in friendship patterns observed between samples. Overprotective parental practices, as well as the limited friendship pool available to adolescents with retardation, restricted opportunities to learn the social skills necessary for establishing and maintaining intimate and mutually responsive relationships. Because peer relationships during adolescence serve as foundations for relationships with spouses, neighbors, and co-workers during adulthood, it is of critical importance that the social opportunities of adolescents with mild retardation be broadened. Shapiro and Friedman (1987) warn that unless substantial efforts are made to develop social skills, it is inevitable that adolescents with retardation will remain isolated and unaccepted by their peers and will continue to have difficult social adjustments.

School and Postschool Experience

The school is the environment where the adolescent works on many of the relevant developmental tasks. Identity development, social skills practice, intellectual competence, and vocational preparation are all part of the school experience. Although wholesale indictment of the school's performance is not the theme of this chapter, adolescents with mild retardation have been found to be as bored, alienated, and lacking in motivation for schoolwork as their nonhandicapped peers (Murtaugh & Zetlin, 1989). In this study, only a minority of students from both regular and special education were involved in their schoolwork, but they appeared motivated by the external rewards of obtaining passing grades, a high school diploma, and entrance to college rather than by the intrinsic rewards of learning. Although both groups exhibited little interest in academic subjects, most of the nonhandicapped youths were involved in at least one outside activity (i.e., tennis, art, scuba diving, acting, music composition) that they pursued with rigor and that seemed especially important to their self-esteem (Murtaugh, 1988). In contrast, the adolescents with mild retardation were less likely to have serious interests outside of the classroom, which seemed due to several factors: lack of basic skills (i.e., reading); inability to concentrate on a task over an extended period of time; and low tolerance of frustration for failure.

Another aspect of the school experience is achievement and success in academics. Here, the adolescent with mental retardation is clearly at risk. Studies of school achievement and dropout show higher failure rates for individuals with lower IQs. For example, in a large-sample study of over 2,000 high school students, Bachman, Green, and Wirtanen (1971) found that the dropout rate for students with IQs of 91 or lower was almost six times greater than for those with IQs of 125 or higher (p. 41). In addition, in the same sample, the students with the lowest reading skills scores had a dropout rate of about 45% in contrast to only 5% for students with the highest reading skills scores (pp. 44–45). More recently, the high school competency movement may be having its negative effects on adolescents with mild mental retardation. In Florida, a state with minimum competency exams, only 3.5% of a sample of educable mentally handicapped students passed reading and writing tests; only 2% passed the mathematics exams (Crews, 1988). Konanc and Warren (1984) present compelling case studies that add dimension to these numbers. They describe how exam failure or the anxiety surrounding potential failure can precipitate individual or family crisis at the time of anticipated high school completion. Clearly, the impact of these failures has implications for community adjustment.

A number of recent studies have examined the post-high school adjustment of former students with mild retardation using employment status and/or post-secondary school attendance as criteria for community adjustment. Richardson (1978), in a comprehensive study in Scotland, found only a slightly higher percentage of unemployment among 22-year-olds with retardation in comparison to those without retardation. However, jobs held by the cohort with retardation required less skill, involved less interpersonal contact, and were lower pay than those held by their nonretarded peers. Richardson cautioned that these data were collected during a period of economic boom when there was virtually full employment in their age group. A decade later, Edgar (1987) followed up 39 graduates of programs for the mildly retarded in the state of Washington and found only 41% were working or in some form of vocational training, while the remaining 59% were doing little or nothing at the time of contact. A study conducted by Kerachsky and Thornton (1987) in five major urban areas, found that one-third of the teenagers with mild retardation had no vocational involvement at all.

Zetlin and Hosseini (1989) presented case studies of six special education graduates, and Zetlin and Murtaugh (1990) described the post-school lives of 20 adolescents with mild retardation. Almost all of the young people described experienced a great deal of instability after high school, drifting without direction between jobs and educational programs. Their "roller-coaster-like" experiences did little to enhance their self-esteem and in many cases left them depressed and open to self-doubt. Feelings of anxiety, frustration over limitations, and uncertainty of their future appeared to place them at risk for developing socioemotional problems that could further impact their community adjustments.

Additionally, even those individuals who may appear to be achieving a normalized life may be relatively poorly adjusted in the community. For example, studies of adults with and without mental retardation demonstrate little social integration in the workplace even when there is physical integration (Chadsey-Rusch, Gonzalez, Tines, & Johnson, 1989; Lignugaris/Kraft, Salzberg, Rule, & Stowitschek, 1988). Dudley (1983), after a multiyear study of 27 adults with mental retardation, emphasized the separateness of the worlds of those with mental retardation and those without. He claimed that, "These two worlds typically exist side by side as separate entities with only occasional points of intersection" and that, "The two worlds are divided on a social basis" rather than on a physical basis (p. 24).

Low-Functioning Adolescents With Mental Retardation

The high-functioning adolescent with mental retardation may share a physical world with the nonretarded adolescent, but the low-functioning adolescent only occasionally shares even that. For the most part, individuals with severe or profound mental retardation are segregated from the nonretarded. They are educated in separate classrooms and frequently in separate schools. Their worlds may intersect only briefly as neighbors, as fellow consumers in a restaurant or bowling alley, or as co-participants in a school or church-related activity. The most important issue regarding community adjustment for the low-functioning adolescent who will never be independent or achieve any of the important developmental milestones of adolescence or adulthood is the issue of societal attitudes and policy regarding normalization and least restrictive environment principles.

A component of societal attitude is that of family attitude. Family stress and distress may deepen during adolescence. Although physical growth and maturation may be delayed or reduced for some adolescents with severe or profound disabilities, for others, larger size may significantly increase the burden of caretaking (Brotherson, Backus, Summers, & Turnbull, 1986). Sexuality and menstruation become issues, and although higher functioning adolescents can be expected to be fully independent in the maintenance of adequate hygiene (Pueschel, 1988), others will need supervision. The family may also come into conflict with the community regarding freedom of sexual expression and protection from sexual exploitation. For example, some parents may want sterilization for their adolescent children, but the courts may see this request as infringing on the rights of the person to be sterilized, regardless of that person's level of functioning (Drew, Logan, & Hardman, 1988).

Perhaps the most difficult but also crucial issues that surface during adolescence are those of lifelong care and training. As age 21 approaches, so does the time when public education will cease. For many families, the transition from school to whatever may come after school is the most difficult transition to be made. Normal routines will need to shift; an aging family may need to consider alternative residences; service availability and accessibility become major foci for the family. And a major adjustment difficulty may ensue with the realization that the educational rights guaranteed for their children from birth to 21 years no longer pertain to adult service programs (Turnbull, Turnbull, Bronicki, Summers, & Roeder-Gordon, 1989).

In sum, for both the family and the rest of the community, adolescence brings with it a rather final facing of the facts with regard to the very disabled person. No longer can the individual be viewed as a child whose development may show a sudden spurt. Physical maturation brings with it the reality of lifelong dependence and the need to confront the issues of family and community responsibility for the person's well-being. How the family and the larger community will respond in the year 2000 is addressed in the next, and concluding, section of this chapter.

Adolescence and Mental Retardation in the Year 2000

Futurism is a risky but necessary business. Planning for the future involves predicting it, and prediction demands examination of past trends and present events. Based on the issues that we have explored in this chapter, we believe that during the next decade the following important developments will take place with regard to adolescence and mental retardation:

1. Adolescents with mental retardation will be studied with increasing frequency. The larger size of the cohort groups will draw attention, as will the recognition that the developmental and related adjustment issues of all adolescents are crucial issues for most adolescents with mental retardation.
2. Continuing review of public education initiatives and how they impact on adolescents with mental retardation will force reexamination of benefits and liabilities of mainstreaming. If higher functioning adolescents with mental retardation fail to graduate from high school, or do not receive the kinds of vocational preparation that are necessary to compete in the adult world of work, the cry for a return to special education may become more strident. In addition, if the recent findings on social segregation despite physical integration are reliable, another reputed value of mainstreaming can be called into question.
3. A focus on life-span issues, borrowed from general developmental psychology, has also become paramount in mental retardation (e.g., Lerner, 1987; Petersen, 1987). We think this focus will receive even more attention in the next decade. This emphasis has special significance for adolescence and mental retardation, and we expect that late adolescence, as the transition between childhood and adulthood, between school and work, will attract more interest from both theoreticians and service providers.
4. The life-span focus is relevant for the lower functioning individual with mental retardation, as well as the higher functioning one. For adolescents who will remain dependent as adults, family versus community responsibilities may engender major controversy. A recent attempt in Maryland to charge parents for costs of group home living may be an augur of what we can expect from governors and state legislatures trying to balance fiscal health against social service principles.

In conclusion, predictions of the future are tenuous, whether they be a prognosis for an individual, a class of individuals, or a society. What is not tenuous, however, is that the life of the future is based on seeds planted in the present. We are already on the trajectory that will take us into the 21st century. What the year 2000 has to offer will be based on current research and policy initiatives. Futurism may be a risky business, but the failure to look and plan ahead is even more dangerous.

Acknowledgment. This manuscript was written while the first author was supported, in part, by National Institute of Child Health and Human Development Grant No. HD 21993.

References

Allen, D. A., & Hudd, S. S. (1987). Are we professionalizing parents? Weighing the benefits and pitfalls. *Mental Retardation, 25*, 133–139.

Bachman, J. G., Green, S., & Wirtanen, I. D. (1971). *Youth in transition: Vol. 3. Dropping out—problem or symptom?* Ann Arbor, MI: Institute for Social Research.

Brier, N. (1986). The mildly retarded adolescent: A psychosocial perspective. *Journal of Developmental & Behavioral Pediatrics, 7*, 320–323.

Brotherson, M. J., Backus, L. H., Summers, J. A., & Turnbull, A. P. (1986). Transition to adulthood. In J. A. Summers (Ed.), *The right to grow up* (pp. 17–44). Baltimore MD: Brookes.

Chadsey-Rusch, J., Gonzalez, P., Tines, J., & Johnson, J. R. (1989). Social ecology of the workplace: Contextual variables affecting social interactions of employees with and without mental retardation. *American Journal on Mental Retardation, 94*, 141–151.

Chess, S. (1977). Evolution of behavior disorder in a group of mentally retarded children. *Journal of the American Academy of Child Psychiatry, 16*, 4–18.

Crews, W. B. (1988). Performance of students classified as educable mentally handicapped on Florida's State Student Assessment Test, Part II. *Education and Training in Mental Retardation, 23*, 186–191.

Drew, C. J., Logan, D. R., & Hardman, M. L. (1988). *Mental retardation: A life cycle approach* (4th ed.). Columbus, OH: Merrill.

Dudley, J. R. (1983). *Living with stigma: The plight of the people who we label mentally retarded.* Springfield, IL: Charles C. Thomas.

Edgar, E. (1987). Secondary programs in special education: Are many of them justifiable? *Exceptional Children, 53*, 555–561.

Edgerton, R. B. (Ed.). (1984). *Lives in process: Mildly retarded adults in a large city.* Monographs of the American Association on Mental Deficiency, No. 6. Washington, DC: American Association on Mental Deficiency.

Edgerton, R. B. (1986). Alcohol and drug use by mentally retarded adults. *American Journal of Mental Deficiency, 90*, 602–609.

Fuhrmann, B. S. (1986). *Adolescence, adolescents.* Boston: Little, Brown.

Glidden, L. M. (1988). Mental retardation: The future. *Mental Retardation, 26*, 318–321.

Grossman, H. J. (1983). *Classification in mental retardation.* Washington, DC: American Association on Mental Deficiency.

Havighurst, R. J. (1953). *Human development and education.* New York: David McKay.

Hopkins, J. R. (1983). *Adolescence, the transitional years.* New York: Academic Press.

Kaufman, S. Z. (1986). Life history in progress: A retarded daughter educates her mother. In L. L. Langness & H. G. Levine (Eds.), *Culture and retardation* (pp. 33–45). Dordrecht, Holland: D. Reidel.

Kerachsky, S., & Thornton, C. (1987). Findings from the STETS Transitional Employment Demonstration. *Exceptional Children, 53*, 515–521.

Koller, H., Richardson, S. A., Katz, M., & McLaren, J. (1982). Behavior disturbance in childhood and early adult years in populations who were and were not mentally retarded. *Journal of Preventive Psychiatry, 1*, 453–469.

Koller, H., Richardson, S. A., Katz, M., & McLaren, J. (1983). Behavior disturbance since childhood among a 5-year birth cohort of all mentally retarded young adults in a city. *American Journal of Mental Deficiency, 87*, 386–395.

Konanc, J. T., & Warren, N. J. (1984). Graduation: Transitional crisis for mildly developmentally disabled adolescents and their families. *Family Relations*, *33*, 135–142.

Lerner, R. M. (1987). A life-span perspective for early adolescence. In R. M. Lerner & T. T. Foch (Eds.), *Biological–psychosocial interactions in early adolescence* (pp. 9–34). Hillsdale, NJ: Erlbaum.

Lignugaris/Kraft, B., Salzberg, C. L., Rule, S., & Stowitschek, J. J. (1988). Social–vocational skills of workers with and without mental retardation in two community employment sites. *Mental Retardation*, *26*, 297–305.

MacMillan, D. L. (1982). *Mental retardation in school and society* (2nd ed.). Boston: Little, Brown.

MacMillan, D. L. (1989). Equality, excellence, and the EMR populations: 1970–1989. *Psychology in Mental Retardation and Developmental Disabilities*, *15*(2), 1, 3–10.

Madden, N. A., & Slavin, R. E. (1983). Mainstreaming students with mild handicaps: Academic and social outcomes. *Review of Educational Research*, *53*, 519–569.

Manaster, G. J. (1989). *Adolescent development, a psychological interpretation*. Itasca, IL: Peacock.

Morrison, G. M., & Zetlin, A. G. (1988). Perception of communication, cohesion and adaptability in families of adolescents with and without handicaps. *Journal of Abnormal Child Psychology*, *16*, 675–685.

Murtaugh, M. (1988). Achievement outside the classroom: The role of non-academic activities in the lives of high school students. *Anthropology and Education Quarterly*, *19*, 381–394.

Murtaugh, M., & Zetlin, A. G. (1988). Achievement of autonomy by non-handicapped and mildly handicapped adolescents. *Journal of Youth and Adolescence*, *17*, 445–460.

Murtaugh, M., & Zetlin, A. G. (1989). How serious is the motivation problem in secondary special education? *The High School Teacher*, *72*, 151–159.

Paulson, M. J., & Stone, D. (1973). Specialist-professional intervention: An expanding role in the care and treatment of the retarded and their families. In R. K. Eyman, C. E. Meyers, & G. Tarjan (Eds.), *Socio-behavioral studies in mental retardation* (Monograph No. 1). Washington, DC: American Association on Mental Deficiency.

Petersen, A. C. (1987). The nature of biological–psychosocial interactions: The sample case of early adolescence. In R. M. Lerner & T. T. Foch (Eds.), *Biological–psychosocial interactions in early adolescence* (pp. 35-61). Hillsdale, NJ: Erlbaum.

Petersen, A. C. (1988). Adolescent development. *Annual Review of Psychology*, *39*, 583–607.

Polloway, E. A. (1985). Identification and placement in mild mental retardation programs: Recommendations for professional practice. *Education and Training of the Mentally Retarded*, *20*, 218–221.

Pueschel, S. M. (1988). The biology of the maturing person with Down syndrome. In S. M. Pueschel (Ed.), *The young person with Down syndrome: Transition from adolescence to adulthood* (pp. 23–34). Baltimore: Brookes.

Richardson, S. A. (1978). Careers of mentally retarded young persons: Services, jobs and interpersonal relations. *American Journal of Mental Deficiency*, *82*, 349–358.

Rowitz, L. (1988). The forgotten ones: Adolescence and mental retardation. *Mental Retardation, 26,* 115–117.

Samuelson, R. J. (1989, October 25). Politics and poverty. *The Washington Post,* p. A27.

Shapiro, E. S., & Friedman, J. (1987). Mental retardation. In V. B. Van Hasselt & M. Hersen (Eds.), *Handbook of adolescent psychology* (pp. 381–397). New York: Pergamon Press.

Siperstein, G. N., & Bak, J. J. (1989). Social relationships of adolescents with moderate mental retardation. *Mental Retardation, 27,* 5–10.

Siperstein, G. N., Bak, J. J., & O'Keefe, P. (1988). Relationship between children's attitudes toward and their social acceptance of mentally retarded peers. *American Journal of Mental Retardation, 93,* 24–27.

Szymanski, L. S. (1977). Psychiatric diagnostic evaluation of mentally retarded individuals. *Journal of the American Academy of Child Psychiatry, 16,* 67–87.

Tingey, C. (1988). Cutting the umbilical cord: Parental perspectives. In S. M. Pueschel (Ed.), *The young person with Down syndrome: Transition from adolescence to adulthood* (pp. 5–22). Baltimore MD: Brookes.

Turnbull, H. R., Turnbull, A. P., Bronicki, G. J., Summers, J. A., & Roeder-Gordon, C. (1989). *Disability and the family: A guide to decisions for adulthood.* Baltimore MD: Brookes.

U.S. Bureau of the Census. (1990). *Statistical abstract of the United States: 1990* (110th ed.). Washington, DC: U.S. Government Printing Office.

Wayment, H. A., & Zetlin, A. G. (1989). Coping responses of mildly learning handicapped and nonhandicapped adolescents. *Mental Retardation, 27,* 311–316.

Zetlin, A. G. (1985). Mentally retarded teenagers: Adolescent behavior disturbance and its relation to family environment. *Child Psychiatry and Human Development, 15,* 243–254.

Zetlin, A. G. (1987). The social status of mildly learning handicapped high school students. *Psychology in the Schools, 24,* 165–173.

Zetlin, A. G. (1989). Managing conflict: Interactional strategies of learning handicapped and nonhandicapped high school students. *Journal of Youth and Adolescence, 18,* 263–272.

Zetlin, A. G., & Hosseini, A. (1989). Moving toward adult status: Six case studies of mildly learning handicapped young adults who have left school. *Exceptional Children, 55,* 405–411.

Zetlin, A. G., & Murtaugh, M. (1988). Friendship patterns of mildly learning handicapped and nonhandicapped high school students. *American Journal on Mental Retardation, 92,* 447–454.

Zetlin, A. G., & Murtaugh, M. (1990). Whatever happened to those with borderline IQ's? *American Journal on Mental Retardation, 94,* 463–469.

Zetlin, A. G., & Turner, J. L. (1985). Transition from adolescence to adulthood: Perspectives of mentally retarded individuals and their families. *American Journal of Mental Deficiency, 89,* 570–579.

8
Lifelong Disability and Aging

Matthew P. Janicki

In the early 1970s, advocacy for equal educational opportunities led to the passage of PL 94-142, the Education for All Handicapped Children Act. With the implementation of this Act (and its amendments), expectations are that children and adolescents with handicapping conditions can be fully integrated within the mainstream of society's opportunities and activities. In the late 1970s, revisions to this and the Rehabilitation Act of 1973 have done the same for preschoolers and work-age adults, respectively. With the inclusion of disability-related provisions in amendments to the Older Americans Act (PL 100-175), the same expectations have been set for older individuals with lifelong disabilities.

For persons with mental retardation, reaching old age always was a readily, albeit a reality that was subordinated to other developmental concerns. In the past, many persons with severe mental retardation had a relatively short life span, and most adults with mental retardation spent much of their lives in public institutions. Consequently, their aging was not of immediate concern. Now, however, increased longevity, resulting in part from more readily available social and residential services and improved health status, and added visibility, as a result of living in the community, have contributed to a raised awareness of life-span development and aging issues (Janicki & Seltzer, 1991).

In this sense, the field of mental retardation has come to full maturity with the acceptance by its workers that their efforts must include all facets of the life span. When early writers first begin to raise the issue of aging (e.g., Dybwad, 1962), the focus was not so much on gerontological issues, but on adult development, especially up to the middle-age years. Contemporary workers are now concerned with all facets of the aging process among adults with mental retardation, in particular, because it is evident that provider agencies serve many individuals from among those in the third age, and even from among the old-old, including some centenarians. Further, another indication of the breadth of these concerns is that the aging of persons with mental retardation and other lifelong disabilities has become a cross-cutting issue among various governmental agencies in the United States and abroad (Davidson et al., 1987; Hogg, Moss & Cooke, 1987).

In the late 1980s, at the behest of Congress, the National Institute on Aging published a report on the assessment of the need for personnel to provide for future populations of the elderly. The report noted that the nation's population of older persons with mental retardation is expected to grow considerably over the next 30 years (National Institute on Aging, 1987). This led the Institute to initiate a broad agenda for aging and mental retardation research (NIH, 1989). The report also identified three major groups of older individuals with mental retardation, each with a different set of needs with clinical and programmatic implications for the future.

The first group represents older adults with *minimal cognitive or physical handicap* who have been fairly independent all their adult lives, and only because of impairments associated with aging is it expected that they again will become dependent on special assistance from social services agencies or the aging network.

The second group represents older adults with *moderate cognitive or physical impairments* who have a need for supervision or special training, and as they age, it is expected that they again will become dependent on a range of special mental retardation–developmental disabilities social services and aging network services.

The third group represents older adults with *severe or profound cognitive and/or physical impairments* whose gross dependency will necessitate a range of very specialized long-term care and habilitation services, and it is expected that they will continue, as they age, to be the life-long responsibility of mental retardation–developmental disabilities agencies.

In anticipation of the future needs of older persons with mental retardation, Congress in the late 1980s amended two distinct federal statutes to include disability-related provisions. The first included the addition of a number of provisions to the Developmental Disabilities Act (PL 100-146). One directed the state developmental disabilities planning councils to appoint to the council the state aging agency administrator, and another required the councils to consider aging-related planning issues. In addition, amendments related to the nation's "university-affiliated programs" called for the addition to the mission of these programs to be expanded to include training and education in the areas of gerontology and/or geriatrics and disability.

The other set of amendments included the addition of numerous special provisions for "individuals with disabilities," including mental retardation, to the Older Americans Act (PL 100-175). These provisions recognized that older persons with disabilities have special needs, which require close collaboration and coordination of planning activities and services between the aging network and disability agencies at the federal, state, and local levels. These provisions were added to ensure the inclusion of persons with lifelong disabilities within the gamut of special services available to other needy elderly persons. They set the expectation that mainstream aging network services would be accessible to all elderly persons irrespective of the nature of their disability (i.e., whether it is late life or lifelong).

Policy and Programmatic Considerations for the Future

Much of the growth of interest in this segment of the life span is attributed to the changing demographics within the United States and other developed nations. Among the general population, currently, about one out of every nine persons is an older adult. Within the next 30 years, that number will increase to one out of every five. These same population changes are expected among older persons with mental retardation. Indeed, in one study, it was noted that for every older person currently in service, three to four would be seeking services within the next 10 to 20 years (Janicki, 1989a). There is no doubt that the number of older Americans with mental retardation has increased in size, as well as visibility, and will continue to grow markedly in the years to come. Changes in health care, nutrition, early childhood services, and social and housing conditions have led to decreases in mortality and morbidity and increases in the older age survivor rate of persons with lifelong disabilities. Expectations are that these trends will continue, particularly given the confluence of federal statutes promoting enriched programs, service entitlements, and general improved health status.

Notwithstanding these expectations, however, older persons with mental retardation, their families, public policy makers, and the myriad of agencies providing services will continue to face a number of problems and considerations for the future related to the aging of persons with lifelong disabilities. Thus, the service end of our field is faced with a number of broad policy dilemmas. One stems from concerns related to *intergenerational equity*—or the competition for resources among workers serving various points on the age span. This competition mirrors that found in the greater society, pitting advocates of children's services against advocates for the disabled and elderly.

Another stems from *intragenerational equity*: unresolved policy decisions among disability program administrators about whether to fund and operate segregated or integrated senior services for persons with lifelong disabilities and questions among administrators of aging network programs about whether to open and share existing scarce community services for the elderly to similarly needy persons with lifelong or other disabilities. Many mental retardation agency administrators with an aging clientele are faced with the choice of whether, when they have to begin to fund and/or provide some older age-related services, they should move to fully develop their programs already in place for older persons with mental retardation or to transfer funds and seek collaborative relationships with aging network programs that may have the capacity to serve some of their clientele. However, with tight budgets prevalent in most the states' human services agencies, fiscal considerations certainly will have more of an influence than "territoriality" in resolving these issues.

Added to these policy dilemmas is the consideration attributed to *increased longevity*, which has created a demand for services and special attention that many states and localities are ill prepared to address. Whereas many states had developed child-oriented developmental and remedial educational services, and adult-oriented vocational and social developmental services, the new demand for senior-oriented retardation services has been unanticipated. Further impacting is the reality that the increased longevity of many older adults has also resulted in unexpected public health concerns. For example, in the instance of older persons with Down syndrome, both the occurrence of premature aging and the co-occurrence of Alzheimer's disease have left agencies with unique challenges in the area of developing transitional services to accommodate middle-aged adults who are aging prematurely and/or who are experiencing progressive mental debilitation.

Another consideration relates to the *two-generation elderly family*, consisting of an elderly parent (or parents) who has (have) continued to bear the burden of care for an aging adult son or daughter with mental retardation. This situation is expected to increase in occurrence as a greater number of older parents continue to provide care within their homes for their aging adult sons or daughters with mental retardation. Added to this will be the enhanced expectations that both families and the adults with a disability will have as a result of having grown older in a service climate in the latter 20th century that was much more abiding to their needs. Certainly, one challenge for these families in the future will be the difficulty shown by their governments in meeting their demands, because many states have yet to link the services generally available to the at-need elderly with more traditional mental retardation services in such special situations or to be sufficiently robust in their service offerings to address this special situation.

Yet another consideration is the *"aging in place"* of older adults with mental retardation currently living at home or in a variety of community residential situations (e.g., foster family care homes, group homes, board and care homes, supportive apartments, and the like) and who, to prevent unnecessary institutionalization, need either a shifting in the types of service provided or new and broader support services. These numbers are continually growing, and as states place a greater emphasis on community care, they will only continue to grow. However, many states have not yet developed the flexibility to adapt their current service models to preclude having seniors move from their home by virtue of their age and/or the lack of preparedness on the part of the staff or inability by the home's administrators to effect program changes or simple building adaptations. Certainly, one major consideration for the year 2000 and beyond is the addressing of long-term care needs on a stable and humane basis (Estes, 1990) and to recognize that "aging in place" will necessitate agencies to rethink their configuration of services.

Another consideration relates to the realization within small communities that *duplicative day services are expensive* and counterproductive. Consequently, local health or aging officials need to look to consolidate day and residential services for age-similar dependent populations with common needs operated by different human services agencies. This would mean, for example, that existing adult day-care programs that may only take in individuals with age-related impairments, may need to open their doors to age peers with lifelong disabilities who require similar types of care. Conversely, disability providers who run adult day-service–type programs should also serve persons with age-associated impairments who have similar care needs.

Another consideration is how to provide transitions to *retirement-oriented senior programs* from vocational services (Cotten & Casey, 1990). Although it is easy to effect "retirement from" it is not that easy to effect "retirement to." In the general population, the primary gain associated with work, a salary, is usually substituted by Social Security old age benefits or a pension. Further, when most persons consider what to do on leaving the workforce, they also think in terms of what will replace work and the secondary gains associated with the work place, such as friendships, a place to go, and the personal identity that is defined by one's job. This notion of replacement leads to "retiring to." Often, the social and personal changes associated with retirement can be traumatic when bridging does not occur. As with other age-peers, older persons with mental retardation also find that the loss or change of friends when moving to a new program can pose a significant barrier. Most agencies are finding that the available alternatives may not compensate seniors for the loss of the social and financial supports associated with continued involvement in vocational services. Many seniors demure on retiring to senior programs because of the fear of losing their workshop or job income and close network of friends made in the workplace. Further, the transition supports normally available to nondisabled persons (such as pre-retirement counseling, pensions, and bridging opportunities) have not been readily available to sheltered workers and those in developmental training programs (DDPC, 1989).

Closely tied to this consideration is how to augment or present a useful service *model for day services* for older adults with continued needs for special services who have retired from vocational services or work.

Workers (e.g., Catapano, Levy, & Levy, 1985; Janicki, 1989b; Thurman, 1988) addressing this issue are finding that the program content within particular sites varies. However, the common theme is that persons with mental retardation should have options and should be able to choose from a range of activities offered in a relaxed and comfortable atmosphere. Program components need to account for health and sensory concern features; recreation and physical fitness; a variety of activities to stimulate cognitive skills, range of motion, socialization, and creativity; and individual or group counseling. Expectations are that as these program models and activities are more fully developed, they will be designed in a manner that is generally in the same vein as those activities provided to other seniors. As states expand their senior service offerings, however, care needs to be taken that program models are constantly reviewed and new creative models entertained.

These policy considerations are a few of the ones that will confront service providers as we move into the next century. Others, albeit more attuned to programmatic concerns, will also need to be addressed. For example, in some circumstances, living at home or in other settings may lead to a need for a change of residential setting. These needs will include a range of residential options. However, many states are wrestling with changes in programmatic regulations or policies that did not anticipate the aging of a large population of dependent adults. Current practices often include requirements for full day program involvement and termination of housing arrangement when the older adult becomes exceedingly frail. These barriers to continued living in the community—and more importantly, to living in one's long-term home—often vex service providers, because state regulations and policies are linked to the financing of the housing program, and once the residence is out of compliance with regard to a particular older resident, that resident's financial supports are undermined. Some states have begun to adapt their regulations and funding to these situations; others have yet to address the problem.

A significant programmatic concern relates to the philosophy of *rehabilitation intent* inherent in a state's clinical and program practices. Most states have supported their community housing through participation in the federal Medicaid program. The participating residences are certified as Intermediate Care Facilities for the Mentally Retarded (ICFs/MR) under Title XIX of the Social Security Act. Because of this, federal and state regulations are based on consistency with the "developmental model," that is, viewing each and every activity in which the participant is involved as leading to building or strengthening skills (Sparr & Smith, 1990). This emphasis on continued development and production of skills consistent with independence has come in conflict with the age-associated capabilities and typical involvements of persons of advanced age.

Gerontologists and workers in mental retardation and aging are beginning to conceive of the programmatic services for seniors with lifelong disabilities as being grounded in several basic tenets (Cotten & Casey, 1990). One is the availability of *"options and choices,"* whereby an older individual can pick from many things that he or she may wish to do, and being able to make a freely conceived choice as to whether to participate in an option or not (in contrast to the more "programmed" approach taken with work-age adults, where choice is subjugated to necessity). A second is the notion of *"interdependence"*—in contrast to independence. With advanced age, rehabilitation intent is no longer directed toward being able to work competitively and being as fully independent in society as possible. The intent is directed toward teaching how to become mutually reliant on others, in particular age peers, thus interdependent. A third is the concept of *"successful aging"*; borrowed from the aging field and meant to connote the learning to grow or capability of growing old with dignity, the term connotes a shift to a life-style typical of the third age, thus learning how to draw on the necessary supports to maintain one's ability to be as fully functional for as long as possible.

The Challenges for the Future

Much was accomplished in the latter 1980s with regard to aging and disability. A number of textbooks were published that examined aging and posited means for delivering services (e.g., Hogg, Moss, & Cooke, 1987; Howell, Gavin, Cabrera, & Beyer, 1989; Janicki, & Wisniewski, 1985; Roboul, Comte, & Jeantet, 1985; Seltzer, & Krauss, 1987; Stroud, Sutton, & Roberts, 1988); special research service initiatives were announced by federal research institutes and federal administrations (e.g., NIH, 1989); special journal issues were dedicated to a compendium of articles on this topic (e.g., Janicki, 1988; Rose & Ansello, 1988; Cotten & Spirrison, 1989; Janicki & Hugg, 1989); and workbooks and manuals were developed for specific guidance related to this area (LePore & Janicki, 1990; Sailer, 1987; Thurman, 1988).

Many state and local plans also were developed and issued (e.g., Woods, 1990); worker-affiliative groups organized, such as the aging and disability special interest groups in the American Psychological Association, the Gerontological Society of America, and the American Association on Mental Retardation; state and regional provider networks developed (LePore & Janicki, 1990), federal and state agreements were signed (e.g., the federal agreement between the Administration on Developmental Disabilities and the Administration on Aging, and the state agreement within New York (LePore & Janicki, 1990). Federal legislation, such as amendments to the Older Americans Act, was enacted; a series of new university training centers in aging and developmental disabilities were established ("ADD Aging Training Projects," 1990); and major national, state, and local conferences gave evidence to a marked interest for cross-training in the fields of gerontology, geriatrics, and mental retardation.

Notwithstanding all these accomplishments, however, realism gives witness to barriers that will serve as impediments to continued development and innovations. There will be barriers that are intrinsic to problems faced by families, to agencies confronted with an aging clientele, and to the lack of legislative and regulatory remedies to address the problems of a service system that has not yet realistically accommodated aging. Some will be systemic and become evident when attempting to collaborate with the aging network, yet others will only become evident when we attempt to develop specialized senior services within the mental retardation system.

Systemic barriers within the aging network include those related to a lack of acceptance of persons with handicapping conditions, program restrictions resulting from limited financial resources, and the lack of staff competent to work with individuals who are disabled. Similarly, there are systemic barriers within the mental retardation system that are based on exclusivity, a sense of superiority, or simply an unwillingness to face the problems that aging presents to an agency (Janicki, 1989b).

Eventual frailty will force agencies to confront the challenge of developing long-term care settings that provide specialized age-related services. There are solutions to these problems. For example, activities directed toward adapting the residence and retraining staff members, rather than forcing movement, are a much more functional means of addressing the transition associated with aging in place. Further, relief from regulatory constrictions to effect such changes can go far to ensure that a home remains a home.

Some barriers remain however, to be more fully addressed. For example, the future will need to address a number of challenges. The biggest is programmatic, and it involves retirement. How can we redesign our services, regulations, laws, and professional ideology and practices to accommodate the final stage of the lifespan? How to accommodate the third age in our thinking? Retirement brings with it its own particular dilemmas. How do persons who are dependent on public support retire? How do we justify a restructuring of programs? How do we provide for pensions or other retirement benefits that bring older persons with disabilities into the mainstream (DDPC, 1989)? What about pensions? When your financial status is set for life and the benefits do not change with age, what has pension to do with it? What about dignity and self-esteem?

Another challenge to address will be the deficits in housing availability. In many situations, the aging of a resident is associated with the thought that "*Well, So-and-so is getting old and needs a nursing home . . .*" However, the question should be: "*Why does he need a nursing home?*" Is it because the home is not barrier free? Is it because he can't retire at the group home or other residence were he lives? Is it because staff are not trained to work with older residents and don't understand the physical effects of aging? Is it because the home is not barrier free? Is it because he is becoming frail and needs more specialized services related to his health care?

What happens when a person with a disability grows old? Do we still need to concern ourselves only with the fact that this is a "*disabled person*"? Or do we now need to think that this is an "*older person*"? Is that lifetime label needed, necessary, or important? The challenge for the future is for us to reorient our thinking when we think about the older clientele of our agencies.

What about services? What are the services that will be needed? One is housing that is comfortable, barrier free, personal, and provides the opportunity to be in the company of other adults of one's choosing. Another is appropriate and adequate health maintenance and care, including nutrition, physical exercise, medical and dental visits, and periodic vision and hearing examinations. Yet another is day service that offers work—if that's what the person wants—or provides for a range of retirement activities and socialization opportunities.

In looking toward the future, one needs to ask, "When I get older, what will I need and under what conditions do I want it?" Do you want to be "*placed*" in a nursing home—when your needs are primarily driven by health care? Do you want to be isolated, lose your autonomy, and have nowhere to go to spend time with other people and do the things that you'd find enjoyable? What would you like? These are the same questions that need to be addressed when discussing options with a person with a lifelong disability. This type of introspection should be on the bases for arriving at what the future will be like in terms of providing housing and other types of supportive care. If services in the community, available to meet your needs and of the sort that you'd find comfort with, are what you decide on, then how do we arrive at these?

One is through building partnerships between community organizations. As we *construct* (or *reconstruct*, depending on your point of view) the services for older adults with disabilities—into and past the year 2000—we must both build on what we've learned and done and stretch ourselves to enter new areas. The population of older Americans is continually growing. The numbers of older Americans with disabilities is continually growing. Longevity and improved health status will take many more to the third age, which previously was an improbability.

In the United States, the weight of Congress and the federal government is behind these efforts. The disability provisions of the Older Americans Act and the interagency agreement between the Administration on Aging (AoA) and the Administration on Developmental Disabilities (ADD) in Washington are excellent examples of this. National organizations, such as the National Council on the Aging and the various gerontological and mental retardation–disability associations have developed strong supports for these initiatives. The federally funded (by ADD) university-based training centers in aging and developmental disabilities have done much to give us the technology and training resources we need. Indeed, many states have taken to heart the call, within the Older Americans Act, to work in concert to bridge the disability and aging networks. We have the benefit of their experiences to build on.

For the future, what needs to be done? We need a well-developed system of adult day and residential services that support seniors with special needs. We need to ensure that all seniors, irrespective of disability, can enjoy the activities and services available in the nation's senior citizens centers. We need to ensure that more seniors with disabilities know about the congregate meal sites in their communities and use them. We need adequate and appropriate housing that will accept and provide for seniors with lifelong disabilities.

States need to develop cooperative agreements spelling how each of the state agencies, the disability and aging agencies, will work to help one another in developing partnerships. This can be done by cooperative planning for services, cooperation in developing and providing services, and ensurances that seniors with disabilities have free and equal access to appropriate aging network programs. To accomplish this, many states will need to work out financial cost-sharing arrangements to help pay for the additional costs associated with providing services—be they residential or day. In many instances, senior services can absorb new seniors with lifelong disabilities; in other instances, the special needs of these seniors may involve additional costs, and these should be borne by the disability agencies.

Localities need to ensure that all providers network and work out arrangements to back each other up and facilitate entry into senior services, yet at the same time draw on the resources available with the disability network and work out arrangements to cooperatively serve the needs of families with aging parents and older sons or daughters with special needs. Further, states and localities need to ensure that cross-training is offered to workers of programs serving older persons with lifelong disabilities. This type of training should involve fundamentals on the aging process, fundamentals about lifelong disabilities, a "walk through" the local services available and who provides them (i.e., a *"who to call approach"*), and some approaches to networking, clinical care, and treatment practices.

States and localities need to ensure that networking efforts are undertaken. This can involve a meeting of providers from both systems, a *"show and tell"* approach whereby each shows its wares, interagency agreements and/or services planning and coordination committees, work-shops, meetings, conferences, public education campaigns, information dissemination efforts, and the like. States and localities need to undertake outreach efforts to families. This can involve understanding that many families are aging themselves and have lifelong care responsibilities for a disabled son or daughter and that they themselves may need services. The use of a partnership whereby the aging agency helps the parents and the disability agency helps the senior might be a consideration. Another is sharing information and referral resources and assisting one another with respite supports.

States and localities need to coordinate their adult day-care services. This can be accomplished by sharing information and referral, cross-funding or staff sharing arrangements, opening disability-based senior programs to all community seniors with similar care needs, cross-certification and provision of technical assistance, and co-location and sharing meals. Last, special efforts need to be undertaken by states and localities to promote and undertake program integration efforts. This means linking agencies that are concerned with elderly persons, working out means to help persons with lifelong disabilities to access generic senior services, collaboration, sharing of resources, technologies, cross-training, planning and program development, and most important, it means burying *"territoriality."*

Closing Commentary

The present realities are that we are just starting to be become prepared for the "greying" of America. Indeed, the disability system may be better prepared than society in general because it is at least acknowledging the problems associated with its elderly. We know that there will be sub-stantially more older and elderly persons among those individuals with mental retardation than ever before in our history. We also know that the character of persons who will become older or elderly over the next 20 to 30 years will be decidedly different than that of age-peers today.

Within this decade, and well beyond the year 2000, we are faced with three substantial challenges. The problems and challenges faced regarding the aging of a significant population of adults with disabilities within the United States are not unique. Most other nations face them or will shortly face them as well. The differences in approaches will be tempered by the political and legislative climate, the organization and structure of social agencies, and the financing schemes inherent in each nation's old-age support systems.

The basic challenges, however, remain constant and include the following:

Challenge of education: We must have a more educated public and concern about the needs of older persons with special needs, we must have a capable and trained staff who work in programs for older persons with special needs, we must have universities with a commitment to a critical mass of informed and specialized faculty in gerontology and disability, and we must have an educated legislature and executive.

Challenge of services: We must have community services that are appropriate and available in adequate numbers, we must have a caring system of long-term care that is free of warehousing and indifference, we must have suitable and accessible housing that minimizes transfers, and most important, we must have the financing schemes to underwrite and support these services.

Challenge of knowledge: We must have an extensive body of research that tells about aging and its interaction with disability, we must have technologies that help us design appropriate services that focus on needs, and we must have information and means to underwrite the costs of the services as we redesign their very structures.

References

ADD aging training projects: Plans for 1991. (1990, Fall). *Aging/MR IG Newsletter*, *4*(2–3). Washington, DC: American Association on Mental Retardation Special Interest Group in Aging.

Catapano, P., Levy, J., & Levy, P. (1985). Day activity and vocational program services. In M. P. Janicki & H. M. Wisniewski (Eds.), *Aging and developmental disabilities: Issues and approaches* (pp. 305–316). Baltimore: Paul H. Brookes.

Cotten, P. D., & Spirrison, C. L. (1989). Issue devoted to elderly persons with mental retardation. *Journal of Applied Gerontology*, *8*(2), 149–270.

Cotten, P. D., & Casey, J. (1990). *Pre-retirement training curriculum guide*. Sanatorium, MS: Boswell Retardation Center.

Davidson, P. W., Calkins, C. F., Harper, D., Hawkins, B. A., McClain, J. W., & Offner, R. B. (1987). *A decade of commitment to elderly persons with developmental disabilities*. Silver Spring, MD: American Association of University Affiliated Programs.

Developmental Disabilities Planning Council. (1989). *A working paper of the committee on adult issues of the New York State Developmental Disabilities Planning Council on the Feasibility of Different Pension Support Options for New York state residents with a developmental disability*. Albany, NY: Developmental Disabilities Planning Council.

Dybwad, G. (1962). Administrative and legislative problems in the care of the adult and aged mental retardates. *American Journal of Mental Deficiency*, *66*, 716–722.

Estes, C. L. (1990). Long-term care *is* mainstream. Why isolate it from acute care? *Perspectives in Aging*, *19*(4), 4–8.

Hogg, J., Moss, S., & Cooke, D. (1987). *Ageing and mental handicap*. New York: Routledge Chapman & Hall.

Howell, M. C., Gavin, D. G., Cabrera, G. A., & Beyer, H. (1989). *Serving the underserved: Caring for people who are both old and mentally retarded.* Boston: Exceptional Parent Press.

Janicki, M. P. (1988). Symposium on aging. *Mental Retardation, 26*(4), 179–216.

Janicki, M. P. (1989a). *Challenges for public health statistics in the 1990's: Proceedings of the 1989 public health conference on records and statistics.* Washington, DC: Public Health Service.

Janicki, M. P. (1989b). Transition from worklife to retirement for older persons with mental retardation. *Proceedings of a Presidential Forum: Citizens with Mental Retardation and Community Integration.* Washington: President's Committee on Mental Retardation.

Janicki, M. P. (1990, January) Building partnerships between community organizations. Keynote address given at conference on partners in aging and disability, Philadelphia.

Janicki, M. P., & Hogg, J. H. (1989). Special aging issue, *Australia and New Zealand Journal of Developmental Disabilities, 15*(4/5), 163–337.

Janicki, M. P., & Seltzer, M. M. (1991). *Aging and developmental disabilities: Challenges for the 1990s (Proceedings of the Boston Roundtable on Research Issues and Applications in Aging and Developmental Disabilities).* Washington: Aging Special Interest Group (American Association on Mental Retardation).

Janicki, M. P., & Wisniewski, H. M. (1985). *Aging and developmental disabilities: Issues and approaches.* Baltimore, MD: Paul H. Brookes.

Lepore, P., & Janicki, M. P. (1990). *The wit to win: How to integrate older persons with developmental disabilities into aging network programs.* Albany, NY: State Office of the Aging.

National Institute on Aging. (1987). *Personnel for the health needs of the elderly.* Washington, DC: National Institute on Aging.

National Institute of Health. (1989, June 2). The aging of retarded adults (program announcement). *NIH Guide for Grants and Contracts, 18*(19).

Roboul, H., Comte, P., & Jeantet, M.-C. (1985). *Les handicapes mentaux vieillissant.* Vanves, France: Centre Technique National d'Etudes et de Recherches sur les Handicaps et les Inadaptations.

Rose, T., & Ansello, E. F. (1988). Special issue on aging and disabilities. *Educational Gerontology, 14*(5), 351–469.

Sailer, M. F. (1987). *Working with developmentally disabled older adults: A training and resource manual.* Elwyn, PA: Southeast Pennsylvania Rehabilitation Center.

Seltzer, M. M., & Krauss, M. W. (1987). *Aging and mental retardation: Extending the continuum.* Washington, DC: AAMR.

Sparr, M. P., & Smith, W. (1990). Regulating professional services in ICFs/MR: Remembering the past and looking to the future. *Mental Retardation, 28,* 95–99.

Stroud, M., Sutton, E., & Roberts. R. (1988). *Expanding options for older adults with developmental disabilities: A practical guide to achieving community access.* Baltimore, MD: Paul H. Brookes.

Thurman, E. (1988). *All of us: Strategies and activity ideas for integrating older adults with developmental disabilities into senior centers.* Grand Rapids, MI: Kent Client Services.

Woods, J. (1990). *Aged and aging Virginians with developmental disabilities.* Richmond, VA: Virginia Department for the Aging.

Part 3
Trends on Health and Services

9
HIV Infection and Mental Retardation

HERBERT J. COHEN

The exponential growth in the number of persons infected with human immunodeficiency virus (HIV) in the United States and in several other areas of the world represents a major challenge to those planning or providing services to the developmentally disabled.

Studies of infants and children with congenital HIV infection—acquired through a transplacental route, which is the most common source of infection in children—indicate that close to 90% of such children have neurodevelopmental abnormalities (Belman et al., 1985; Epstein & Sharer, 1988; Ultmann et al., 1987). Continued follow-up of such children indicates that eventually virtually all infected children will have neurological or developmental disabilities (Diamond & Cohen, 1989). This has resulted, based on the current projections of future cases, in a prediction that HIV will become the most common infectious cause of developmental disability (Diamond & Cohen, 1987).

Those involved with service, training, and research related to mental retardation and developmental disabilities must also be concerned about the anticipated effects of HIV infection on the teenage and adult population. For teenagers without developmental disabilities, the fear is that there will be a rapid explosion in the number of cases among these adolescents and that more infected infants will be produced as a result of the concomitant adolescent pregnancies that are the result of promiscuity. There is also a considerable degree of anxiety about the potential spread of HIV into the population of adolescents and adults who are developmentally disabled. This will create an additional burden for families of such adolescents and adults, as well as other caretakers and service providers.

The total number of persons infected with HIV is unknown. The Centers for Disease Control estimates that 1.5 million persons in the United States may be infected. By 1989, over 100,000 human cases had already been reported and 61,000 had died of AIDS (Centers for Disease Control, 1989). The General Accounting Office predicts that, by the end of 1991, 480,000 Americans will have contracted AIDS (General

131

Accounting Office, 1989). Worldwide, at least 600,000 people have had AIDS, and up to 6 million may be infected (World Health Organization, 1989). Exactly how many will be infected in the United States by the year 2000 is unknown. The World Health Organization, however, conservatively estimates that up to 10 million people will have been infected worldwide by the year 2000 (World Health Organization, 1989).

Demographics of HIV Infection

The geographical distribution of HIV infection in the United States clearly indicates that the highest concentrations of this disease are on the East and West coasts. New York, New Jersey, California, Florida, Maryland, Texas, and Massachusetts are among the states with higher incidences of pediatric HIV infection and, to a major extent, of adult HIV infection. The major means of transmission to children, the predominant group with associated developmental disability, is through direct transmission from the mother to the developing fetus. Most mothers acquire the infection through intravenous (IV) drug use or sexual activity with an HIV-infected drug user. The adolescent or adult with a developmental disability who becomes infected with HIV usually does so through the same mechanism as other adolescents and adults, namely, through sexual contact or IV drug use.

The cause of HIV infection in adults has shown substantial change in the last few years. Before 1985, 63% of those infected were homosexual or bisexual men with no history of IV drug use, 18% were heterosexual men and women with reported IV drug use, and 2% were sex partners or children of IV drug users (Editorial, *American Journal of Diseases of Children*, 1989). In the first 6 months of 1989, 56% were reported to be homosexual or bisexual men, 23% were male or female IV drug users, and 4% were sex partners of IV drug users or children. The proportion of women in that time span had grown from 7% to 11%. African Americans and Hispanics continue to be disproportionately represented, especially among the IV drug-user population.

The demographic data illustrate the fact that an increasing number of women are infected and, as a result, there is an increasing risk of perinatal transmission of the disease. Estimates are that as many as 20,000 infants may be HIV infected by 1991 (Novello, Wise, Willoughby, & Pizzo, 1989).

The critical questions for the year 2000 will be the following:

1. Will the exponential growth of the disease continue and pour additional new HIV-infected mentally retarded or developmentally disabled (MR/DD) children into the service-delivery system? No one knows whether a vaccine to prevent the disease will be developed in the 1990s, though there have been predictions that such a vaccine may be available

in the next few years. However, because of the high mutation rate or adaptability of the virus, many investigators view the development of a widely effective vaccine as unlikely in the near future. Unfortunately, prevention efforts through education have not clearly demonstrated a substantial impact among the heterosexual, susceptible populations and those at high risk of IV drug use.

2. Will new treatments either arrest the course of the disease or cure it? At this point, cures appear unlikely in the immediate future, but improved treatment will definitely have an impact. The net result of treatment with currently available drugs, such as Azidothymidine (otherwise known as Zidovudine or AZT), gamma-globulin or possibly Dideoxyinosine (DDI), as well as other medications that may be developed, will be to increase the number of infected children whose progression of HIV disease, or the related neurodevelopmental abnormalities, may have slowed down or arrested. However, despite this, these children with HIV infections in increasing numbers will need a range of developmental and rehabilitative services.

The Impact of HIV Infection on Service Providers

Optimally, care for the mentally retarded and developmentally disabled requires considerable interagency cooperation and collaboration. Health, education, social service, mental health, and vocational training systems have important roles in the care of the disabled, with the ideal approach an interdisciplinary one that is complemented by well-established linkages between program providers and includes a high level of family (parental) and direct consumer input into the planning process and program delivery. The system of care for the developmentally disabled has favorably evolved over the past two decades from a treatment or service-planning model based on medical diagnoses, where medical management issues coupled with a sometimes unfortunate authoritarian approach dictated future management, to a shared model of decision making based on a broad consideration of the client's and family's need.

The advent of HIV on the MR/DD service scene has created a new series of challenges for the service provider. Children with HIV infection, like the increasing number of seriously chronically ill and/or technology dependent children who require services, have substantial medical needs. Unlike most children with MR/DD, they are frequently ill and generate substantial concern about their susceptibility to infections that they may acquire from others. In addition, there is the unsubstantiated but real fear that the HIV-infected person may pose a risk of spreading HIV or other infections to their peers or to staff.

The implications for the service-delivery system are obvious. This is a population that requires considerable medical monitoring, has substantial health-care requirements, and though their profile and locations for services should not be primarily dictated by medical concerns, humanistic developmental services for them may require a substantial amount of medical participation in the decision-making process. As well, health-care professionals have to participate in the development of procedures, staff training, and required liaison activities with other agencies caring for the child and family. Cooperation with health, MR/DD, education and social service programs and staff is an absolute necessity to appropriately manage the care for children with HIV infection and developmental disabilities. In addition, given the changing demographics of HIV in adults, especially women in the childbearing years, delivery of services, including prevention, tracking, diagnosis, and intervention for high-risk infants, plus family service planning and provision, will also involve agencies treating adolescents and adults who are substance abusers. In addition, there must be outreach to unserved or underserved minority group populations who are at high risk of HIV infection for themselves and their offspring. Management of clients with an HIV infection in the 1990s and beyond will require service providers to form new linkages to agencies serving substance abusers, pregnant teenagers, and minority infants from poor families who attend day-care or head-start programs.

One other substantial challenge posed for the service provider to the child with HIV infection is that traditional models of working with biological families are usually not applicable. First, because many of the parents are themselves infected, the parents may be chronically ill, disabled, or dying. The mother may have already died from HIV disease or its complications. Second, many children with HIV infection are cared for by foster parents, grandparents, friends of the parents, or other relatives. The Individual Family Service Plan may assume a new dimension for programs emphasizing family involvement in preschool or day-training programs, when there are alternate caretakers involved or when the biological parents are unreliable, are substance abusers, or are ill.

In the year 2000, with the projected continuing expansion of the number of women in the work force and the development of many varied day-care models, agencies providing services for children with or without disabilities, HIV infected or not, will no doubt have to acclimate to working with parents who are limited in their ability to offer daytime parenting and home-based treatment. Therefore, specialized service delivery in day-care settings for children with special needs, including those with HIV infections, will have to substantially increase. On the other hand, if some futurists are correct and the use of computers in networking arrangements may encourage more work at home for some professionals, then the challenge may be a different one. There may be parents whose home environment is their work environment. This may also be the child's treatment environment. However, this model is a more middle-class one and is unlikely to substantially apply to most of the HIV-infected population.

Agencies serving adolescents and adults with MR/DD must also be prepared to forge new linkages with service providers outside of the traditional spectrum of collaborators. This may include the provider of care to substance abusers and the experts in infectious disease. Issues such as contraception, homosexuality, confidentiality of medical information, and restriction of sexual expression create new challenges and take on enhanced significance when confronting the threat of spread of HIV infection to and among clients whom they serve.

Issues in Training

Those providers who have dealt firsthand with the HIV epidemic have important lessons to transmit to others. Given the considerable anticipated growth of the HIV-infected population and the probable changing nature of the disease as a result of improved treatment and/or prevention measures, there will be a need to adopt new training strategies. An important issue that must be dealt with not only for the HIV, but for other infectious agents, is the basic requirement to improve health and hygienic practices in child-care, day-programs, and residential settings where dependent persons are cared for or participate in programs. Surveys indicate that routine hygienic practices in day-care settings are poor, as are standards to prevent spread of infectious disease and to promote occupational health and safety (APHA/AAP Project, 1990). It is likely that similar problems occur in settings that provide services to older children and adults. Therefore, training in preventive health and hygiene, occupational safety, and teaching staff how to promote safe-sex practices for older clients will be essential ingredients in future program settings.

Other important issues that will likely grow in importance as training requirements in the coming decade, at least in part provoked by the lessons of the HIV epidemic, include developing and setting appropriate behavioral goals and objectives for persons with chronic illness who are unlikely to make substantial progress or who may, if arrest of progressive deterioration from HIV disease cannot be fully achieved, be likely to lose milestones or functional capabilities. A rethinking of the developmental model and its application will be imperative. As a result, service professionals will require retraining to assume different roles within the interdisciplinary model. As noted, there will have to be more integrated participation of medical and health professionals than has been current practice in most settings. It will, therefore, be necessary to modify current interdisciplinary training practices, change the content of training materials, and engage in considerable outreach to generic providers in the entire spectrum of the service system.

The Challenge in Research

Scientists and practitioners have certainly been taken by surprise at the unexpected emergence of a new major infectious cause of mental retardation, especially in the era of advancement of immunizations that have provided substantial protection against the formerly common scourges, such as measles and rubella. These previously ubiquitous childhood illnesses, acquired during pregnancy in the case of rubella or during early childhood in the case of measles, have left many children with MR/DD in their wake. The implications for the expert in infectious disease are that new troublesome viral or possibly drug-resistant bacterial agents will likely continue to emerge and that some of these organisms may wreak havoc among the susceptible population and could result in a new population of neurologically impaired persons. Continued research to identify the emergence of new dangerous organisms will be vital, as will development of new generations of antiviral and antibacterial agents. This quest will undoubtedly be aided by advances in genetic engineering techniques and the lessons learned from the battle against HIV.

It is too early to judge all of the scientific benefits that will results from the current HIV epidemic. It is reasonable to predict, however, that critically important scientific knowledge will be gleaned from both the current targeted and the adjunctive research involving HIV. Advances in the understanding of complex retroviruses are certain, along with better insight about the precise methods and techniques involved when agents act to stimulate or undermine the human immune system. Fundamental progress is likely in cell biology and in defining the mechanisms through which viruses interact with the human intracellular genetic material. As well, the effects of "slow viruses" on the nervous system will be further elucidated, as will the role of HIV and related viruses in producing progressive encephalopathy.

One need not be a delphic prophet to also realize that the predicted research advances will, as have past achievements, themselves stimulate many new fundamental questions in molecular biology, about the pathogenesis of neurological disease, and in determining the impact of treatment modalities and other interventions, including genetic engineering. All of these advances will in turn create new ethical and legal dilemmas. With each advance in technology and with its respective application, profound new challenges are generated that must be considered by those conducting the research and those offering human services. HIV has posed many initial challenges, and the scientific progress it will have stimulated by year 2000 will undoubtedly create many new moral and ethical concerns.

Issues for the Policy Maker

The emergence of HIV as a new entity in the MR/DD service system should have taught humility to the service planners, none of whom could have anticipated it. The issue of infectivity, the required interagency collaboration, and the development and implementation of rational policies should all have been dealt with in 1990s. What then will the issues be in the year 2000? Assuming that the growth of HIV disease will have leveled off, and that medical treatment will have improved, there is still the likelihood that there will be a large number of children with HIV infection, and resultant neurological impairment who, much like the rubella babies produced in the 1960s, will age into the service-delivery system in the subsequent decades. The persons with HIV infection will have a wide range of disability, including some severely and multiply handicapped as a result of the devastating early pathological effects of the virus. The needs of this HIV-infected population will have to be met. Making it more complicated is the inability to predict what the long-term course of HIV disease will be and how effective medical treatment and other therapies will be. This may inhibit the capability of making reasonable predictions about the HIV infected person's future general health and developmental status.

It is hoped, of course, that HIV will reach the level of acceptability that rubella has—namely, a disease that has largely done its damage to children, and then these children will require specific help later on without undue concern about confidentiality and special infectious precautions. However, given the current fatal nature of HIV, public concern and wariness about infectivity are unlikely to be easily mitigated. Therefore, program planners may have to continue to make special provisions in planning new programs, including emphasizing the health, hygiene, and safety concerns elaborated on previously. There also will be the continuing need to deal with a large number of children and young adults with HIV disease who have no available biological parent but who may have other concerned caretakers. The models for service delivery may have to be modified to deal with the special needs and requirements of this population.

Summary and Conclusions

HIV infection is spreading rapidly in the United States and the world. Its neurodevelopmental consequences are creating a sizable population of children with progressive disabilities but whose future course is less certain. Improved treatment is likely to avert the deterioration in many children. It is hoped and felt that preventive measures, including new vaccines to immunize susceptible persons, will reduce the rapid rate of increase in the number of cases of HIV disease in both children and adults.

Those infected with HIV will create new dilemmas for service and training providers, as well as scientists engaged in research. Though the exact problems and issues that will dominate the year 2000 are not clearly predictable, there are likely to be continuing concerns about health and safety of both the infected clients and their caretakers, uncertainty about the natural long-term course of the disease, how treatment will modify it, and what will be the specific service requirements for those who are both infected and have neurodevelopmental dysfunction. Ultimately, however, it is likely that HIV disease will be treated more like a common chronic illness rather than a unique disease. As with other such illnesses associated with a developmental disability, to provide optimal services, an interdisciplinary approach will be required that assures adequate medical and health input into the service plan, collaborative planning between service system components, and a strong interdisciplinary training effort. A continuing basic science commitment is mandatory to expand on the likely discoveries in the fields of virology, immunology, and neuropathology that will emerge from the concentrated research efforts stimulated by the interest and concern about HIV in the 1980s and 1990s.

References

American Public Health Association/American Academy of Pediatrics Project to Development of Health Standards for Day Care. (1990). *Survey of State Child Care Facilities*. American Public Health Association, Washington, DC.

Belman, A. L., Ultmann, N. H., Horoupian, D., Novick, B. D., Spiro, A. J., Rubinstein, A., Kurtzberg, D., & Cone-Wesson, B. (1985). Neurological complications in infants and children with acquired immunodeficiency syndrome. *Annals of Neurology, 18*, 560–566.

Centers for Disease Control. (1989). AIDS Program, Center for Infectious Diseases. *Morbidity and Mortality Weekly Report, 38*, 496–499.

Diamond, G., & Cohen, H. J. (1987). *AIDS and developmental disabilities. Prevention Update*. National Coalition on Prevention of Mental Retardation.

Diamond, G., & Cohen, H. J. (1989). *HIV infection in children: Medical and neurological aspects. Technical report: Number 1*. Silver Springs, MD, American Association of University Affiliated Programs Consortium Project.

Editorial. (1989). First 100,000 cases of acquired immunodeficiency syndrome—United States. *American Journal of Diseases of Children, 143*, 1274–1275.

Epstein, L. G., & Sharer, L. R. (1988). Neurology of human immunodeficiency virus infection in children. In M. L. Rosenblum, R. M. Levy, & D. E. Bredeson (Eds.), *AIDS and the nervous system* (pp. 79–101). New York: Raven Press.

General Accounting Office. (1989). AIDS forecasts. Underestimating of cases and lack of key data weakens existing estimates. *PEMD, 89–13*.

Novello, A., Wise, P., Willoughby, A., & Pizzo, P. (1989). Final report of the United States Department of Health and Human Services Secretary's work group on pediatric human immunodeficiency virus infection and disease: Content and implications. *Pediatrics, 84*, 547–555.

Ultmann, M. H., Diamond, G. W., Ruff, H. A., Belman, A. L., Novick, B. E., Rubinstein, A., & Cohen, H. J. (1987). Developmental abnormalities in children with acquired immunodeficiency syndrome (AIDS). A followup study. *International Journal of Neuroscience*, *32*, 661–667.

World Health Organization. (1989). *Projections of worldwide AIDS statistics*. Geneva, Switzerland: Author.

10
Prevention of Mental Retardation (Genetics)

Hugo W. Moser

More than half of severe mental retardation is caused by genetically determined disorders. Advances in genetics are proceeding at an accelerating pace, which is primarily due to advances in DNA technology. It is likely that DNA markers for all of the major genetic causes of mental retardation will be available by the year 2000, or not long thereafter. These advances provide an almost awesome potential for the prevention of severe mental retardation. Unlike so many other issues covered in other chapters in this book, the main limitation will *not* be financial: It is anticipated that technical advances will diminish the cost of the "unit of detection" of a preventable genetic cause of severe mental retardation. On the other hand, financial issues will surely arise in respect to administration of therapies that are beginning to be available and will surely "explode" in the future. Probably the most difficult problems will arise from ethical issues, which will dwarf those that we are not resolving well at the present time.

The potential of DNA technology for the prevention of mental retardation is greater than the majority of our professionals currently recognize. If this chapter can highlight this potential as well as the social and ethical issues it will generate, then it will have served a useful purpose.

Genetic Causes of Severe Mental Retardation

An analysis of studies of the causes of severe mental retardation reveals that 35% to 60% are assigned to genetic causes (Moser, Ramey, & Leonard, 1983). This analysis was based on three surveys that displayed a high degree of medical sophistication and also were reasonably representative. Two of the surveys were regional and community based, in Sweden (Gustavson, Hagberg, Hagberg, & Sars, 1977) and the United Kingdom (Laxova et al., 1967), and one was based in a residential institution in the United States (Kaveggia, Durkin, Pendleton, & Opitz, 1975).

The term *severe mental retardation* here refers to persons with an IQ of less than 50. The majority of persons in this category have demonstrable brain pathology (Crome, 1960). For the purpose of this discussion, we omit consideration of the larger group of persons with mild mental retardation, where environmental and genetic factors interact in a manner too complex to permit precise delineation of genetic aspects (Moser, et al., 1983).

The genetic causes of severe mental retardation include the most frequent single cause, Down syndrome, which accounts for 30% of severe mental retardation. A more recently recognized cause is the fragile-X syndrome (Turner & Jacobs, 1983) with an estimated incidence of 1:2000 (approximately half that of Down syndrome). These two disorders together may account for 45% of severe mental retardation. In addition, there are other known disorders with abnormalities of the number or structure of chromosome (1%–4%) and the inborn errors of metabolism (5%–7%). Summation of these causes leads to the conclusion that more than 50% of severe mental retardation is genetically determined.

This summation excludes other disorders, some already known, others yet to be defined, that are associated with mental retardation. McKusick's (1988) catalogue of Mendelian inheritance in man lists 4,344 distinct genetic disorders that affect humans. A computer analysis of this catalogue revealed that mental retardation was a prominent feature in 448 of these 4,434 disorders (H. W. Moser, 1991, unpublished observation). These disorders include disorders previously classified as multiple congenital anomalies syndromes, such as Zellweger (Kelley, 1983) and Rubinstein-Taybi syndrome (Rubinstein & Taybi, 1963). Zellweger syndrome has now been defined in biochemical terms and can be prevented by genetic counseling. Also included are recently recognized disorders such as Rett syndrome, a disorder with a unique behavioral phenotype that leads to severe mental retardation in approximately 1 in 15,000 females (Hagberg, 1989). While a listing and appraisal of this bewildering number of genetic disorders is beyond the scope of this chapter, this brief listing illustrates the complexity of the topic. Until now, the large number of disorders, the difficulty in categorizing the multiple clinical manifestations, and the imperfection and expense of diagnostic assays interfered with precise diagnosis and the application of preventive techniques. In the next section we will describe new technologies which are expected to overcome these limitations by the year 2000 or not long thereafter.

Present and Future Diagnostic Techniques that will Facilitate the Prevention of Severe Mental Retardation that is Due to Genetic Causes

Present Strategies

Allen Crocker (1985) described "1985" strategies for the prevention of mental retardation. For the genetic disorders, "flagship status" should be assigned to programs that screen newborns for phenylketonuria (Guthrie & Susi, 1963) and hypothyroidism (Burrows & Dussault, 1980) and to techniques that can identify pregnancies at risk for Down syndrome (Wald et al., 1988) and neural tube defects (Wald, Brock, & Bonnar, 1974).

Mass metabolic screening for phenylketonuria (incidence, 1:11,000) and hypothyroidism (incidence, 1:3,500) are now routine in many parts of the world. Hundreds of millions of infants have been screened. Early therapy in infants identified with these metabolic abnormalities prevents severe mental retardation, and a favorable benefit/cost ratio has been proven beyond doubt, both in human and financial terms. A recent careful statistical study has defined a set of analytical techniques applied to maternal serum samples that now permit identification of 60% of pregnancies in which the fetus has Down syndrome (Wald et al., 1988). This is a significant improvement over the 30% that could be identified when maternal age above 35 years was the only criterion for the identification of pregnancies at high risk for Down syndrome. Measurement of alpha-fetoprotein levels in maternal serum (Wald et al., 1974) and ultrasound studies can detect the majority of fetuses with neural tube defects. An exciting new dimension to prevention is added by the recent report by Milunsky et al. (1989) that multivitamin and folic acid supplementation in early pregnancy reduces the prevalence of neural tube defects.

Technical Advances that will Revolutionize Genetic Studies of Mental Retardation

Two recent publications summarize the advances in DNA technology that will revolutionize genetic studies of mental retardation (Eisenstein, 1990; Landegren, Kaiser, Caskey, & Hood, 1988). The polymerase chain reaction permits the amplification of truly minute amounts of DNA—the carrier of genetic information. It requires only minimal amounts of material and can be applied to materials stored under adverse conditions, even to a 7,000-year-old mummy (Eisenstein, 1990). New techniques of analysis will make it possible to automate analyses, to test simultaneously for groups of disorders, and to do so with relatively inexpensive non-radioactive reagents (Landegren et al., 1988). It is thus conceivable, and indeed likely, that large-scale screening for genetic disorders associated with mental retardation will become feasible at an affordable cost.

Applying These New Techniques to the Study of Mental Retardation

Application of DNA technology to the study of mental retardation requires that we identify the DNA abnormalities that are associated with the major, and eventually all, genetic causes of mental retardation. This is a Herculean task, because there are at least 1,000, and probably many more, distinct genetic causes of mental retardation. This task will coincide with the new national and international commitment to map and sequence the human genome (McKusick, 1989). This remarkable national and international undertaking aims to determine in the next 15 years the sequence of the 3 billion base pairs that make up the human genome. McKusick calculates that a mere printing of that number of base pairs would require 13 sets of the *Encyclopedia Britannica*. Overwhelming as the task appears, it may well be accomplished by the year 2005, not far beyond the scope of enquiry of this present volume. It is estimated that the human genome contains 50,000 to 100,000 genes. At this time, 1,500 have been mapped to specific chromosomes and chromosomes regions; 600 have been cloned and sequenced (McKusick, 1989).

Even though it is evident that the major task lies ahead, significant advances toward the DNA analysis of mental retardation have already been achieved. The genes of disorders that are often associated with mental retardation have been mapped or even isolated. For example, the gene that is defective in Prader-Willi syndrome has been mapped to chromosome 15 (Mattei, Soviah, & Mattei, 1984); lissencephaly syndrome (in which the brain lacks the normal convolutional pattern), to chromosome 17 (Greenberg et al., 1986), and at least one form of tuberous sclerosis to chromosome 9 (Fryer et al., 1987). All persons with Prader-Willi and lissencephaly syndromes and approximately 50% of persons with tuberous sclerosis are mentally retarded. Many of these gene localizations depend on studies that use mathematical techniques to determine the relationship in a given family between a particular disease state and other genetic markers. As the number of available DNA markers is increasing, the technique is becoming increasingly powerful, as described in a recent editorial entitled the "triumph of linkage analysis" (Rosenberg, 1990). The studies referred to so far have mapped the abnormal gene to a specific chromosome region. The ultimate aim is to study the abnormal gene itself and to define exactly the DNA alteration that causes it to malfunction. This goal has now been achieved in respect to Duchenne muscular dystrophy, and the protein product that is defective has been identified (Hoffman, Brown, & Kunkel, 1987). Approximately 30% of patients with Duchenne muscular dystrophy are mentally retarded.

It is beyond the scope of this chapter to list all the advances in biochemistry, genetics, and neuroscience that contribute to our understanding of the causes of mental retardation. However, two areas are of particular pertinence to prevention. One is the continued refinement of high-resolution cytogenetic techniques and the probability that it will become possible to automate these techniques at least in part through computer-assisted technology. It has already been noted that approximately 50% of severe mental retardation is associated with disorders that can be identified by cytogenetic techniques.

A second finding that is pertinent to the prevention of mental retardation is the report of a recent collaborative study of chorionic villus sampling for the early prenatal diagnosis of cytogenetic abnormalities (Rhoads, Jackson, Schlesselman, de la Cruz, Desnick, et al., 1989). This study analyzed the results of 2,278 first-trimester chorionic villus samplings. Cytogenetic diagnoses results in 97.8% of the studies, and the fetal loss rate was only 0.8% higher than for second-trimester amniocentesis. This study indicates that first-trimester prenatal diagnosis is accurate and carries only minimal risk to mother and fetus.

Issues for the Future

It is likely that not far beyond the year 2000 it will become possible to develop DNA markers for all or most of the genetic disorders associated with mental retardation. This will be accomplished either by linkage analysis (Rosenberg, 1990) or by demonstration of the abnormality in the gene itself (Friedman, 1990). This anticipated new capacity inspires hope and fear simultaneously. Hope derives from the fact that an understanding will be gained of the causes of many conditions that lead to severe mental retardation and the capacity to provide precise and person-specific information about the risk of the condition in a person's children or family members. Persons at risk can make informed reproductive decisions. Perhaps the most pleasing result is that it will be possible to identify with certainty those family members who in fact are *not* at risk. Because of the limitation of our present knowledge, many individuals who are considered to be *possibly* at risk (but if we had better diagnostic techniques could be shown *not* to be), either elect not to reproduce, or live under a cloud for years because of the fear that their children may be affected.

The Cost of Therapy of Genetic Disorders may be Prohibitive

Other reasons for hope include the possibility that the acquisition of knowledge about the exact nature of the genetic abnormality may lead to effective therapy (Friedman, 1989). This hope must be tempered with realism. Successful delivery of gene therapy requires the solution of many technical problems (Friedman, 1989). It is not certain that these can be solved, and it will take a long time to assess safety and effectiveness. Furthermore, while the capacity to *detect* genetic disorders associated with mental retardation may well become financially feasible, the cost of the large-scale application of complex therapies might well exceed current health expenditures by an order of magnitude. This will require careful analysis of benefit–cost ratios, and priority setting.

Policy Implications of the Capacity to Identify Genetic Disorders Associated with Mental Retardation

Holtzman (1988) has reviewed the general public policy implications of recombinant DNA technology and genetic tests. While he addressed himself to the field as a whole, virtually all of the concerns apply to mental retardation. The major concerns follow:

1. The validity of the tests and methods to ensure quality control: Curiously, legal and operational problems in relation to quality control multiply when a test becomes simplified.

2. The need to develop a network of laboratories capable of performing large numbers of tests in a reliable fashion, and perhaps even more important, to train a cadre of personnel who can transmit complex information and provide genetic counseling accurately and in a manner that can be understood by the client, and that will lead to truly informed decisions: Holtzman estimates that the number of qualified personnel presently available for all genetic tests can serve 500,000 individuals annually. He estimates that in the future as many as 18 million persons may be involved in some type of genetic tests each year. New strategies will be needed to meet these greatly increased needs. I believe that genetic issues related to mental retardation will constitute a significant proportion of this new need.

3. Special problems associated with the capacity to detect serious disorders for which there is no effective therapy: As already noted, this may be a not infrequent outcome for genetic disorders associated with mental retardation. The problem may be especially vexing for progressive disorders that lead to handicaps only in adulthood. Special care will need to

be taken to ensure that decisions are truly informed and based only on the individual's well-being. A risk to be avoided is that these decisions not be contaminated with misguided thoughts about eugenics as practiced in this country at the beginning of this century and too long thereafter; or the criminal policies of the Third Reich.

4. Testing for insurance purposes and by employers: These issues arise particularly with disorders such as sickle cell disease, glucose 6 phosphate dehydrogenase deficiency, Huntington's chorea, and nongenetic disorders such as acquired immune deficiency syndrome (AIDS). The above-mentioned disorders (except for congenital AIDS) are not associated with mental retardation, and this issue may not be as pertinent to mental retardation as those discussed previously. In my view, the priority must always be the best interests of the individual rather than society as a whole.

Conclusion

Genetic disorders are estimated to account for more than half of severe mental retardation in developed countries. Advances in DNA technology are proceeding at a rapid and accelerating pace. It is likely that not long after the year 2000, it will be possible to define all of the more than 1,000 genetic disorders that are associated with severe mental retardation. It is also likely that early, and often prenatal, diagnosis will become feasible at an affordable cost, with noninvasive procedures. While this new capacity will open up new and effective approaches toward genetic counseling and prevention, many new and difficult issues will be raised. These include the need for additional technically qualified personnel who also have the capacity to communicate with accuracy, understanding, and humanity. While the capacity to diagnose will almost surely develop, avenues of therapy may be limited by technical difficulties and cost. It is anticipated that major new ethical and policy issues will arise within a decade and that there is an urgent need for preparation to meet them. This discussion has focused on developed countries. The causes of severe mental retardation in developing countries are related to a greater extent to infectious diseases, nutritional deprivation, and deficient prenatal care, and different approaches and priorities are indicated in these countries.

References

Burrows, G. N., & Dussault, J. (Eds.). (1980). *Neonatal thyroid screening*. New York: Raven Press.

Crocker, A. C. (1985). Prevention of mental retardation. *Annals of the New York Academy of Sciences, 477*, 329–337.

Crome, L. (1960). The brain and mental retardation. *British Medical Journal, 1,* 897.

Eisenstein, B. I. (1990). The polymerase chain reaction. A new method of using molecular genetics for medical diagnosis. *New England Journal of Medicine, 322,* 178–183.

Friedman, T. (1989). Progress toward human gene therapy. *Science, 244,* 1275–1281.

Friedman, T. (1990). The human genome project—Some implications of extensive "reverse genetic" medicine. *American Journal of Human Genetics, 46,* 407–414.

Fryer, A. E., Connor, J. M., Povey, S., Yates, J. W. R., Chalmers, A., Fraser, I., Yates, A. D., & Osborne, J. P. (1987). Evidence that the gene for Tuberous Sclerosis is on chromosome 9. *Lancet, 1,* 659–661.

Greenberg, F., Stratton, R. F., Lockhart, L. H., Elder, E. F. B., Dobyns, W. B., & Leabetter, D. H. (1986). Familial Miller-Dieker Syndrome associated with pericentric inversion of chromosome 17. *American Journal of Medical Genetics, 23,* 853–859.

Gustavson, K. H., Hagberg, B., Hagberg, G., & Sars, K. (1977). Severe mental retardation in a Swedish county: II. Etiological and pathogenetic aspects of children born 1959–1970. *Neuropadiatrie, 8,* 293–304.

Guthrie, R., & Susi, A. (1963). A simple phenylalanine method for detecting phenylketonuria in large populations of newborn infants. *Pediatrics, 32,* 338–343.

Hagberg, B. A. (1989). Rett syndrome: Clinical peculiarities, diagnostic approach, and possible cause. *Pediatric Neurology, 5,* 75–83.

Hoffman, E. P., Brown, R. H., Jr., & Kunkel, L. M. (1987). The protein product of the Duchenne muscular dystrophy locus. *Cell, 51,* 919–928.

Holtzman, N. A. (1988). Recombinant DNA technology, genetic tests, and public policy. *American Journal of Human Genetics, 42,* 624–632.

Kaveggia, E. G., Durkin, M. V., Pendleton, E., & Opitz, J. M. (1975). Diagnostic/genetic studies on 1224 patients with severe mental retardation. *Proceedings of the 3rd Conqress of the International Association for the Scientific Study of Mental Deficiency* (pp. 82–93). Warsaw: Polish Medical Publishers.

Kelley, R. I. (1983). The cerebrohepatorenal syndrome of Zellweger. Morphological and metabolic aspects. *American Journal of Medical Genetics, 16,* 503–517.

Landegren, U., Kaiser, R., Caskey, C. T., & Hood, L. (1988). DNA diagnostics— molecular techniques and automation. *Science, 242,* 229–237.

Laxova, R., Ridler, M. A. C., & Bowen-Bravery, M. (1967). An etiological survey of the severely retarded Hertfordshire children who were born between January 1, 1965 and December 31, 1967. *American Journal of Medical Genetics, 1,* 75–86.

Mattei, M. G., Soviah, N., & Mattei, J. F. (1984). Chromosome 15 anomalies and the Prader-Willi syndrome: Cytogenetic analysis. *Human Genetics, 66,* 313–334.

McKusick, V. A. (1988). *Mendelian inheritance in man. Catalogs of autosomal dominant, autosomal recessive and x-linked phenotypes.* Baltimore: The Johns Hopkins University Press.

McKusick, V. A. (1989). Mapping and sequencing the human genome. *New England Journal of Medicine*, *320*, 910–915.

Milunsky, A., Jick, H., Jick, S. S., Bruell, C. L., Maclaughlin, D. S., Rothman, K. J., & Willett, W. (1989). Multivitamin/folic acid supplementation in early pregnancy reduced the prevalence of neural tube defects. *Journal of the American Medical Association*, *262*, 2847–2852.

Moser, H. W., Ramey, C. T., & Leonard, C. O. (1983). Mental retardation. In A. E. H. Emery & D. L. Rimoin (Eds.), *Principles and practice of medical genetics* (pp. 352–366). Edinburgh: Churchill-Livingstone.

Rhoads, G. G., Jackson, L. G., Schlesselman, S. E., de la Cruz, F. F., Desnick, R. J., et al. (1989). The safety and efficacy of chorionic villus sampling for early prenatal diagnosis of cytogenetic abnormalities. *New England Journal of Medicine*, *320*, 609–617.

Rosenberg, R. (1990). The triumph of linkage analysis. *Annals of Neurology*, *27*, 111–113.

Rubinstein, J. H., & Taybi, H. (1963). Broad thumbs and toes and facial abnormalities. *American Journal of Diseases and Childhood*, *105*, 588–608.

Turner, G., & Jacobs, P. (1983). Marker (X) linked mental retardation. In H. Harris & K. Hirschhorn (Eds.), *Advances in human genetics* (Vol. 13, pp. 38–112). New York: Plenum.

Wald, N. J., Brock, D. J. H., & Bonnar, J. (1974). Prenatal diagnosis of spina bifida and anencephaly by maternal serum-alpha-fetoprotein measurement. *Lancet*, *1*, 765–767.

Wald, N. J., Cuckle, H. S., Densem, J. W., Nanchahal, K., Royston, P., Chard, T., Haddow, J. E., Knight, G. J., Palomaki, G. E., & Canick, J. A. (1988). Maternal serum screening for Down's syndrome in early pregnancy. *British Medical Journal*, *297*, 883–887.

11
Mental Retardation and Mental Illness in the Year 2000: Issues and Trends

JACK A. STARK and FRANK J. MENOLASCINO

Identifying the issues, trends, and events that will affect persons with mental retardation and mental illness by the year 2000 presents the authors of this chapter, who bring 50 years of combined experience of specialization with this subpopulation, a challenging and unique opportunity to present what we feel could and should happen to this group of individuals.

Of all the subpopulations of persons with mental retardation who continue to be underserved (viz., the medically fragile, the aged, the offender, and persons with mental retardation and mental illness), the dually diagnosed are an especially complex group to serve for economic, social, and political reasons. Persons with mental retardation and mental illness often are expensive to treat, particularly if inpatient care is required or if 1:1 staffing around the clock is mandated. Cost can be double, and even quadruple, the average cost of serving persons with mental retardation who do not display a behavioral disorder. It has also been our experience that there is a disproportionate number of persons with mental retardation and mental illness in large institutional settings as a result of our inability to integrate this group into the confluence of community programs because of the lack of trained personnel and political concerns about having "these" individuals in group homes. Yet, despite these reasons why this group should be a high priority, there exists a paucity of services and research findings to guide us.

The materials presented in this chapter, therefore, are intended to provide the reader with a blueprint of the future directions of services to persons with mental retardation and mental illness based on the predictions during the next decade for our society in general and how this will specifically impact on this unique population.

Future Predictions

It is extremely difficult to predict where programs and services will be in 10 years, particularly during this time of so much political, economic, and social change. Indeed, with the globalization of America, it is more and more difficult to predict international changes that are having profound effects on America. Take, for instance, the recent changes in Communist bloc countries; the impact that this is having on our economy and the defense industry in particular is unprecedented.

A review of the research in this field (Menolascino, Neman, & Stark, 1983) reveals that we are in a period of rapidly accelerating research in the entire field of developmental disabilities. Although research heretofore with the dually diagnosed population has been disappointing, we anticipate that the research data base as in all young scientific fields, will double in the next 7 years, and possibly triple in 10 years.

A similar project to predict issues and trends in the year 2000, as it relates to persons with mental retardation, was undertaken by the President's Committee on Mental Retardation in conjunction with six futurist consultants via the "Future's Project." Their resulting publication (Plog, & Santamour, 1980) focused on the conceptual approaches and actual projected living situations for persons with mental retardation. Components of this "future's project" also centered on the technological advances, which were extremely insightful, although the biomedical areas were perhaps underestimated. Predicting the human ecological factors for society in the future proved to be much more challenging in this book. The findings of this well-written text point out the critical and complex process that the reader of this chapter should keep in mind, that is, predicting how our society will be in the future (year 2000) as it relates to persons with mental retardation. It is so intricately intertwined with all of the political, economic, social, and biological factors that need to be fully understood if we are to build the programs and services that will be meaningful and last well into the 21st century for persons with developmental disabilities.

Therefore, to design programs that will be state-of-the-art in the year 2000, we discuss the many larger trends in society that will basically dictate these services. The remaining part of this chapter will focus on two major sections. The first section will present changes that will reflect more of a "macrochange" in terms of "society in general" as well as its implications for persons with mental retardation. The second section of this chapter will focus more specifically on issues relating to persons with mental retardation and mental illness, specifically as it relates to the epidemiological research training and services.

Macrotrends

Political Trend

In mid-1990, the Senate passed and the President signed the most historic legislation ever to protect the civil rights of disabled people. The signing of the Americans With Disabilities Act is a profound rethinking of how this country views disabled people, defined as "anyone with a physical or mental impairment that substantially limits everyday living." Essentially, for the first time, America is saying that the biggest problem facing disabled people is not their own disability but that of discrimination. The bill has been hailed as an Emancipation Proclamation for persons with disabilities that will fundamentally change their lives, by getting more of them out of their homes and institutions and into the full participation of society. This political milestone, affecting some 43 million disabled individuals, or approximately one-fifth of the national population, impacts every family. In short, the political power of persons with disabilities will continue to be critical in the allocation of resources and maintenance of quality services and programs for persons with disabilities throughout the 1990s, particularly at the state and local levels.

Economic Trends

In the 1980s, the United States changed from being the greatest creditor in the world to being the greatest debtor in the world. Foreign debt is anticipated to increase to more than two trillion by the mid-1990s, which could seriously erode the American standard of living as reported by the Congressional Research Services in 1988. The second major variable in our economy is the trade deficit. The trade deficit ballooned to between 150 to 200 billion in each year in the late 1980s. In addition, many economists are predicting that it will rise even more sharply in the 1990s. We could see a trade deficit that could hit more than $300 billion by the mid-1990s. If our trade balance continues at this rate, the total foreign debt could be one fourth of this country's Gross National Product. In essence, this foreign debt means that foreigners now own more U.S. investments than we own in overseas investments.

The third major component that has had a major impact on our economy is the federal debt. The inability to balance the budget has resulted in the federal deficit of approximately $12,000 for every person in this country. Even if we are able to balance the budget soon, it would take two to three decades to pay off the enormous deficits accumulated during the 1980s alone. More than 10% of our total federal budget each year goes toward interest payments alone on our national debt. This further erodes our ability to fund critical social services programs.

The chief concern of financial markets in this country continues to be the worry over inflation. Certainly, the double-digit inflation of the late 1970s significantly eroded funding for research, training, services, and programs for persons with developmental disabilities. We also realize that funding has not kept pace with the inflationary pressures. The major economic issue we are currently facing is a strong possibility of a recession in the early 1990s. The Federal Reserve Board (Stark & Goldsbury,

1988) indicates that operating rates in the American factories, mines, utilities, and the like rose to almost 85%, which is the highest level in 10 years. This high operating rate of 85% is considered by analysts to represent a strong possibility of an increase in inflation. The concern is that if companies have a difficult time meeting production demands, it is considered by economists to be the level that would ignite inflation, which will in turn be passed on to consumers. In addition, imports had a tremendous impact on this country, particularly in the area of manufacturing, which has been flooded with cheaper products resulting in the loss of jobs, many of which are relatively easy to teach, even to persons with severe disabilities.

Societal Trends

There seems to be a growing acceptance of cultural diversity, resulting in the growth of a multicultural and integrated national society. Minorities will exert more influence over our national agenda as the population of African Americans, Hispanics, and Asians increases to more than 25% by the year 2000. Regional differences, attitudes, incomes, and life-styles are diminishing as people shift from one region to another. There will also be an increase in the middle class, as the United States will have less and less very poor and less very rich individuals. Our society is also witnessing more mobility in our personal, physical, occupational endeavors. Indeed, in a 5-year period, more than 40% of the population is expected to move, steadily increasing during the 1980s, and will significantly increase more in the 1990s. The population migration via work force shifts will lead to a concentration of the population (including those with developmental disabilities) in western and southern states. Higher divorce rates, smaller family size, and a large portion (60%) of women in the work force will dramatically alter the nature of families in which developmentally disabled families live. Today, more than two thirds of women between 25 and 44 are employed, and 60% of working women have children—a 35% increase in the last 20 years. This dramatic alteration in the traditional nuclear family will have a big impact on persons with developmental disabilities who are growing up in the natural family and in the community. There will also be a growing need to provide more in-home care while parents work. In addition, we are seeing an increase in the older population in that for the first time in history there are more Americans over the age of 65 than there are teenagers. There will be a greater emphasis on serving developmentally disabled individuals in the 1990s. However, they will need to speak for themselves through legislative activism, particularly via the formation of grass-root coalitions at both the local and state levels.

The tremendous changes within the family during the 1990s will dramatically impact persons with disabilities. Families in the year 2000 will average 1.81 children, down from 1.84 in the 1990s, because 60% of the children born in the 1980s will live for a time with one parent. One child in four will live with a stepparent by age 16, and one third of all households will be childless. The parents will work longer hours, perhaps 60 hours per week in the year 2000. In addition, the major breadwinner in the family can expect to change jobs 10 times in his or her lifetime and to change careers three times. The cost for the American taxpayer for the health-care system will be double what the nation spends on defense and 50% more than it will devote for education. Medicare and federal programs for the elderly and disabled are growing so fast that they will outstrip the defense budget by the year 2005. The major concern in the health-care field is that we will have more than half a million physicians in the year 2000. Yet we will continue to see a shortage of mental health workers, psychiatrists, psychologists, and psychiatric social workers who are willing to devote their life to working with the concerns of persons with mental retardation and mental illness (Dentzer, 1990; Findlay & Silberner, 1989–1990).

Educational Trends

Educational trends in the 1990s will be the most significant of all trends to change. Improvements in our educational system, particularly in higher education, will lead to a higher educational index. These changes, however, will not be commensurate with the changes in occupational demands. Improved educational opportunities for special education students have led to an increase in the proportion of American population that has graduated from high school. Because of fundamental changes in our economy, however, there will be fewer and fewer well-paying jobs not requiring advanced training. Tremendous infusion of new monies will be needed to help adequately fund reeducation programs and programs for disadvantaged students. Schools will dramatically change in their academic days and calendar years via a need to constantly upgrade and provide ongoing training to the American work force. For example, 85% of the information in the National Institute of Health computers is upgraded every 5 years. National testing services indicated that the United States has one of the worst systems in the industrialized world in helping high school graduates into the work force. Only 50% of individuals go to college. The General Accounting Office report of June 1990 indicated that 9 million of the United States' 33 million youth, aged 16 to 24, do not have the skills needed to meet employer's requirements for entry-level positions. In short, there will be a major refocusing of our educational institutions to provide emphasis on vocational training at the high school level to provide functional skills training for disabled individuals to help work in the service industries, which is where 85% of all the jobs will be in the year 2000.

Job and Labor Trends

The civilian labor force is predicted to reach approximately 140 million people in the year 2000. This projected increase will be up 15% during the 1990s and represents a significant slowing in both the number joining the labor force and the rate of growth. The eligibility pool of young workers fell below 8 million by 1990, resulting in an unemployment rate of 5.3% in 1990—a 14-year low. It is important to note that the commerce and labor specialists consider the employment rate of 5% to be a "full-employment" figure (US Department of Labor Statistical Report, June 1990). They have indicated that we will continue to have tremendous shortage of workers both in the skilled and unskilled areas throughout the 1990s. We will continue to have an acute shortage of workers, particularly in those areas in which persons with dual diagnosis have been most successful in the past. These areas include low-skilled, low-paying jobs. For example, the National Restaurant Association says that their industry is short by 200,000 workers (Stark, & Goldsbury, 1988). The shift from a goods-producing to a service-producing economy will be evident in the year 2000, when nearly 85% of all jobs will be in the service industry such as health care, education, food preparation, hotel and motel services, and janitorial and maintenance care. The drop in birth rates will also contribute to a shortage of workers (Kelly, 1990; Little, 1988). Some 130 million people, or over 70% of the total working age population, held jobs by the 1990s, and this is anticipated to increase, representing a 2½ million increase each year in the 1990s (Bureau of the Census, 1987). Despite the increase in jobs, we are witnessing a decline in the number of middle-class workers as a result of a decrease in high-wage union jobs, causing a polarization into high- and low-wage paying jobs (Stark, Bredar, & Goldsbury, 1989). National surveys taken in 1990 revealed that more than half the individuals with a disability were prevented from working who wanted to. Two thirds of those working felt that they were underemployed. The vocational implication for persons with mental retardation is indeed promising but will require, particularly in the early 1990s, creative approaches in working more with the private sector with more local and state funding. The private sector is being increasingly forced to train its workers, particularly in the services industry. Private industry spent over $80 billion in 1990, and this is expected to double by the year 2000. Most of the new jobs were generated by small businesses who can't afford training. This will require businesses to be more involved in schools, job-training programs, and community resource programs. Over 1 million people drop out of high school each year, and the dropout rates in some school areas is close to 50%. Added to this is the fact that 70 million adults are functionally illiterate or borderline illiterate (Templin, 1988). As a result, job-training programs in the private sector should expand rapidly, with a third of the eligible workers by the year 2000 attributing the skill they need to obtain their jobs by training acquired informally or on the job.

Technology Trends

The impact of computer technology will be felt most dramatically in the workplace, particularly in the service sector. Futurists predict that tele-communication devices via the use of computers will provide developmentally disabled adults with the first tools to extend their cognitive capabilities. Computer-aided instructions, videotapes, and video terminals may lead to (a) allowing students to proceed at a more individual pace, thereby reducing their stigma; (b) enable developmentally disabled individuals to work at home or wherever convenient; and (c) provide learning aids specifically designed for the developmentally disabled population to learn more individualized techniques. Of the 85% of the people working in service industry by the year 2000, 43% will work in the information industry and 22% will work at home. Computer competence will be required of almost everyone, with some 70% of U.S. homes having computers in the year 2000 compared with just 20% in the year 1990.

Health Care

The United States spent almost $700 billion in health care in 1990. The U.S. Commerce Department estimates that this represents almost 12% of the Gross National Product. Costs in health care have accelerated significantly over the past several years and will continue at a 10% to 14% annual clip to the year 2000. These rising costs provide concerns for the approximately 37 million uninsured Americans and pressure for long-term coverage for the elderly and disabled, which will put a great deal of pressure on the U.S. health-care system and which seems inevitable by the end of the century. We predict that we will see a modified version of a national health system, which will be an improvement over that seen in Canada and the United Kingdom. This will particularly affect persons with developmental disabilities as it relates to their health care and more specifically to the mental health needs, which will be incorporated more and more into the general health-care system of package of services, particularly in the private industry. In addition, this shift to Health Maintenance Organizations and Preferred Provider Organizations (referred to as "managed care") will most likely replace the traditional health-care plans.

Microtrends

Definitional Trends

A great deal of confusion exists as to what constitutes mental illness in individuals who are mentally retarded, which has led to inappropriate assumptions, equivocation, and teleological arguments (e.g., the term *dual diagnosis*). The definition of mental retardation is accepted with wide consensus, (Grossman, 1983). However, there is considerable debate about the difficulty as it relates to functional areas in mental retardation, particularly the area of adaptive behavior and our ability to measure it precisely. Certainly, the new definitional issues that will be discussed in the terminology and classification manual scheduled to be completed in 1992 should shed further light on the entire definitional aspects of mental retardation. However, the definition of mental illness, which refers to "abnormality of behavior, emotions, or reactions sufficiently marked or prolonged so as to require specialized care" (DSM-III-R American Psychiatric Association, 1980), engenders a considerable amount of discussion when concern is focused on individuals who exhibit both diagnoses. Mental illness includes a considerable number of categories, and yet there is seldom more than a 50% to 60% consensus agreement to what constitutes a specific mental illness (i.e., depression, schizophrenia, etc.). In essence, the major need in the next 10 years will be to come up with a national standard that will clearly define this group and allow persons with mental retardation/mental illness to be accurately measured so as to allow for a more precise way to determine eligibility, which is critical for future funding needs.

Epidemiological Factors

The whole area of epidemiology will undergo a radical expansion and improvement, which is a much-needed area of research in the entire field of developmental disabilities. Certainly, epidemiologists who have conducted research thus far have played a major role in helping us to understand broad trends and the prevalence of some of the more common and easily defined conditions associated with cognitive disability. Epidemiologists have, however, been frustrated at not being able to make larger contributions to the study of the frequency of different syndromes as it relates to biological impairment. There is clearly a need for a more coherent and satisfactory system of classification if epidemiologists are to make a greater contribution. With the new developments in genetic research in the 1990s as it relates to the mapping of the human genome is clearly important that these diagnostic advances be based on sound epidemiological research (Russell & Menolascino, 1989). In essence, a considerable amount of research thus far would indicate (Menolascino &

Stark, 1984) that people with mental retardation are at risk to develop an allied mental illness that is due to neurological, language, memory, or learning deficits, as well as vulnerability to crises and social demands.

Current epidemiological studies, although lacking in solid methodology, indicate an occurrence rate of mental illness in those who are mentally retarded that is significantly higher. Studies of mental illness in the mentally retarded range from 10% to 60% with an average of 25% to 35% versus that found in the nonretarded population of 18%. As Stark points out, it is an interesting note that Diagnostic and Statistical Manual, III-R states that "the prevalence of mental disorders is at least 3 or 4 times greater among persons with mental retardation than the general population" (Stark, 1989). Recent research by Reiss (1990) suggested an overall rate of 39%, which was high primarily because personality disorders were very common. Of this group, only 11.7% of the subjects had a psychiatric diagnosis in their case files, suggesting that the diagnosis was underdiagnosed for the sample group. Perhaps the most comprehensive study ever conducted in North America was done by Sharon Borthwick-Duffy and Richard Eyman (1990) who evaluated the mental health problems among persons with mental retardation using a state data base of 78,000+ individuals who received services in the state. These two superb researchers found that approximately 10% of persons with mental retardation also had a psychiatric disorder that was diagnosed by the state (Bruininks, Hill, & Morreau, 1988). In short, via continued epidemiological research, we predict this type of research will reach a much higher level of respect and reliance that will be demanded by Congress, state, and local funding agencies in order to accurately qualify individuals seeking funding, particularly in community-based programs (Jacobson, 1990).

Current prevalence research (DSM-III-R) indicates that some 60% of the 2 million Americans with disabling mental illness (without mental retardation) live with their families at least part of the time, and hundreds of thousands more reside in nursing homes and private-run "board and cares." Some $17 billion plus each year are spent annually in the United States on Mental Health care. Yet, this money is not funneled for those who need it most, particularly in the form of coordinated community services, crisis centers, outreach team, housing, and job-training programs (Goode, 1989).

Diagnostic Trends

Studies to date (Stark, et al., 1988) indicate that individuals who are mentally retarded may display the same range of psychiatric disorders as others. Certainly, by the year 2000, we predict that we will see a significant increase into the diagnosis of persons with dual diagnosis. We also know that some psychiatric symptoms are unique to this subpopulation, such as entrenched self-injurious behavior seen in persons with more severe retardation. However, the complexity and heterogeneity make the diagnostic process a real challenge. The major variables that influence the diagnostic process, which should be multidisciplinary and team based, are (a) cognitive/adaptive/functional levels; (b) age; (c) gender; (d) severity, duration, and type of symptom presentation; (e) health and physical impairments, including seizures; (f) medication; (g) environmental and caretaker history; and (h) professional perspective and data needs, that is, policy making, reimbursement, service, or research based (Stark, 1989).

Evaluation

The development of assessment instruments has been woefully lacking during the 1980s. Attempts have been made with limited success to adapt instruments that are generally used with the population as a whole and administered to persons with mental retardation. The major difficulty has been in developing devices for those who are more severely retarded and who may exhibit the higher frequency of more severe forms of mental illness.

Undoubtedly, the greatest area of enthusiasm is the development of new scientific advancements in our diagnostic instrumentation, particularly in the biomedical sciences. A quiet revolution is taking place, particularly in the area of neuroanatomy with the use of new, sophisticated equipment. The development of neuroimaging technology will have a major impact on our efforts to understand the basic neuroanatomic systems and will provide rationales for treatment that can ultimately reduce the manifestations of mental retardation and also mental illness (Stark, Menolascino, & Goldsbury, 1988). Following are some of the more exciting pieces of technology.

Positron-Emission Tomography

Positron-emission tomography (PET) uses an injection of short-lived chemical substances containing radioactive atoms that emit positrons, which result in the recording of multiple radiographic films, which can be converted into sophisticated computer images of the multiple metabolic events that are occurring in an organ. This new PET technology gives us remarkable information about organ function and organ anatomy. Neuroscientists believe that PET will do for the behavioral sciences what CT scanners have done for the physical medicine. It will not only help to record the brain's chemistry but will allow us to examine the interaction of other neurochemical factors within the brain and changes secondary to external psychological factors. In this sense, PET will give us a "scientific window" into the causes of emotional states in an individual.

Contemporary brain imaging techniques can be divided into two main areas and five disciplines. The first area emphasizes brain structure and anatomy and uses computerized tomography (CT) and magnetic resonance imaging (MRI). The second area emphasizes different ways of examining brain function and blood flow metabolism and receptor status using PET and single-positron-emission computerized tomography (SPECT) and electrophysiologically using computerized electroencephalography (CEEG).

All methods examine the brain in different ways and have inherent strengths and weaknesses (Kuperman, Gaffney, Hamdan-Allen, Preston, & Venkatesh, 1990). All of this research is available because of the tremendous breakthroughs occurring in the computer chip industry. We are seeing a tremendous reduction in the cost of computers, which by the year 2000 will be purchased at approximately 1/100th of the cost and will be able to process 10 million bits of data per second. Much of this is due to the tremendous development of the static random-access memory chip (SRAM), which is so fast it can read an entire 75-volume encyclopedia in 1 S. In addition, optic discs will become commonplace with computers and will play a larger role as our technology develops. For example, these large optic discs and their technology will allow researchers to develop wallet-size cards for $1.50 that can store a 1,000-page novel. These breakthroughs will allow us to simplify many of the learning and training techniques for individuals with mental retardation and mental illness.

Services and Model Programs

We predict the development of model programs and funding for this population will be significantly increased in the mid-1990s, resulting in a tremendous and rapid growth in establishing model programs. We do have a small number of established model programs throughout the country ranging from inpatient and outpatient day programs to specialized community services programs focusing on certain treatment aspects in working with this population. However, above all, we lack a national mandate from Congress with a responsibility to assign a federal agency for coordinating services, training, research, and policies for this neglected group of individuals. If we are going to be successful in developing these programs, a specific federal agency will need to be identified to help develop and establish a national research and training center devoted exclusively to the area of dual diagnosis. This will require many federal agencies coming together, helping to coordinate and cooperatively fund these types of programs. We think model service centers will also be established throughout the country, at least at a regional level and then later at the state level when expertise is available to conduct evaluation, treatment, and follow-up of individuals. These will be interdisciplinary treatment centers, which can be specialized in working with this population and can be easily worked into current treatment centers such as the university affiliated programs throughout the country. We also see a significant increase in the training of critical personnel, particularly in the area of psychiatry, psychology, and the entire mental health field who have cross training and feel comfortable working with both systems.

Last, we predict that by the year 2000 the amount of research will significantly increase. We predict that this will involve a five-phase process, which will need to be funded by the federal government. These phases are (a) identification of available services and resources as a prelude to phase 2; (b) establishment of a national data-collection system focusing on the epidemiological characteristics of this population; (c) development of a differential diagnostic system that would include valid assessment instruments; (d) research and advocacy of treatment approaches and techniques; and (e) community integration with a comprehensive care system and a fully operational prevention process.

Treatment

Of course, treatment will depend on the development of all of the trends mentioned here. We will need epidemiological data, adequate diagnostic processes, and valid assessment instruments. We also need to establish program evaluation of the models used in providing services throughout the country. Many areas in the treatment process will enhance our successful efforts. There has been a virtual explosion in the development of psychopharmacology with new drugs helping to provide a tremendous relief for such areas as depression and anxiety (Goode, Lennin, & Burke, 1990). In addition, we are finding tremendous breakthroughs in the neuroscience areas in understanding the brain's biology using microscopic probes to sample electrical pulses from the 100 billion neurons that make up the brain. And, by the year 2000, we will be able to say that "We do understand how the brain really works."

Additional areas of excitement will involve the use of gene therapy and more specifically a newer technique called *gene targeting*, which will be used to cure inherited diseases that cause mental retardation and mental illness in the beginning. We will then be able to prevent and/or reverse numerous causes of mental retardation and mental illness.

In addition, with the ongoing development of the knowledge in such areas as supported employment, we feel that research and programs will be developed to provide a greater integration of these individuals into community-based programs, which has been an area of virtually no research (Wehman, 1990).

Summary

In this chapter we have focused on two major trend areas. The first involved the more "macrotrends" involving societal changes of which those of us in the human services field need to become more knowledgeable because they will have a tremendous impact on research, training, and services. In the second part of the chapter, we directed our attention to the "microtrends" involving definitional, epidemiological, diagnostic and evaluational, and treatment issues specific to this population. We remain committed to our work with these individuals and their families and are optimistic about where we will be by the year 2000 despite the disappointing decade of the 1980s (Cetron & Davies, 1989).

References

American Psychiatric Association. (1980). *Diagnostic and statistical manual of mental disorders*. Washington, DC: American Psychiatric Association.

Borthwick-Duffy, S. A., & Eyman, R. K. (1990). Who are the dually diagnosed? *American Journal of Mental Retardation*, 94(6), 586–595.

Braddock, D., & Hemp, R. (1986). Government spending for mental retardation and developmental disabilities. *Hospital and Community Psychiatry*, 37, 702–707.

Bruininks, R. H., Hill, B. K., & Morreau, V. (1988). Prevalence and implications of maladaptive behaviors and dual diagnosis in residential and other service programs. In J. A. Stark, F. J. Menolascino, M. H. Albarelli, & V. Gray (Eds.), *Mental retardation/mental health: Classification, diagnosis, treatment, services* (pp. 3–29). New York: Springer-Verlag.

Bureau of the Census. (1987). *Statistical abstract of the United States* (107th ed.). Washington, DC: U.S. Department of Commerce.

Cetron, M., & Davies, O. (1989). *American Renaissance. Our life at the turn of the 21st century*. New York: St. Martin's Press.

Dentzer, S. (1990, March 12). America's scandalous health care: Here's how to fix it. *U.S. News and World Report*, pp. 24–30.

Editor. Foreign debt could crimp our lifestyle (Special Report). (1988). *USA Today*, February 12, 1988.

Editor. (1990). Federal Reserve Board. *US News & World Report*, October 23, 1990.

Editor. (1990). General Accounting Office. *US News & World Report*, August 13, 1990.

Findlay, S., & Silberner, J. (1989–1990, December 25–January 1). Outlook 1990. Cost and cures. *U.S. News and World Report*, pp. 68–69.

Goode, E. C. (1989, April 24). When mental illness hits home. *U.S. News and World Report*, pp. 54–65.

Goode, E., Linnon, N., & Burke, S. (1990, March 5). Tailoring treatment for depression's many forms. *U.S. News and World Report,* pp. 54–56.

Grossman, H. J. (Ed.). (1983). *Manual on terminology and classification in mental retardation*. Washington, DC: American Association on Mental Deficiency.

Jacobson, J. W. (1990). Do some mental disorders occur less frequently among persons with mental retardation? *American Journal of Mental Retardation*, *94*(6), 596–602.

Kelly, D. (1990, July 31). Making ends meet is an uphill battle. *USA Today*, p. D1.

Kuperman, S., Gaffney, G. R., Hamdan-Allen, G., Preston, D. F., & Venkatesh, L. (1990). Neuroimaging in child and adolescent psychiatry. *Journal of American Academy of Child and Adolescent Psychiatry*, *29*(2), 159–172.

Little, R. (1988, July 20). Working for a living. *USA Today*, p. D1.

Menolascino, F. J., Neman, R., & Stark, J. A. (Eds.). (1983). *Curative aspects of mental retardation: Biomedical and behavioral advances*. Baltimore, MD: Paul H. Brookes.

Menolascino, F. J., & Stark, J. A. (1984). *Handbook of mental illness in the mentally retarded*. New York: Plenum Press.

National Surveys. (1990). *USA Today*, September 5, 1990.

Plog, S. C., & Santamour, M. B. (Eds.). (1980). *The year 2000 and mental retardation*. New York: Plenum Press.

Reiss, S. (1990). Prevalence of dual diagnosis in community-based day programs in the Chicago metropolitan area. *American Journal of Mental Retardation*, *94*(6), 578–585.

Russell, J. A. O., & Menolascino, F. J. (1989). Mental retardation: Editorial overview. *Current Opinion in Psychiatry*, *2*(5), 591–592.

Stark, J. Viewpoint. (1989). Mental illness in persons with mental retardation. *News & Notes* (American Association on Mental Retardation), 6, pp. 1–2.

Stark, J. A., Kiernan, W. E., Goldsbury, T. L., & McGee, J. J. (1986). Not entering employment: A system dilemma. In W. E. Kiernan & J. A. Stark, (Eds.), *Pathways to employment for adults with developmental disabilities*. Baltimore, MD: Paul H. Brookes Publishing Company.

Stark, J. A., Menolascino, F. J., Albarelli, M. & Gray, V. (Eds.). (1987). *Mental retardation/mental health: Classification, diagnosis, treatment, services*. New York: Springer-Verlag, Inc.

Stark, J. A., Brader, M., & Goldsbury, T. L. (1989). Injured and well worker: Interface between industry, insurance, and government. In W. E. Kiernan & R. L. Schalock (Eds.), *Economics, industry, and disability: A look ahead* (pp. 237–251). Baltimore, MD: Paul H. Brookes Publishing.

Stark, J. A., & Goldsbury, T. (1988). Analysis of labor and economics need for the next decade. *Mental Retardation*. *26*(6), 363–368.

Stark, J. A., Menolascino, F. J., & Goldsbury, T. (1988). An updated search for the prevention of mental retardation. In J. A. Stark & F. J. Menolascino (Eds.), *Preventive and curative intervention in mental retardation* (pp. 3–29). Baltimore: Paul H. Brookes Publishing.

Strauss, G. (1988). The rush to fill jobs. *USA Today*, July 12, 1988.

U.S. Dept. of Labor, Statistical Report, June, 1990.

Templin, S. (1988, July 12). Young workers lack skills. *USA Today*, p. D1.

Wehman, P. (1990). *A national analysis of supported employment growth and implementation*. Richmond: Virginia Comonwealth University, Rehabilitation Research and Training Center on Supported Employment.

12
Expansion of the Health-Care Delivery System

ALLEN C. CROCKER

Efforts undertaken in the 1980s secured critically valuable foundations from which it should be possible to establish a generally satisfactory health-care delivery system for persons with mental retardation by the year 2000. Much of this work centered initially on small children, and even infants, but in the development idiom, one can insinuate progression to older children, youth, and adults. Some of the relevant and important phenomena of this past decade are discussed in the following paragraphs.

1. *Diminution of the institutional focus:* The numbers of persons living in large congregate-care facilities, originally well over 200,000, fell to 93,000 by 1989. The quality of medical care in the institutions underwent substantial improvement as the population reduced, reinforced especially by provisions of the approximately 50 class action suits that sought amelioration in treatment and programs. Medical care was commonly a central element in the concerns of the courts, and this concentration served to bring new resolves and personnel into the field. Some of the knowledge and experience proved to be transferable.

2. *Early analysis of access to health care in the community:* The devotion and availability of medical supports for persons with mental retardation in community circumstances began to receive systematic consideration in this period, including in the reviews by McDonald (1985), Minihan (1986), Minihan and Dean, (1990), Crocker and Yankauer (1987), Rowitz (1988), Nowell, Baker, and Conroy (1989), and Birenbaum, Guyot, and Cohen (1989). These works served also to provide better understanding of acute and chronic health-care needs and the patterns in which service is sought.

3. *Growth in professional identification and commitment:* A cohort of physicians with major involvement in the delivery of health care for children and adults with mental retardation now exists. This development

Preparation of this material was supported in part by the U.S. Department of Health and Human Services, Maternal and Child Health Bureau (Project MCJ-259150), and Administration on Developmental Disabilities (Project 03DD00135).

is assisted and promoted by many professional organizations—including the American Association on Mental Retardation (Medicine Division), American Association of University Affiliated Programs for Persons With Developmental Disabilities, the Society for Behavioral Pediatrics, the Society for Developmental Pediatrics, and the American Academy of Pediatrics. Increased professional opportunities stimulated by the previously mentioned court actions have also favored recruitment of new persons.

4. *Rise of consumerism (and parent–professional partnership):* The 1980s can assuredly be said to have been the time when parents, and family members generally, established their rightful place as central contributors to the planning and implementation of health-care systems. Many professionals welcomed this and had worked for it; others were surprised and reluctant as parents became true partners in determining the style and deployment of health-care resources. Parent action was aided by many large and effective organizations, such as the National Down Syndrome Congress, the Association of Retarded Citizens/US, The Association for Persons With Severe Handicaps, the Federation for Children With Special Needs, the Alliance of Genetics Support Groups, the Association for the Care of Children's Health, and many others. We can never go back again to the era of exclusive professional domination.

5. *Emergence of value systems in health care:* A large debt is owed to the Maternal and Child Health Bureau (or Division or Office, at different times) of the United States Public Health Service, to the American Academy of Pediatrics, and, above all, to C. Everett Koop as Surgeon General, for promoting the thoughtful enumeration of the values that should characterize the provision of care for children generally, and particularly those with disabilities and chronic illness. This was spurred, to some extent, by an urgency following the Baby Doe dilemma but had already been begun in a series of national conferences hosted by the Maternal and Child Health Bureau (MCH) starting in 1982. Some elements featured were that such care must be comprehensive, developmentally oriented, continuous, integrated, nondiscriminatory, and payment ensured. The most critical components of this earnest consideration of values were captured in the simple phrase, "family-centered, community-based, coordinated care." The authorship of this cogent slogan for the times is not precisely known, but contributions were made by McPherson, MacQueen, Koop, Magrab, Bishop, and Berman (Heron, 1989). The implications are well discussed by Brewer, McPherson, Magrab, and Hutchins (1989). Equivalent listings for values in the delivery of care for adults can be readily formulated.

6. *Modern standards of care:* Once the tabulation of fundamental values has been carried out, it was possible to proceed with conversion of these ideas to modern operational principles—or standards. The traditional references of the Accreditation Council of Services for People with Developmental Disabilities (AC/DD) and Title XIX guidelines have been

of substantial value regarding the minimum levels of service acceptable for certification. Ideal schemes have also been devised for individual disorders. A broader system has now been proposed by New England SERVE, as "Enhancing Quality—Standards and Indicators of Quality Care for Children With Special Health Care Needs" (Epstein et al., 1989). In this pioneering effort, desired behaviors and characteristics are considered for health-care teams, facilities, health departments, and the social setting. Again, adult-care applications can be developed.

7. *A more demanding look at payment methods:* The plight of persons who are uninsured or underinsured finally became the base of much discussion and assistance in recent years. The arbitrariness of private insurance coverage and the patchwork nature of Medicaid have obviously left many families and individuals with suboptimal access to satisfactory care or with debilitating penalties. These matters will be given considerable commentary later in this chapter.

Consideration of Health Care for Adults

The Knowledge Base

Our ability in current times to provide accurate health care for adults with mental retardation is improved but incomplete. Taken as a class, these persons are obviously of diverse personal and clinical background, and generalizations should be approached cautiously. For the majority, the medical needs can be expected to approximate those of average persons, although influences may occur because of altered personal independence and self-care practices and from particular past experiences and supports. Others have special vulnerabilities deserving preventive and therapeutic assistance.

When significant disability exists, it is important to know about the basic nature or cause of the disorder. One's hopes for appropriate anticipatory care and interventions depend in some regards on insights about probable natural history and/or health-related complications. Information about causation can usually be induced, although a significant number of "unknown" situations occur (Crocker, 1989a). In recent years, the traditional statements about mortality for various disorders have been substantially revised, and a greater diligence and accountability have been brought to medical support activities (Eyman et al., 1990, 1991).

Surveys have been conducted of identified medical problems for residents of state residential facilities (Nelson & Crocker, 1978; Rubin, 1987), where seizures, orthopedic problems, and adjustment or behavioral difficulties are the most prominent, with infections, gastrointestinal problems, and cardiac issues also significant. These findings are obviously skewed by the population characteristics there, featuring persons with multiple disabilities. In recent times, survey information has also become available from community origins. The Morristown (NJ) Developmental Disabilities Center reported on 729 persons, again with prominent seizures and orthopedic problems (Ziring, 1987; Ziring et al., 1988). Inclusion of genetic study in that program uncovered or corrected many syndromic diagnoses. Reported medical problems in a Pennsylvania project were, in order of prevalence, seizures; behavioral; ear, nose, and throat; cardiac; and gastrointestinal for clients living in supported community facilities; for adults still living with their families, the major frequencies were for seizures, allergies, skin problems, cardiac issues, and foot problems (Nowell et al., 1989).

More information should be gathered on the expectations in health-care needs in the coming decade, particularly in a longitudinal fashion by use of departmental data systems and problem-oriented medical records. Our understanding of life course issues and special susceptibilities and correlations must be strengthened. A recent text has reported much of what is presently known in this regard (Rubin & Crocker, 1989).

As we progress toward the year 2000, departments of mental retardation/ developmental disabilities have an obligation to establish information systems that will allow more accurate planning for health-care resources in this population; university centers must share in this work. From such information, it will be possible to design protocols for preventive and supportive care, related to specific diagnoses and situations, plus reasonable mortality tables.

Standards of Care

Persons with significant mental retardation constitute a "special" group in our society, identified as requiring planning and support by public agencies. On a cultural basis, they are likely to have fewer options in the self-determination of medical care. Hence, there should be more nearly an entitlement rather than merely an expectation for the procurement of quality care. In that situation, it would be fitting for programs to be guided by standards derived from established values, and formulated by the joint consideration of consumers, advocates, and professionals. Accreditation of facilities, including for reimbursement with public funds, does exist, but these processes often lack a more conceptual framework or concurrent quality assurance. As mentioned, the drive for family-centered, community-based, coordinated care has become a public and private concern in the last several years relating to children with disability. The adult equivalent would look to the same personalized, supportive, and integrated goals. In the MCH-sponsored "Enhancing Quality" document of New England SERVE, one can find many standards applicable to adult care programs—especially as these involve written plans, individualized evaluation, continuity, use of specialty care as needed, attention to prevention, family partnership, and alliance with habilitative resources (Epstein et al., 1989).

In the coming years, professional, governmental, and consumer groups should establish standards of health care for serving adults with mental retardation; lessons can be gained from the experience with children's programs.

Factors in Community Medical Practice

Necessary Agency Commitment to the Conduct of Office Practice

The primary medical care for persons with mental retardation in the community will preeminently rest with generic community-based physicians for the decade to come. It is to be hoped (and anticipated) that in this setting the majority of persons can truly find a "medical home," where some personalization and continuity can be assured. Certain innovative designs for centers and projects will be mentioned later in this chapter, but it is both inevitable and desirable that the normalized circumstance of local care serves the majority. Specialty care has other issues involved, as will be discussed. For such patients, especially those who have behavioral atypicality, the office or clinic assignment may be a larger one than average. An open interest, and even a degree of outreach, on behalf of community physicians is more broadly present than is often insinuated (see, e.g., results of the survey in Maine, Minihan, Dean, & Lyons, 1989; and in Pennsylvania, Nowell et al., 1989).

In this setting, however, a major limitation in effectiveness is created by difficulties in information transfer. This refers to the scattered medical records available for most community clients, unfamiliarity or naivete of the accompanying residence or program personnel, and problems in achieving follow-through collaboration or information. These hindrances can be enormously modulated by the assumption of a more active role by the "department" that has responsibility for the "client." These next years should see widespread use of a truly problem-oriented and portable health and habilitative services record that can accompany the person to medical visits. This must include information on past health-care events and interventions in a convenient (accessible) and accountable (standardized) format.

A further, and even more strategic, contribution by the department would be that of enhanced "service coordination" by dedicated persons who maintain current familiarity with clients and join them for medical encounters. They would simultaneously assist in completion of necessary paper work and assurances for follow-up components. These activities can be a part of so-called "case management." The process of coordination of care, as it relates to health issues, is even more effective when nursing personnel become part of the team, provide regular contact and review, and join in the care decisions. The past record of performance by such nurses (or nurse practitioners) is superior. They may be working out of state regional offices, be deployed with vendor groups, be part of

Visiting Nurse Association programs, or be affiliated with special health-care projects. Their good judgment and advocacy should, but often do not, protect them from the constraints of departmental budget cuts; one hopes that this decade will provide reinforcement for these valuable professionals.

Issues in Medical Education

It has assuredly been true that conventional physician training includes sparse information about the world of persons with mental retardation, in spite of the fact that such individuals constitute 2% to 3% of the population. Selected scientific material on hereditary or chromosomal aberrations may be introduced in pediatric curricula at the undergraduate level, but traditionally, little is discussed about coordinated long-term care needs. Pediatric residents encounter children with special needs episodically; trainees in internal medicine receive very little contact with involved adults. The coming decade should rectify this lapse. Medical schools and training programs related to university-affiliated programs (UAPs) may do more in this regard, with lectures, practica, and elective courses, and this should be reinforced. Legislation currently under consideration in Massachusetts would require teaching about issues in mental retardation within the medical schools. Programs at the Dartmouth-Mary Hitchcock Hospital in New Hampshire and the University of North Carolina at Chapel Hill require that each pediatric resident provide a day of respite home care for a child with serious developmental disabilities, and these have proven to be popular.

The American Academy of Pediatrics and many of the UAPs offer continuing education regarding children with disabilities; few internists or general practitioners are reached in this way. Two new serial publications are now available to provide information and interest for physicians who have patients with developmental disabilities—*Exceptional Physician*, published by New England INDEX in Waltham, Massachusetts, and *Exceptional Health Care* from the Developmental Disabilities Center at the Morristown (NJ) Memorial Hospital.

Medical Referral Systems and Resource Centers

There may be difficulty in finding experienced and responsive specialty providers in the community for referral. Surveys of mental retardation program administrators have indicated problems in locating appropriate dentists, gynecologists, allergists, neurologists, and orthopedists, in that order, in eastern Pennsylvania (Nowell et al., 1989), and psychiatrists, dentists, gynecologists, and neurologists in Massachusetts (Howard & Autor, 1989). A highly relevant assistance for this dilemma has been begun by New England INDEX, an information center for individuals with disabilities (in Waltham, Massachusetts). This program has launched a computer-based, call-in Physician Registry, which lists doctors who have signed on to such a referral service in response to a selected inquiry by mail. Requests received in the first months from families and program administrators were most frequent regarding primary care physicians, and then (in order) for psychiatrists, neurologists, orthopedists, ophthalmologists, and gynecologists (Damon, Gould, Bass, & Jones, 1990). Some effort will be made by subsequent query to identify the satisfactoriness of these referrals. This type of public service should be extended to other geographic areas. Using a similar physician mailing list, and other outreach, New England INDEX has also begun a Medical Education Program for interested physicians, where in regularly scheduled meetings, key clinical topics are presented (with continuing medical education [CME] credits), and circumstances of practice are discussed.

For persons with mental retardation and complex or multisystem disorders, primary care physicians may wish to use the backup and coordination services of a specialized resource center. Such a facility would be staffed by clinicians with familiarity and expertise in the complications of developmental disabilities. These could be based in a UAP, for example, or could be an outreach function of the care team in a modern state residential facility. These workers could provide periodic update on the care plans for seriously affected clients, and assist in new interventions where necessary (Crocker et al., 1987).

Recommendations

As we progress toward the year 2000, some specific recommendations include the following:

1. Responsible state agencies of mental retardation and developmental disabilities must acknowledge the key role of appropriate health-care provision as a right for persons who are eligible for their services and assume responsibility for assistance in the process.
2. Of particular relevance is the creation of portable, problem-oriented health-care records, and assured care coordination by nurses and/or other experienced persons.
3. Compassionate and accurate education on the circumstances and needs of persons with developmental disabilities would appropriately be incorporated in the medical school and postgraduate training of all physicians. A generation of internists and family practitioners must be developed who have been trained in issues of care relating to adults with mental retardation.
4. Reinforcement for the requirements of families and of primary care physicians should be provided by assisted referral systems for specialty care and the availability of expert resource centers.

Areas of Particular Concern

Continuing Care and the Prevention of Secondary Disability

In discussions of medical care supports for adults with mental retardation in the community, it is usually concluded that current systems are satisfactory regarding the responses available for acute issues. Infections, injuries, and other emergency matters generally find appropriate response in the generic system. Quite another level of concern rests with the consideration of chronic problems. A number of the disorders in which mental retardation is a counterpart also have taxing health-related cumulative effects. Examples include gastroesophageal reflux, recurrent aspiration, and chronic pulmonary disease in persons with profound disability; and recurrent urinary tract infection, with renal damage, in severe cerebral palsy and in spina bifida. Nutritional failure, obesity, hypothyroidism, periodontal disease, chronic middle ear disease, arthritis, and mitral valve prolapse all occur with increased prevalence in persons with developmental disabilities. Any other chronic disorder of mankind may also occur, of course, and not be identified because symptoms are not enunciated. These matters require monitoring and inquiry for detection.

A valuable component of the Disability Prevention Programs, begun with state grants in 1988 from the Centers for Disease Control, has been an earnest focus on prevention of secondary disability, an area that previously had not received systematic attention. This has also been included prominently in the "National Agenda for the Prevention of Disabilities" formulated by a special task force in the Institute of Medicine, National Academy of Sciences (Pope & Tarlov, 1991). Their concerns include potential complicating respiratory, vascular, cardiac, renal, skin, gastrointestinal, and musculoskeletal developments, as well as issues such as substance abuse, psychologic problems, and recurrent injury. Attention to these matters, not notably significant for the person with mild expression of disability, has major relevance for persons who are more seriously involved.

Our ability to provide best long-term care in the circumstances of developmental disabilities is somewhat limited by features of the natural history of certain syndromes, which are as yet poorly tabulated. Progressive diminution in vision, hearing, language, or, most specifically, in cognition, occurs in certain persons with serious mental retardation, and the cause may be unclear. Functional losses in motor function, such as loss of ambulation, are frequently seen in individuals with spastic quadriplegia as the decades pass, and our capacity to prevent this is not known (though probably is considerable). There is much we must learn in the coming decade.

The Potential for Rehabilitation

For occasional individuals, the improvement of function or comfort is possible by means of special surgical (surgery of the back, joints, eye, ear, palate, etc.) or medical (growth hormone, anti-inflammatory agents, relaxants, etc.) intervention. One can hope that by 2000, there will be new wisdom and experience here. Also, assistive technologies are a growing area for help in communication, learning, mobility, self-care, and other capabilities (see Chapter 16). One looks to well-developed resource centers, as described, and to university programs, for leadership.

Behavioral Issues and/or Mental Illness

The substantial prevalence of "challenging behaviors" in persons with significant mental retardation may testify to our frequent ineptness in creating desirable living and learning circumstances. Our understanding in this area, and our training of mental health personnel with necessary insights, will assuredly grow in this decade. Szymanski (1987) has spoken well for preventive measures.

The Pursuit of Wellness

Much of the material in the previous pages of this chapter can be considered as unduly preoccupied with a "disease model." There has been an attempt in the foregoing suggestions to provide a secure stewardship for the health, safety, and best personal progress, of the person with mental retardation, but predominantly in the reference frame of sound medical membership on the treatment team. Physicians, however, must guard against schedules, interventions, or medications that inhibit other program considerations. They should also advocate for those supports that work toward the person's wholeness and peace, such as good sleep, relaxation, exercise, appropriate nutrition, and stress control. Further, when medical disorders are in good compensation (such as seizures well controlled), one should celebrate basic wellness. Health education for the client, and self-understanding, can assist in achieving greater self-esteem. We must all be devoted to the precious goal of the person maintaining or reaching happiness.

Recommendations

As we progress toward the year 2000, some specific recommendations include the following:

1. A medical review for each person, at least annually, should look to possible chronic care challenges, and these health matters should be succinctly featured in the updated Individualized Service Plan (ISP).
2. All worsening of disability with time should be thoughtfully inves-

tigated, with consultation obtained as needed regarding possible supports or interventions.
3. A preventive program for best health and the creative use of rehabilitative measures (when values are balanced) are responsibilities of the medical care team.
4. A sense of wellness, even in the presence of substantial disability, should be sought.

Financing Community Health Care

Usage Levels and Patterns of Coverage

The presence of multisystem medical disorders, and the concern about health-related secondary disabilities, has been described here for persons in the community with serious mental retardation. When one views the population as a whole, however, such as the total of those enrolled in services with state mental retardation agencies, it becomes apparent that medical problems are commonly modest in degree, and usage of medical resources is often at or near that for the general public. Cole (1987) estimated that for persons in Massachusetts 45% were in a "Level I, low consuming group," with one to three medical visits per year, 40% were at an intermediate Level II, occasionally using specialty consultants, and only 15% could be considered to be at Level III, a high-consuming group needing ongoing monitoring and access to tertiary care. Minihan and Dean (1990) also report that a minority of clients can be expected to require high levels of special medical services. Adams, Ellwood, and Pine (1989) analyzed Medicaid usage tapes for California, Georgia, Michigan, and Tennessee. Among persons with Supplemental Security Income Program (SSI) disability coverage, those with mental retardation were below the average for Medicaid expenditures in all of the states except California. In a Pennsylvania study, adults with mental retardation living with their families had an average of 5.9 medical visits per year, compared to 3.0 for the general population; those in community living arrangements had 14.8 visits, more often because of agency patterns of monitoring and response rather than a higher level of illness (Nowell et al., 1989). Requirements for mental health services constituted a specific exception. For the most part, the urgency for special planning regarding medical care derives particularly from the higher usage group of clients.

The overwhelming majority of adults with significant mental retardation are Medicaid eligible. Concern about coverage is based not so much on eligibility as from the complications of that system. Reimbursement levels are substandard for the usual fees in community practice, limitations commonly exist for important elements of the whole care package, and support does not exist for the essential activities of care coordination. These factors have led to a situation where there is often a lack of a devoted alliance for continuing care, the presence of attitudinal and other barriers, failure to carry out preventive programs, incomplete referral for specialty care, reliance on emergency rooms, and poor coordination. Dental care, mental health care, and use of the habilitative therapies (physical, occupational, and speech therapy) are commonly difficult to obtain in a Medicaid-driven system. Private health insurance is infrequently active or available for adults no longer with their families, and it, too, may have serious restrictions in coverage.

Alternative Designs

There is general agreement that reliance on Medicaid coverage in the setting of the generic health-care system, without other supports or interventions, is inadequate to fulfill the service obligations for adults with significant mental retardation (Crocker, 1988). Elements that must be secured include (a) more realistic levels of reimbursement; (b) more comprehensive access to a spread of necessary benefits and allied services; (c) enhanced involvement of training, new information, and consultation for providers; and, most significantly, (d) supporting nurses and other personnel who can supply coordination, continuity, assistance, and quality control on the activities. These components would then allow formation of a "health-care network" (Crocker et al., 1987), or, in modern language, a "managed health-care network" (Henderson, Howard, & Porell, 1990).

Certain experiments have been conceived in this regard, representing views of the potential for improved year-2000-type systems. A more secured and anticipatory coverage has been planned by providing Medicaid funds to be used for private health-maintenance organization (HMO) enrollment in the Massachusetts "Health Choices" design (Master, 1987), or combined state agency–Medicaid funding for a "university-based Health Maintenance Organization for Developmentally Disabled Persons" in Buffalo (Griswold, Msall, & Cooke, 1987). The previously mentioned Developmental Disabilities Center at the Morristown (NJ) Memorial Hospital has carried out a valuable program for 7 years, with the support of a state contract (plus involvement of Medicaid funds), and with physician training and strong professional contributions by nurse practitioners.

Is There a Prescription?

It is clear that in this coming decade we have an obligation to address the fiscally related limitations in the health-care delivery system. Because it is improbable that state agencies for mental retardation will be able to assume the base costs for medical care, we must then look to other public monies to be combined in an inspired fashion with agency leadership and quality-control responsibility. For adults in the community, requirements that employers be pressed for more adequate insurance coverage for their work force have only remote relevance. More reasonable at the moment is that Medicaid's provisions encompass more comprehensive benefits, including those of competitive reimbursement for providers, coverage for care coordination costs, and assistance to aspects of information management. Central to this will be the diversion of substantially larger proportions of Medicaid resources into the community, in contrast to institutional supports. The various "Chafee bills," now 7 years into the Medicaid reform process, are the principal hope here. Currently, S. 384 (Medicaid Home and Community Quality Services Act) would work toward an entitlement for a spread of key services, including health costs and case management. Patchwork revisions of Medicaid coverage, including the proliferation of waiver components, have been helpful but have not begun to grasp the larger issues.

Seven years ago, when the Vanderbilt study commented on options for the support of chronic illness programs, it seemed politically remote that a national health insurance plan could be developed (Hobbs, Perrin, & Ireys, 1985). Now such ideas have achieved astonishing levels of general support, somewhat in reaction to disturbing care costs in the free enterprise system and the irregular coverage existing for key groups of people. One could hope for achievement of universal access to health care, uniform standards for use of related services, and a move toward true entitlement that would benefit all sections of the population. It would be very gratifying to have predictable and assured resources for full care.

Recommendations

As we progress toward the year 2000, the following recommendations are proposed:

1. It is essential that a "managed health-care network" be established to ensure effective provision of medical and allied services for adults in the community with significant mental retardation. This should have the attributes of access to stable primary care, appropriate use of referral services, resource centers as needed, normal reimbursement levels for providers, data collection and appropriate records, personnel training and reinforcement, and most especially, reimbursed care coordination, and/or case management services.
2. Leadership for the network would appropriately rest with the state mental retardation agency, with enrollment of involved clients from the community at a full and equitable level. An advisory council composed of consumers, providers, and planners should monitor the system.
3. For the immediate upcoming years, reimbursement for services within the network should be based on an expanded Medicaid scheme (with passage of S. 384).
4. The significant advantages of a full national health insurance system

suggest that such a plan would be an improvement to the continuing readjustment of Medicaid coverage.

The Health-Care System for Children

Values and Standards

The statements regarding values and attributes in the provision of health care for adults with mental retardation, posited in the previous sections, are rigorously applicable to children as well (and were often first conceptualized in relation to systems for children). Here, one encounters the parents as preeminent care givers, the urgency is present for home-centered and developmentally supportive patterns of care, and the requirement is strong to bring correlation to services in the schools and child advocacy programs. Hence, there is special cogency to the affirmation of care plans that are "family centered, community based, and coordinated." While the need exists to enhance accuracy in the knowledge base about children with disabilities, and to ensure dedicated specialized services, there is also an obligation to acknowledge a nurturant balance in the "alike–unalike" dialectic in the provision of care. Most children with special health-care needs will receive most care within the generic system, or with moderate supplements to it. The New England SERVE document, "Enhancing Quality," has a strategic use in suggesting the favorable characteristics for supportive health care (Epstein et al., 1989). An example of a modern pattern of treatment assurances, the "Declaration of Health Care Rights for the Person With Down Syndrome," is given in Appendix 12.1 (Crocker, 1991).

As we progress toward the year 2000, the design, promulgation, and monitoring of health-care systems for children with mental retardation should be built on increasingly accurate knowledge about the involved disabilities, and should ensure that such services are family centered, community based, and coordinated.

Provision of Services for Children

Within pediatric practice, there are several levels of identification and preparation for provision of care for children with developmental disabilities (Crocker, 1989b). The most extensive involvement is with the primary care doctor in the community ("Physician A"), who attends to acute illness and guides (sometimes with consultative help) the chronic issues. Some primary care pediatricians bring further training to the work and have a partial concentration in this area ("Physician B"); they require difficult adaptations in office schedules to meet this special interest. Others work in child development centers, following specialty study, and serve to provide backup support for complex children or special families ("Physician C"). A survey of the Massachusetts Chapter of the American Academy of Pediatrics (mostly Physician A's) showed that current office practice for each member has, on average, a moderate number of children with mental retardation (14), but small numbers with other disabilities including cerebral palsy (10), severe hearing impairment (3), severe visual impairment (2), spina bifida (2), autism (2), and muscular dystrophy (1). A review of health-care access for children in special education programs in five sites in different states by Palfrey's group (Singer, Butler, & Palfrey, 1986) demonstrated wide regional variation in the patterns, with considerable correlation to economic and social factors. From 48% to 85% of the children were followed in doctors' offices, 9% to 29% in hospital outpatient clinics, 3% to 22% in various governmental or school clinics, 0% to 4% in emergency rooms, and 2% to 15% had no regular source of care.

Enactment of PL 94-142 (the "Education for All Handicapped Children Act") in 1975, and its implementation in 1977, placed a requirement on public schools to provide therapeutic services within the school setting for children with developmental disabilities for whom an Individual Education Plan had been established. These were designated as "such developmental, corrective, and other supportive services as are required to assist a handicapped child to benefit from special education." The extent to which these therapies are currently carried out has been reported by Palfrey, Singer, Ralphael, and Walker (1990) for the five school districts in the Collaborative Study of Children With Special Needs. In this review, an average of 18% of children whose primary disability was mental retardation were receiving occupational or physical therapy; 34%, counseling services; and 57%, speech/language therapy. In the category of physical or multiple disabilities, these figures were 74%, 38%, and 54%, respectively. These levels of investment are gratifying and reflect the enormous strategy of the entitlement mechanism. As Palfrey notes, "schools are likely to continue as major providers of therapeutic services to children during the next decade."

Also of great importance is the gradually increasing agreement of school systems to incorporate direct nursing and medical supports within the classroom for children with serious continuing illnesses, including those who are "technology dependent." Many of these young persons did not survive in earlier times (before modern medical interventions), or were consigned to existence in a clinical or home environment only. The pioneering work of Palfrey's "Project School Care" (Haynie, Porter, & Palfrey, 1989) in assisting schools to establish supportive care plans for children with requirements for intravenous lines, catheterization, ostomy or tube feeding, or oxygen or other respiratory care has brought critical new opportunities for educational progress. See also the text of Graff, Ault, Guess, Taylor, and Thompson (1990).

Finally, it should be noted that the role of parents and other family members as "care providers" has become substantially enlarged in recent years (Taylor, Epstein, & Crocker, 1990). This now involves a wide range of activities and expectations that were formerly less completely offered or provided in some degree by other personnel or agencies. Included are assignments in the following:

Physical maintenance (diets, adaptive equipment, home adaptations, treatments)
Emotional and psychological support (training in independence, socialization, work with brothers and sisters)
Ensuring access to education (advocacy, conferencing, monitoring)
Social and recreational opportunities (finding possibilities for groups, camps, sports, etc.)
Ensuring the transition to adulthood (living, vocational, and personal components)

Though assistance in carrying out these elements is, of course, available, it is often scattered, and parents have been pressed into becoming the ultimate case managers. Coordination of medical care may be prominent in these responsibilities. The professions have traditionally under-estimated the magnitude of parental contributions to the success of a child's course with disabilities or chronic illness.

During the 1990s, it will be necessary to progress toward the following:

1. Pediatric training and continuing education still require enhanced attention to the care requirements for children with mental retardation and other developmental disabilities. The concern of professional groups is needed regarding the present and future adequacy and availability of care, such as the "Access to Care" project of the American Academy of Pediatrics.
2. The provision of "related services" in schools, per the requirements of PL 94-142, should be rigorously defended. Further interdisciplinary studies of content and effectiveness should be undertaken.
3. Classroom supports for children with special medical needs are enormously strategic; there should be national replication of Project School Care.
4. Parents as caregivers deserve more respect, training, and support.

The Financing of Care for Children With Disabilities

The present system for securing reimbursement for health-care costs for children with mental retardation is multifaceted, opportunistic, and incomplete. As a result, there are frequent situations of family stress, suboptimal usage of services, and institutional predicaments. The principal issues are the availability and adequacy of private insurance, and the unsure role and responsibility of the backup by Medicaid. Statistics on the routes for payment by families vary predictably by the setting of the survey. One representation can be seen from the experience of the Developmental Evaluation Center in the Boston Children's Hospital, where the author works. A recent review showed that for children arriving at this tertiary facility for developmental services (but not necessarily those who should be considered eligible), 24% had Blue Cross coverage, 22% had other private insurance, 7% came by way of an HMO or other prepayment plan referral, 29% were on Medicaid, and 5% were "self-pay."

The various private insurance plans, usually obtained via parental employment, have been much analyzed in current times (see discussion in Taylor et al., 1990). For children with serious constitutional disorders, there are often substantial barriers—including exclusions, waiting periods, restricted benefits, deductibles, co-payment requirements, and caps (annual or lifetime). Resultant out-of-pocket costs for families are extensive and almost universal; notable elements include medications, bills after insurance, special equipment, physical changes in the home, parking for appointments, and lost wages. Newacheck and McManus (1988) report that these elements are two to three times higher on average for children with disabilities, compared with other children.

Limitations also exist within the design of the usual HMOs. These are driven in part by the fundamental motivation for cost containment, and by certain intrinsic constrictions in freedom of choice for the subscriber. The range of services, access to specialists, and assistance for medical equipment are commonly incomplete (Horwitz & Stein, 1990).

The coverage by Medicaid is relatively broad, but eligibility for entry into the system can be quite rigorous. Recent legislation has moved the family means test to 133% of the "poverty level" (this level now is $8,420 for a family of two, $12,700 for a family of four). Other access is through qualification for the disability criteria of SSI or by means of specific waivers. The latter include various "medically needy" definitions, "home and community based" provisions, or certain individual state conceptions. Their usage has not been extensive in the country as a whole. Medicaid remains the ultimate "catastrophic" coverage for families who have children with disabilities, but obstacles exist for many families in learning about or securing enrollment.

Exclusion from the preceding systems is surprisingly widespread. Estimates vary considerably in different surveys, but most indicate that between 10% and 20% of families of children with disabilities have no insurance (Taylor et al., 1990). Less than a quarter of these situations are based on unemployment; more commonly insurance is not available because the work is part-time, in certain service jobs, self-employed, or with small employers. As a group, uninsured families are often identified as the "near-poor," and their ability to access public fiscal supports is limited. The public policy challenge in this unjust phenomenon is well described by Oberg (1990). Underuse of medical services is usual for such families.

As we progress toward the year 2000, some specific recommendations include the following:

1. State-based review of the adequacy of private insurance coverage is needed, with uniform criteria applied for addressing family requirements in the circumstances of disability.
2. Federal leadership must continue in defining the true role of reimbursement through Medicaid. If it remains the principal insurance for low-income families, then enrollment procedures need simplification, and the benefits coverage should be reviewed. If it is instead to be the core of reimbursement for all families who have children with developmental disabilities, then the waiver systems need standardization and liberalization. Passage of S. 384 would greatly assist this situation.
3. Coordination of care for families who have children with significant disabilities should be provided through the Title V (Children With Special Health Care Needs) programs in each state Department of Health. Financial counseling is an element of good case management.
4. A universally applied national health insurance system is unquestionably the best resolution for fair, equitable, and effective support for children and families with developmental disabilities (including mental retardation). It seems not too much to hope that this will be secured by the year 2000.

Epilogue

In recording one's anticipations for enhanced health-care services in the year 2000, it is difficult to separate elements of *conviction* from those of *prediction*. Hopefully, by that time they will be quite similar.

For adults with mental retardation, one can expect that the relevant state agency will assume leadership in securing the right for appropriate health care. Components of commitment will constitute a network, including supported care coordination by nurses, a problem-oriented and portable health record, an information and referral system, specialty resource centers, consideration of chronic and secondary health issues in the ISP, and a sound data base. Preservice and postgraduate education for physicians (including internists and family medicine doctors) and other health service providers will feature accurate insights regarding the needs of persons with developmental disabilities. There will be either extensive Medicaid reform or the final achievement of universal national health insurance.

Care for children with mental retardation, other disabilities, and chronic illness will be assisted by enhanced professional training, use of quality therapeutic services within special education, and classroom assistance for those with special direct medical needs. Supports will be strengthened for the family role as care giver, including through care-coordination services. There will have been rectification of the presently incomplete aspects of insurance coverage, regarding both eligibility and benefits.

The outlook for these good actions derives from both professional guidance and inspired public policy.

References

Adams, E. K., Ellwood, M. R., & Pine, P. L. (1989). Utilization and expenditures under Medicaid for Supplemental Security Income disabled. *Health Care Financing Review, 11*, 1–24.

Birenbaum, A., Guyot, D., & Cohen, H. J. (1989). *Reality and policy in financing the health care of children and young adults with serious chronic conditions.* Bronx: Rose F. Kennedy Center UAP.

Brewer, E. J., Jr., McPherson, M., Magrab, P. R., & Hutchins, V. L. (1989). Family-centered, community-based, coordinated care for children with special health care needs. *Pediatrics, 83*, 1055–1060.

Cole, R. F. (1987). Community-based prepaid medical care for adults with mental retardation: Proposal for a pilot project. *Mental Retardation, 25*, 233–235.

Crocker, A. C. (1988). Medical care for adults with developmental disabilities. *Journal of the American Medical Association, 260*, 1455.

Crocker, A. C. (1989a). The causes of mental retardation. *Pediatric Annals, 18*, 623–636.

Crocker, A. C. (1989b). Systems of health care delivery: Private practice. In I. L. Rubin & A. C. Crocker (Eds.), *Developmental disabilities: Delivery of medical care for children and adults* (pp. 30–34). Philadelphia: Lea & Febiger.

Crocker, A. C. (1991). A declaration of health care rights for the person with Down syndrome. *Down Syndrome News, 15*, 24.

Crocker, A. C., & Yankauer, A. (1987). Symposium on community health care services for adults with mental retardation. *Mental Retardation, 25*, 189–242.

Crocker, A. C., Yankauer, A., & the Conference Steering Committee (1987). Basic issues. *Mental Retardation, 25*, 227–232.

Damon, K., Gould, K. E., Bass, R. W., & Jones, G. H. (1990, May 1). *Impacting on medical services to persons with developmental disabilities and children with special needs: The application of an I&R service to promote systems change.* Paper presented at the 5th Annual National Symposium on Information Technology, Myrtle Beach, SC.

Epstein, S. G., Taylor, A. B., Halberg, A. S., Gardner, J. D., Walker, D. K., & Crocker, A. C. (1989). *Enhancing quality: Standards and indicators of quality care for children with special health care needs.* Boston: New England SERVE.

Eyman, R. K., Grossman, H. J., Chaney, R. H., & Call, T. L. (1990). The life expectancy of profoundly handicapped people with mental retardation. *New England Journal of Medicine, 323*, 584–589.

Eyman, R. K., Call, T. L., & White, J. F. (1991). Life expectancy of persons with Down syndrome. *American Journal on Mental Retardation, 95*, 603–612.

Graff, J. C., Ault, M. M., Guess, D., Taylor, M., & Thompson, B. (1990). *Health care for students with disabilities*. Baltimore, MD: Paul H. Brookes.

Griswold, K. S., Msall, M. E., & Cooke, R. E. (1987). A university-based health maintenance organization for persons with developmental disabilities. *Mental Retardation, 25*, 223–225.

Haynie, M., Porter, S. M., & Palfrey, J. S. (1989). *Children assisted by medical technology in educational settings: Guidelines for care*. Boston: Children's Hospital.

Henderson, M., Howard, A., & Porell, F. (1990). *Managed health care network for adults with mental retardation or other developmental disabilities: A concept paper*. Waltham, MA: Brandeis University.

Hobbs, N., Perrin, J. M., & Ireys, H. T. (1985). *Chronically ill children and their families*. San Francisco: Jossey-Bass.

Horwitz, S. M., & Stein, R. E. K. (1990). Health maintenance organizations vs indemnity insurance for children with chronic illness. *American Journal of Diseases of Childhood, 144*, 581–586.

Howard, A. M., & Autor, S. (1989) *The status of health care services for adults with mental retardation living in DMR region IV residential programs*. Boston: Massachusetts Department of Mental Retardation.

Master, R. J. (1987). Medicaid after 20 years: Promise, problems, potential. *Mental Retardation, 25*, 211–214.

McDonald, E. P. (1985). Medical needs of severely developmentally disabled persons residing in the community. *American Journal of Mental Deficiency, 90*, 171–176.

Minihan, P. M. (1986). Planning for community physician services prior to deinstitutionalization of mentally retarded persons. *American Journal of Public Health, 76*, 1202–1206.

Minihan, P. M., & Dean, D. H. (1990). Meeting the needs for health services of persons with mental retardation living in the community. *American Journal of Public Health, 80*, 1043–1048.

Minihan, P. M., Dean, D. H., & Lyons, C. M. (1989, May 29). *Providing care to patients with mental retardation: A survey of physicians in the State of Maine*. Paper presented at the annual meeting of the American Association on Mental Retardation, Chicago.

Nelson, R. P., & Crocker, A. C. (1978). The medical care of mentally retarded persons in public residential facilities. *New England Journal of Medicine, 299*, 1039–1044.

Newacheck, P. W., & McManus, M. A. (1988). Financing health care for disabled children. *Pediatrics, 81*, 385–394.

Nowell, N., Baker, D., & Conroy, J. (1989). *The provision of community medical care in Philadelphia and Northeastern Pennsylvania for people who live in community living arrangements and with their families*. Philadelphia: Philadelphia Coordinated Health Care.

Oberg, C. N. (1990). Medically uninsured children in the United States: A challenge to public policy. *Pediatrics, 85*, 824–833.

Palfrey, J. S., Singer, J. D., Ralphael, E. S., & Walker, D. K. (1990). Providing therapeutic services to children in special educational placements: An analysis of the related services provisions of Public Law 94-142 in five urban school districts. *Pediatrics*, *85*, 518–525.

Pope, A. M., & Tarlov, A. R., (Eds.) (1991). *Disability in America; Toward a national agenda for prevention*, (pp. 214–241). Washington, DC: National Academy Press.

Rowitz, L. (1988). Health care issues in community residential settings. In M. P. Janicki, M. W. Krauss, & M. M. Seltzer (Eds.), *Community residences for persons with developmental disabilities* (pp. 203–215). Baltimore: Paul H. Brookes.

Rubin, I. L. (1987). Health care needs of adults with mental retardation. *Mental Retardation*, *25*, 201–206.

Rubin, I. L., & Crocker, A. C. (1989). *Developmental disabilities: Delivery of medical care for children and adults*. Philadelphia: Lea & Febiger.

Singer, J. D., Butler, J. A., & Palfrey, J. S. (1986). Health care access and utilization among children with disabilities. *Medical Care*, *24*, 1–13.

Szymanski, L. S. (1987). Prevention of psychosocial dysfunction in persons with mental retardation. *Mental Retardation*, *25*, 215–218.

Taylor, A. B., Epstein, S. G., & Crocker, A. C. (1990). Health care for children with special needs. In M. J. Schlesinger & L. Eisenberg (Eds.), *Children in a changing health system: Assessments and proposals for reform* (pp. 27–48). Baltimore, MD: Johns Hopkins University Press.

Ziring, P. R. (1987). A program that works. *Mental Retardation*, *25*, 207–210.

Ziring, P. R., Kastner, T., Friedman, D. L., Pond, W. S., Barnett, M. L., Sonnenberg, E. M., & Strassburger, K. (1988). Provision of health care for persons with developmental disabilities living in the community. *Journal of the American Medical Association*, *260*, 1439–1444.

Appendix 12.1[1]

Declaration of Health Care Rights for the Person with Down Syndrome

Article I: The person with Down syndrome has the right to have health care furnished earnestly, positively, and creatively by both generic and specialized providers.

Article II: Parents and other family members shall be active partners and contributors in all aspects of planning and accomplishing health care.

Article III: For persons with Down syndrome the initial diagnosis shall be achieved swiftly, and the transfer of information shall then be thoughtfully carried out, with endorsement of the child's personal value and provision of accurate supplementary facts; contact for parent-to-parent support will be offered promptly.

---

[1]*Note.* From Crocker, A. C. (1991) A declaration of health care rights for the person with Down Syndrome. *Down Syndrome News*, *15*, 24. Reprinted by permission.

Article IV: The infant with Down syndrome has the right to have timely professional cardiac evaluation, consultation, and follow through.

Article V: The young child with Down syndrome has the right to early audiologic study by modern methods, otologic consultation as appropriate, and careful consideration of needed intervention.

Article VI: Throughout life a preventive or anticipatory health care approach shall be utilized, including in such areas as visual function, skeletal issues, thyroid function, nutritional guidance, and management of infections.

Article VII: In direct matters of medical care, the person with Down syndrome has the right to have the best and most recent knowledge applied, with generous use of consultation and second opinions.

Article VIII: Means shall be assured so that the special contributions of the habilitative therapies can be richly provided, including physical therapy, occupational therapy, speech/language therapy, adapted physical education, and arts therapies.

Article IX: The person with Down syndrome shall not be subjected to manipulative unconventional treatments; for new or experimental programs great care shall be taken regarding personal and family rights.

Article X: Prime importance shall be given to the achievement of wellness, adjustment, beneficial behaviors, and happiness.

Article XI: The family and the person with Down syndrome have the right to accurate financial counseling regarding available assistance for reimbursing the costs of health care.

Article XII: Research must be diligent in key ares relating to health with special reference to cardiac intervention, protection of hearing function, behavioral guidance, and supports to self-esteem.

13
Policy and Program Development for Infants and Toddlers With Disabilities

MARTY WYNGAARDEN KRAUSS and PENNY HAUSER-CRAM

The passage in 1986 of the Education of the Handicapped Act Amendments (PL 99-457) marked a turning point in public policy commitments to meeting the educational and therapeutic needs of children with disabilities and their families. Described as "the most important legislation ever enacted for developmentally vulnerable young children" (Shonkoff & Meisels, 1990, p. 19), the law consists of three major provisions. First, the law establishes a new discretionary program for family-centered, community-based, multidisciplinary, comprehensive services of early intervention for children with handicaps or developmental delays and their families (Part H of the law and the focus of this chapter). Second, the law reverses the contemporary retrenchment in special education services for children between the ages of 3 and 6 (Mallory, 1981), by mandating entitlements to special educational services beginning at age 3 years. Third, it reauthorizes a variety of discretionary programs under the Education of the Handicapped Act for deaf-blind children, personnel preparation, and early childhood research institutes. Thus, the law begins the task of creating an infrastructure for a national system of early intervention and preschool services that reflects the diverse social, health, educational, and therapeutic needs of young children with known or probable developmental disabilities and their families (Hauser-Cram, Upshur, Krauss, & Shonkoff, 1988).

The law's passage is a tribute to the achievements of early intervention and preschool programs during the latter half of the 20th century. During this period, important research was reported that documented the cognitive gains made by infants and toddlers with disabilities participating in a broad array of early intervention programs (Farran, 1990; Shonkoff & Hauser-Cram, 1987). Moreover, several research efforts fueled general public support for early childhood programs, despite retrenchment in

Support for the preparation of this chapter was provided by grant 250583 from the Maternal and Child Health Bureau, Department of Health and Human Services.

federal funding of other social and educational programs. The most widely publicized early childhood research project for disadvantaged children was the Perry Preschool Project (Berreuta-Clement, Schweinhart, Barnett, Epstein, & Weikart, 1984), which reported significant developmental and socially important long-term benefits for participating children and families. The Perry Preschool results added to a broad base of findings from other early childhood projects on the longitudinal effects of early education (Lazar, Darlington, Murray, Royce, & Snipper, 1982). As a group, such findings marshalled much support for early childhood programs for vulnerable children.

Despite the legacy of accomplishment and public commitment to early intervention and preschool programs in the latter quarter of the 20th century, the provisions of PL 99-457 raise significant issues for programs as they enter the 21st century. This chapter discusses the challenges faced by the early intervention policy and service community in fulfilling the goals expressed by Congress. These challenges include fuller recognition of the changing demographic characteristics of the target population and their families, the development of flexible service models that will respond to the complex and varying needs of the target population, and the changing role of families within the service system. While these issues are not unique to the early intervention service community, there is a general belief that PL 99-457 will create a coherent, equitable, and responsive system of services that will be emulated by other service systems affecting persons with disabilities and their families.

Definition of Early Intervention Services and Target Populations

The term *early intervention services*, as defined by Part H of PL 99-457, includes publicly supported services designed to meet a handicapped infant's or toddler's physical, cognitive, language and speech, psychosocial developmental needs, or self-help skills. The services include family training, counseling and home visits, special instruction, speech pathology and audiology, occupational or physical therapy, psychological services, case management services, medical and health-care services, and early identification, screening, and assessment services. These services must be provided in conformity with an Individualized Family Service Plan (IFSP) that is based on a multidisciplinary assessment of the child's and family's unique strengths and needs and the identification of services appropriate to those needs.

In contrast to the specificity regarding the services to be available within early intervention programs, the law is less definitive about the eligible target population. It states (Sec. 672) that the term *handicapped infants and toddlers* "means individuals from birth to age 2, inclusive, who need early intervention services because they are experiencing developmental delays, as measured by appropriate diagnostic instruments and procedures in one or more of the following areas: cognitive development, physical development, language and speech development, psychosocial development, or self-help skills, or (who) have a diagnosed physical or mental condition which has a high probability of resulting in developmental delay." Further, states are given discretionary authority to serve infants and toddlers who are "at risk of having substantial developmental delays if early intervention services are not provided."

The sanctioning of services to the "at-risk" population has generated considerable controversy regarding the reliability and validity of criteria used to identify this group. Because biological factors alone account for only a small proportion of intellectually delayed children (Broman, Nichols, & Kennedy, 1975; Sameroff & Chandler, 1975), clinicians and researchers have focused on identifying parental or environmental markers that are predictive of poor child outcome (Meisels & Wasik, 1990). For example, Trohanis, Meyer, and Prestridge (1982) found that screening procedures for high-risk infants generally focus on maternal characteristics such as age (advanced or adolescent), history of substance abuse, low education or cognitive functioning, or low income. Others point out, however, that "it is the accumulation of risk variables rather than the action of specific factors that produce [sic] morbidity in a variety of domains" (Sameroff, Seifer, Barocas, Zax, & Greenspan, 1987, p. 349). While there is a deeper understanding of the factors associated with at-risk children's resilience and vulnerability to impoverished environments (Rutter, 1987; Werner, 1990), it is clear that targeting services *within* the at-risk population remains an art rather than a science. States intending to include the at-risk population within their early-intervention programs will continue to face a significant challenge in determining valid outreach and screening criteria. As Werner notes, "Risk factors are not black boxes into which one fits children to be neatly labeled and safely stored away. Like protective factors, they are probability statements, the odds of a gamble whose stakes change with time and place" (1990, p. 112).

Changing Demographics of Target Populations

While we anticipate that knowledge of the effects of various combinations of risk factors will expand during the 1990s, the population of children at risk for atypical development is likely to increase as well. Four general trends in the demographic and social characteristics of families in the United States will have important implications for early intervention services, both in terms of the eligible population and the nature of the services provided. These trends include (a) the increase in the number of children living in poverty, (b) the increase in children afflicted with human immunodeficiency virus (HIV) infection and disabilities caused by maternal substance abuse, (c) the disproportionate increase of minority and non-English-speaking families within the general population, and (d) the increase in the employment rate of women with young children.

First, estimates indicate that about one in every four children lives in poverty at some point during his or her formative years (Newberger, Melnicoe, & Newberger, 1986). The rise in family poverty is attributable to many causes, including increases in births to adolescents (Henshaw, Kenney, Somberg, & Van Vort, 1989), in female-headed households, and in the working poor (Ellwood, 1988). Projections indicate that the number and proportion of children living in poverty and with poorly educated mothers will increase steadily over the next three decades (Halpern, 1987). Although poverty is only one risk factor, it is associated with both prenatal and perinatal effects on the child that make normal development less probable (Parker, Greer, & Zuckerman, 1988). An increase in poverty will result in not only more children with environmental risk factors but also more children with biological or established risk who come from families with multiple critical needs.

Second, several changes in the characteristics of the children served by early intervention programs will have significant impacts on the nature of services. Among the most alarming is the rise in the number of infants born with HIV infection, which is projected to become the largest infectious cause of mental retardation and brain damage in children within the next 5 years. By 1991, the Center for Disease Control estimates that 10,000 to 20,000 infants and children will be infected with HIV (Dokecki, Baumeister, & Kupstas, 1989). Nearly all become developmentally disabled through central nervous system involvement (Diamond, 1989). Their service needs are essentially the same as other children with developmental problems, with the added complications of serious medical considerations and the public concerns about the transmission of infection to others (Crocker, 1989).

Another rising concern is the number of children born to substance-abusing mothers. Although precise figures are difficult to gather, one population-based study in the state of Florida found that 14.8% of pregnant women had positive urine toxicology tests for alcohol, cocaine, opiates, and other similar substances (Chasnoff, Landress, & Barrett, 1990). Cocaine use by pregnant women is associated with a host of structural and neurological defects as well as with preterm labor and low birth weight (Chasnoff, Burns, & Burns, 1987; Hoyme et al., 1990). Because many of these children may begin their lives living in dysfunctional households, the combined risk factors are increased substantially for them. When the basic needs of the family are not being met, the role of other services, such as early intervention, may need to be reshaped.

Third, the population in the United States is increasingly affected by differential fertility rates, which will result in a disproportionate increase in the minority population. Predictions indicate that by the year 2010, one of every three Americans will be African American, Hispanic, or Asian American (Hodgkinson, 1986). Moreover, the proportion of children who speak a primary language other than English is expected to rise from about 2.5% in 1982 to 7.5% in the year 2020 (Pallas, Natriello, & McDill, 1989). Such changes in the population will multiply the need for service providers who represent these various communities.

Finally, estimates indicate that nearly two thirds (63%) of mothers with children under 6 years of age are in the labor force either full-time or part-time (U.S. General Accounting Office, 1990), and projections indicate a continuous rise in this percentage (Bloom & Steen, 1988). The employment of women with young children has had substantial impact on the daily lives of families and created a necessity to restructure the ways that the needs, including service needs, of various family members can be met.

Changing Service Models Within Early Intervention

Changes in the demography of the target population will have a profound effect on the strategies by which programs provide services. The ability of early intervention programs and service personnel to meet the range of complex and multiple needs of families that occur when children live in poverty or when parents are substance abusers will surely be challenged. Meeting these needs will require extensive efforts in interagency co-ordination. The staff time and expertise required to be effective linkages and brokers of services adds a new dimension to the range of resources needed within early intervention programs.

The ability of early intervention programs and service personnel to meet the multicultural needs of a diverse population is also a major challenge for the future. The absence of qualified minority personnel (Baca & Amato, 1989) and the dearth of instructional materials available in different languages limits the capacity of early intervention programs to serve fully minority infants and toddlers with disabilities or to work productively with their families. What is needed is not simply translations of curriculum and learning materials, but rather individuals who have a similar heritage, a common language, and a respect for the cultural values of those they serve. Tempting such individuals to obtain training necessary to become early intervention service providers is a critical challenge for the field as a whole.

Finally, the traditional model of a center-based program to which children and their parents (usually mothers) come once or twice a week for either individualized or group therapies and services may prove to be inadequate for meeting the varied family contexts and child-care arrangements of the 21st century. The use of home visits, another staple early intervention service-delivery mechanism, will be challenged by the increasing labor force participation of women with very young children.

New methods of service delivery that respond to the work lives of both mothers and fathers will be required and will undoubtedly demand greater flexibility on the part of early intervention service providers and programs. Early intervention and day-care services will need to join together more closely in the future to provide the full range of services needed by the child and family. Early intervention service programs will need to seek ways to ensure that the family's role in early intervention services is not diminished, even though the child may be spending less time in the family. Indeed, the family's role in intervention will be a critical challenge to the early intervention system in general.

Changing Context of Family Involvement

The distribution of roles and responsibilities between parents and professionals has been an enduring issue in compensatory or special educational services since the 1960s. In Head Start Programs (PL 89-794) and in demonstration projects authorized by the Handicapped Children's Early Education Program (PL 90-538), parents were encouraged to participate in the development and operation of preschool programs and, in some cases, were eligible for parent training as a component of these programs. The rationale for the planned involvement of parents was that it was a critical ingredient in increasing program effectiveness, both because parents possessed considerable "instructional" time for their children and because their parenting skills would be enhanced through program participation.

The watershed for parent involvement, however, was the passage in 1975 of the Education for All Handicapped Children Act (PL 94-142), which codified a much deeper and more responsible role for parents in the educational planning for their children. Parents are entitled to notification before formal testing of their child, to explanations of the results of testing or proposed services, to participation in formal planning meetings from which educational plans are established, to access to all school records regarding their child, and to appeals procedures if they disagree with the outcomes or process of educational planning. Thus, parental roles shifted from advisory (as authorized in federal compensatory programs passed in the 1960s) to decision makers. The mandates of PL 94–142 reduced professional dominance and control over the lives of young children with disabilities and articulated a parent–professional partnership that had been the goal of many for decades (Turnbull & Turnbull, 1986; Zeitlin, Williamson, & Rosenblatt, 1987).

While parental roles in early childhood programs have evolved considerably over time, IFSPs now required within early intervention programs set a new precedent in public policies for families (Krauss, 1990). Rather than simply enjoying legal rights to participate in educational planning, parents are now potential recipients of services because of their child's handicaps or delays. Although this mandate enables early intervention programs to provide more comprehensive services to the family as a unit, it fundamentally restructures the process and outcomes of child and family assessment procedures and service provision.

The IFSP codifies the prevailing practice within many existing early intervention programs to provide multidisciplinary assessments and to include parental perspectives on the identification of needs and determination of relevant services. It extends current practices, however, in requiring that the service plan focus on the family as a unit rather than the child in isolation from his or her environment and in requiring that a case manager be appointed for each family (McGonigel & Garland, 1988). It requires that the plan contain a statement of the child's present functioning in a variety of areas and of the family's strengths and needs related to enhancing the development of the family's handicapped infant or toddler. Specific goals for the child and family are to be enumerated, along with the criteria and timing to be used to evaluate goal achievement.

Numerous analyses of the implications of the IFSP have focused on the radical shift in the orientation of early intervention programs engendered by this critical provision of the PL 99-457 (Dunst, Trivette, & Deal, 1988; Krauss, 1990; Sheehan & Sites, 1988). For example, the IFSP transforms programs from being family oriented to family focused. Rather than simply acknowledging the importance of the family context, programs are now accountable for "evaluating" or assessing this context with respect to its contribution to the therapeutic needs of the child and the family. As a result, the IFSP requires direct programmatic involvement with families who might not otherwise invite or need professional intervention.

Important issues about the nature and context of family involvement have been generated by the IFSP mandates that will test the flexibility and maturity of early intervention programs. Specifically, the form and process by which family assessment will occur has been subjected to sharp debate. The IFSP provisions have stimulated deep thinking by researchers, early intervention program personnel, and parent-advocacy groups about methods of family assessment that are responsive to the spirit of the legislation while preserving respect for family privacy and avoiding a presumption of family pathology (Dunst et al., 1988; Summers et al., 1990). The perceived potential for intrusive or insensitive questions of family life and parental adjustment has led to formulations of "family-friendly" approaches to family assessment. These strategies are characterized by informality, by emphases on family strengths rather than deficits, and are driven by family preferences rather than professional judgment. The approaches are based on the belief that effective collaboration between professionals and families requires the development of personal relationships, in which informal conversations replace formal processes for client assessment and service planning.

Conversely, the IFSP provisions have also invigorated efforts to develop standardized assessment procedures that enable program personnel to collect information systematically on service recipients. Structured assessment procedures offer service providers more reliable information about the functioning of the family in various domains, its formal and informal resources, and its service needs. They also offer possibilities of group comparisons and more refined testing of important questions about the characteristics and needs of families of children with disabilities. Because most strategies for standardized assessment rely on instruments developed initially for research, rather than programmatic, purposes, their utility for accomplishing the goals of the IFSP process needs further testing (Bailey & Simeonsson, 1986; Fewell, 1986; Krauss & Jacobs, 1990).

Further, the requirement that parents be part of the multidisciplinary team that guides the delivery of services alters traditional divisions of roles between parents (as recipients of services for their children) and professionals (as providers of services). As Healy, Keesee, and Smith (1985) note:

The concepts of parental empowerment and parental involvement in decision making have been increasingly a part of early intervention rhetoric. But a concrete understanding of what these concepts mean for professionals is still evolving and may yet lead to revolutionary changes in practices. (pp. 37–38)

While this is the goal of many early intervention professionals (Dunst et al., 1988) and families served in such programs (Ziegler, 1989), methods for truly integrating parents with widely varying characteristics and resources into the business of assessment and service planning have yet to be fully developed and promulgated. Interestingly, an analysis of the proposed FY 1987 activities of the 50 states and the District of Columbia revealed that few states gave a high priority to developing quality and responsive IFSP procedures (Campbell, Bellamy, & Bishop, 1988).

There is little doubt that Congress's intent was to protect the interests of families as critical decision makers about their own unique needs as well as those of their child with a disability or delay. The benefits attributed to meaningful parental involvement in programs serving very young children and their families have been articulated persuasively in the scientific and applied literature (Bricker & Casuso, 1979; Bronfenbrenner, 1974; Florin & Dokecki, 1983; Peterson & Cooper, 1989). However, the stylistic and philosophical differences between the "family-friendly" and systematic, structured family assessment procedures illustrate one of the basic tensions between professionals and families that have surfaced since the law was passed. On the one hand, there is a strong and vocal community within the early intervention system that advocates for greater family control over the delivery of services. On the other hand, there is concern that the professional skills and expertise of early intervention specialists are being unduly dismissed (Shonkoff & Meisels, 1990). Negotiating the differences between these two communities constitutes an important and fundamental challenge for early intervention programs, which are required to implement an IFSP process that meets both legislative and programmatic objectives.

Summary

Over the last quarter of the 20th century, early intervention programs for very young children with disabilities demonstrated increasing versatility in providing a complex range of therapeutic services to a population about which scientific knowledge was often grossly inadequate. With the passage of PL 99-457 in 1986, the Congress signaled its intention of equalizing the access to early intervention programs nationally, expanding the target population to include children with probable rather than demonstrated delays and respecting the primary role that families play in the lives of such young and vulnerable children. In an era characterized by retrenchment rather than expansion of service systems, the success of the scientific, clinical, and advocacy communities to secure the future of early intervention services can only be described as a major national achievement.

In previewing the challenges facing the early intervention system in each state during the 21st century, it is clear that the ambitions of Congress will stretch existing resources, knowledge, and practices to a significant degree. For example, strategies for identifying children in need of early intervention services become far more complicated when *risk factors* rather than *demonstrated delays* are used as criteria. While much is known about the types of environments and individual characteristics that are associated statistically with developmental problems, the probability of false-positives is still unacceptably high for most clinicians and service providers. Whether states promulgate eligibility policies that cast a wide net (and thus tolerate a high level of false-positives) or seek to limit their responsibility is an issue of considerable importance for the future.

Ambiguity also surrounds the effects on early intervention programs of the projected increases in the number of children whose developmental problems will stem from HIV infection or drug addiction. Meeting the needs of these children and their families will require a much deeper linkage among a variety of community-based service providers and a different range of professional skills than may be typical among existing early intervention programs. This is clearly an area in which college- and university-based professional training programs must assume some leadership in attracting and training new students who are equipped with a multidisciplinary perspective on the social and developmental needs of a large group of children with problems that were unheard of when most practicing clinicians were trained.

The problem of identifying the full range of potentially eligible children and preparing for a group of children with extremely complex social, medical, and developmental needs is matched by the problem of developing service models that are sufficiently flexible to respond to the changing demographics of the American family. Congressional interest was focused on enumerating the types, not the method, of services to be provided. Considerable programmatic experimentation (accompanied by well-designed evaluation studies) will be needed to yield model delivery systems. The array of early-intervention programs that will be available by 2025 may look vastly different from those currently used.

Early intervention programs have also been handed an important responsibility to develop methods for truly integrating a family approach into the human services. The traditional distinction between services for children and services for families should be increasingly blurred by the 21st century, at least within the early intervention network. Whether the benefits of this approach can catalyze other service systems affecting children and adults with disabilities to adopt comparable family-based approaches is of substantial policy and programmatic importance.

Public and professional commitment to enhancing the educational, health, and social opportunities of young children—with and without disabilities—has been galvanized by the passage of PL 99-457 in 1986 and the celebration of the 25th anniversary of the Head Start program in 1990. Whether the popularity of such programs will be sustained into the 21st century depends, to be sure, on adequate resources to meet expanded public expectations. It also depends, however, on a partnership between researchers and program personnel to collaborate in systematic investigation on the efficiency of various screening approaches, the effectiveness of new program models, and the methods for forging new roles between parents and the professionals who serve them and their children.

References

Baca, L., & Amato, C. (1989). Bilingual special education: Training issues. *Exceptional Children, 56*, 168–173.

Bailey, D. B., & Simeonsson, R. J. (1986). Design issues in family impact evaluation. In L. Bickman & D. L. Weatherford (Eds.), *Evaluating early intervention programs for severely handicapped children and their families* (pp. 209–230). Austin, TX: PRO-ED.

Berreuta-Clement, J. R., Schweinhart, L. J., Barnett, W. S., Epstein, A. S., & Weikart, D. P. (1984). *Changed lives: The effects of the Perry Preschool Program on youths through age 19*. Ypsilanti, MI: High/Scope Press.

Bloom, D. E., & Steen, T. P. (1988). Why child care is good for business. *American Demographics, 10*, 22–27.

Bricker, D., & Casuso, V. (1979). Family involvement: A critical component of early intervention. *Exceptional Children, 46*, 108–116.

Broman, S. H., Nichols, P. L., & Kennedy, W. A. (1975). *Preschool IQ: Prenatal and early developmental correlates*. Hillsdale, NJ: Lawrence Erlbaum.

Bronfenbrenner, U. (1974). Is early intervention effective? *Teachers College Record, 76*, 279–303.

Campbell, P. H., Bellamy, G. T., & Bishop, K. K. (1988). Statewide intervention systems: An overview of the new federal program for infants and toddlers with handicaps. *The Journal of Special Education, 22*, 25–40.

Chasnoff, I. J., Burns, K. A., & Burns, W. J. (1987). Cocaine use in pregnancy: Perinatal morbidity and mortality. *Neurotoxicology and Teratology, 9*, 291–293.

Chasnoff, I. J., Landress, H. J., & Barrett, M. E. (1990). The prevalence of illicit-drug or alcohol use during pregnancy and discrepancies in mandatory reporting in Pinellas County, Florida. *The New England Journal of Medicine, 322*, 1202–1206.

Crocker, A. C. (1989). Developmental services for children with HIV infection. *Mental Retardation, 27*, 223–225.

Diamond, G. W. (1989). Developmental problems in children with HIV infection. *Mental Retardation, 27*, 213–217.

Dokecki, P. R., Baumeister, A. A., & Kupstas, F. D. (1989). Biomedical and social aspects of pediatric AIDS. *Journal of Early Intervention, 13*, 99–113.

Dunst, C., Trivette, C., & Deal, A. (1988). *Enabling and empowering families: Principles and guidelines for practice.* Cambridge, MA: Brookline Books.

Ellwood, D. T. (1988). *Poor support: Poverty in the American family.* New York: Basic Books.

Farran, D. (1990). Effects of intervention with disadvantaged and disabled children: A decade review. In S. J. Meisels & J. P. Shonkoff (Eds.), *Handbook of early childhood intervention* (pp. 501–539). New York: Cambridge University Press.

Fewell, R. R. (1986). The measurement of family functioning. In L. Bickman & D. L. Weatherford (Eds.), *Evaluating early intervention programs for severely handicapped children and their families* (pp. 263–307). Austin, TX: PRO-ED.

Florin, P. R., & Dokecki, P. R. (1983). Changing families through parent and family education: Review and analysis. In I. Sigel & L. L. Laosa (Eds.), *Changing families* (pp. 23–61). New York: Plenum.

Halpern, R. (1987). Major social and demographic trends affecting young families: Implications for early childhood care and education. *Young Children, 42*, 34–40.

Hauser-Cram, P., Upshur, C., Krauss, M. W., & Shonkoff, J. P. (1988). Implications of Public Law 99–457 for early intervention services for infants and toddlers with disabilities. *The Social Policy Report of the Society for Research in Child Development, 3*, 1–15.

Healy, A., Keesee, P., & Smith, B. (1985). *Early services for children with special needs: Transactions for family support.* Iowa City: The University of Iowa.

Henshaw, S. K., Kenney, A. M., Somberg, D., & Van Vort, J. (1989). *Teenage pregnancy in the United States: The scope of the problem and state responses.* New York: The Alan Guttmacher Institute.

Hodgkinson, H. L. (1986). What's ahead for education. *Principal, 65*, 6–11.

Hoyme, H. E., Jones, K. L., Dixon, S. D., Jewett, T., Hanson, J. W., Robinson, L. K., Msall, M. E., & Allanson, J. E. (1990). Prenatal cocaine exposure and fetal vascular disruption. *Pediatrics, 85*, 743–747.

Krauss, M. W. (1990). New precedent in family policy: Individualized family service plan. *Exceptional Children*, *56*, 388–395.

Krauss, M. W., & Jacobs, F. (1990). Family assessment: Purposes and techniques. In S. J. Meisels & J. P. Shonkoff (Eds.), *Handbook of early childhood intervention* (pp. 303–325). New York: Cambridge University Press.

Lazar, I., Darlington, R. B., Murray, H. W., Royce, J., & Snipper, A. S. (1982). Lasting effects of early education: A report from the Consortium for Longitudinal Studies. *Monographs of the Society for Research in Child Development*, *47* (2–3, Serial No. 195).

Mallory, B. L. (1981). The impact of public policies on families with young handicapped children. *Topics in Early Childhood Special Education*, *1*, 77–86.

McGonigel, J. J., & Garland, C. W. (1988). The individualized family service plan and the early intervention team: Team and family issues and recommended practices. *Infants and Young Children*, *1*, 10–21.

Meisels, S. J., & Wasik, B. A. (1990). Who should be served? Identifying children in need of early intervention. In S. J. Meisels & J. P. Shonkoff (Eds.), *Handbook of early childhood intervention* (pp. 605–632). New York: Cambridge University Press.

Newberger, C., Melnicoe, L., & Newberger, E. (1986). The American family in crisis: Implications for children. *Current Problems in Pediatrics*, *16*, 671–737.

Pallas, A. M., Natriello, G., & McDill, E. L. (1989). The changing nature of the disadvantaged population: Current dimensions and future trends. *Educational Researcher*, *18*, 16–22.

Parker, S., Greer, S., & Zuckerman, B. (1988). Double jeopardy: The impact of poverty on early child development. *Pediatric Clinics of North America*, *35*, 1–14.

Peterson, N. L., & Cooper, C. S. (1989). Parent education and involvement in early intervention programs for handicapped children: A different perspective on parent needs and the parent–professional relationship. In M. J. Fine (Ed.), *The second handbook on parent education: Contemporary perspectives* (pp. 197–234). New York: Academic Press.

Rutter, M. (1987). Psychosocial resilience and protective mechanisms. *American Journal of Orthopsychiatry*, *57*, 316–331.

Sameroff, A. J., & Chandler, M. (1975). Reproductive risk and the continuum of caretaking casualty. In F. D. Horowitz, M. Hetherington, S. Scarr-Salapatek, & G. Siegel (Eds.), *Review of child development research* (Vol. 4, pp. 187–244). Chicago: University of Chicago Press.

Sameroff, A. J., Seifer, R., Barocas, R., Zax, M., & Greenspan, S. (1987). Intelligence quotient scores of 4-year-old children: Social-environmental risk factors. *Pediatrics*, *79*, 343–350.

Sheehan, R., & Sites, J. (1988). Implications of P.L. 99–457 for assessment. *Topics in Early Childhood Special Education*, *8*, 103–115.

Shonkoff, J. P., & Hauser-Cram, P. (1987). Early intervention for disabled infants and their families: A quantitative analysis. *Pediatrics*, *80*, 650–658,

Shonkoff, J. P., & Meisels, S. J. (1990). Early childhood intervention: The evolution of a concept. In S. J. Meisels & J. P. Shonkoff (Eds.), *Handbook of early childhood intervention* (pp. 3–31). New York: Cambridge University Press.

Summers, J. A., Dell'Oliver, C., Turnbull, A. P., Benson, H. A., Santelli, E., Campbell, M., & Siegel-Causey, E. (1990). Examining the Individualized Family Service Plan process: What are family and practitioner preferences? *Topics in Early Childhood Special Education*, *10*, 78–99.

Trohanis, P. L., Meyer, R. A., & Prestridge, S. (1982). A report on selected screening programs for high-risk and handicapped infants. In C. Ramey & P. L. Trohanis (Eds.), *Finding and educating high-risk and handicapped infants* (pp. 83–100). Baltimore, MD: University Park Press.

Turnbull, A. P., & Turnbull, H. R. (1986). *Families, professionals, and exceptionalities: A special partnership*. Columbus, OH: Charles E. Merrill.

U.S. General Accounting Office (1990). *Early childhood education: What are the costs of high-quality programs?* (Report No. HRD-90-43BR). Washington, DC: Author.

Werner, E. (1990). Protective factors and individual resilience. In S. Meisels & J. P. Shonkoff (Eds.), *Handbook of early childhood intervention* (pp. 97–116). New York: Cambridge University Press.

Zeitlin, S., Williamson, G. G., & Rosenblatt, W. P. (1987). The coping with stress model: A counseling approach for families with a handicapped child. *Journal of Counseling and Development*, *65*, 44–65.

Ziegler, M. (1989). A parent's perspective: Implementing P.L. 99-457. In J. Gallagher, P.L. Trohanis, & R. M. Clifford (Eds.), *Policy implementation and P.L. 99-457: Planning for young children with special needs* (pp. 85–96). Baltimore, MD: Paul H. Brookes.

14
The Changing Face of Residential Services

K. Charlie Lakin, Robert H. Bruininks, and Sheryl A. Larson

This chapter about "residential services" for persons with mental retardation begins with a reminder that what we are really talking about are the homes of over 300,000 people who live neither independently nor with their families. Our use of general terms like *residential services* must not detract from or change how we think about the basic qualities of the homes provided to persons with mental retardation and how well these qualities reflect the cultural standards for desirable home settings. This issue will be examined more fully later in this chapter because we believe that a growing concern about cultural standards of quality of life will substantially alter our perspectives on residential service programs.

Background

The 21st century in the United States will begin with perspectives governing residential services for persons with mental retardation that differ radically from the perspectives that prevailed throughout much of the 20th century. These new perspectives have generated and continue to generate major changes in the nature, purpose, and location of residential services. In the 1950s, when a small group of parents joined together in Minneapolis, Minnesota, to form what is today the Association for Retarded Citizens, they could scarcely have imagined the changes that have taken place since then, much less the ones yet to come. For them, the mental retardation system provided two choices: placement of their children in large, isolated institutional settings, or maintaining them at home without the benefit of the most basic public support, not even schooling. Today, a wide and growing variety of residential and support options are available to persons with mental retardation and to their families.

In the broadest sense, residential services can be defined as the protection and assistance provided to people with mental retardation in their homes, whether those homes are institutions, studio apartments, or the family home; and whether those services are constant care, supervision, and training, or only occasional counseling. Most typically, however, "residential services" have come to be viewed as housing and related services provided to people in out-of-home "placements." Because other chapters in this volume focus on families and family support, we will discuss primarily those residential services called out-of-home placements. If one accepts the estimate that about 1% of the population has mental retardation, the population to which this chapter attends represents only 12% to 15% of persons with mental retardation at any one time, a statistical range of persons in organized residential service programs that has been relatively constant throughout the latter half of the 20th century.

Despite the relatively small proportion of people with mental retardation receiving residential services at any one time, residential services have important social and economic consequences to persons with mental retardation, their families, and their communities. These services involve billions of dollars from federal, state, local, and private expenditures each year and represent the single greatest government financial allocation for persons with mental retardation. What is more, the changing patterns in where and how people with mental retardation live mark the evolution and moral bearing of our society.

In this chapter we review the current status, changing patterns, and our view of the outlook for residential services in the United States as we approach the 21st century. This effort is organized according to five major themes that we believe are presently shaping and will continue to shape the nature of those services. These themes are by no means independent; they are related to broader concepts, such as "normalization," or "full citizenship." Nevertheless, the five themes that we see shaping residential services now and in the near future are (a) increasing presence in real communities, (b) promoting personal growth and development, (c) fostering typical social relationships, (d) providing opportunities for valued community participation, and (e) permitting and encouraging increased personal autonomy. We will examine each of these issues in terms of recent trends, findings and issues of relevance, and prospects for the century's end. Our attention to these subtopics will seek to establish where residential services appear to be heading; what factors and findings appear to be posed to accelerate, sustain, or decelerate current trends; and finally, how the trends and intervening factors may interact on the way to the year 2000.

Increasing Presence in Communities

Recent Trends

Deinstitutionalization has been the term applied to the general social commitment to increase access to real communities for persons with

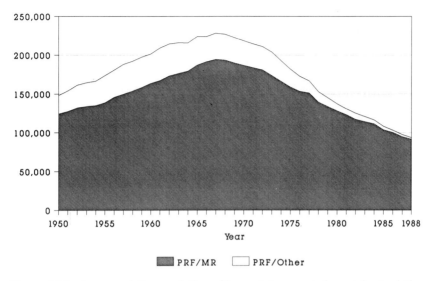

FIGURE 14.1. Average daily population of large state-operated mental retardation facilities, 1950 to 1988. (MR, mentally retarded; PRF, Public Residential Facilities. (White, Lakin & Bruininks, 1989)

mental retardation. Deinstitutionalization is most commonly characterized by the statistics in Figure 14.1, which shows the average daily census of state institutions from 1950 to 1988. Between 1967 and 1988, deinstitutionalization led to a 58% reduction in the average daily population of people with mental retardation living in state-operated mental retardation and psychiatric institutions, from 228,500 to 93,515; populations of state mental retardation institutions decreased from 194,650 to 91,582 (White, Lakin, & Bruininks, 1989).

As a social program, deinstitutionalization has involved both discharging people living in institutions to alternative living arrangements and avoiding initial institutional placements of people already living in the community. To exemplify the changes in placement patterns that have constituted the deinstitutionalization movement, in 1965, with an average daily state mental retardation institution population of 187,305, there were 9.2 admissions and 5.0 discharges per 100 residents; in 1988, with an average daily state mental retardation institution population of 91,582, there were 5.9 admissions and 7.0 discharges per 100 residents (White et al., 1989). These relatively small shifts in placement patterns that led from net increase to net decrease in state institution populations have compounded annually for over 20 years to reduce those populations to less than half of what they once were. Figure 14.2 shows these statistics in terms of actual numbers admitted to and released from state institutions between 1950 and 1988, including the number of people who died in institutions.

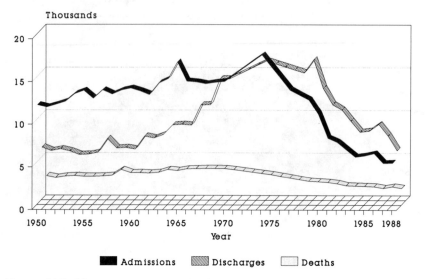

FIGURE 14.2. Movement patterns in large state-operated mental retardation facilities, 1950 to 1988. (White, Lakin & Bruininks, 1989)

Of course, reducing state institution placements has not in itself provided access to community living arrangements. States have undertaken major development of a variety of community residential alternatives, but many of them have not offered appreciably more access to community that did the large, isolated public institutions. Figure 14.3 shows the changing patterns in use of different sizes and types of residential alternatives. Clearly, between 1977 and 1988, notable strides were made in moving people with mental retardation into community living arrangements (i.e., those of 15 and fewer residents), and within the community arrangements generally, into small settings of six or fewer residents (Lakin, White, Hill, Bruininks & Wright, 1990). On the other hand, a large number of people with mental retardation are still housed outside natural communities in this country.

While greater numbers of the people in residential service settings have been provided a physical presence in communities in recent years, greater proportions also appear to be experiencing community living by living independently or staying in their family home. In 1967, there were 130.3 persons in all state and nonstate mental retardation facilities per 100,000 of the general population. This placement rate decreased to 119.9/100,000 by 1977, and to 108.2/100,000 by 1982. Since then, it has generally stabilized, with a reported rate of 109.3/100,000 in 1988 (Lakin, Hill & Bruininks, 1985; Lakin et al., 1990). However, it should be noted that with the general maturing of our population, including both persons with mental retardation and their parents, it is likely that increasing pressure will be generated for higher rates of placement in mental retardation

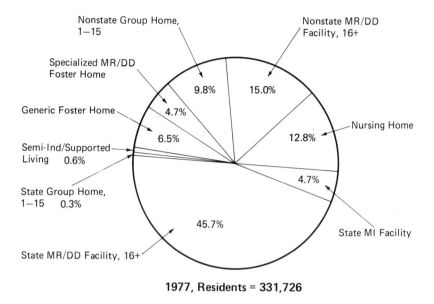

1977, Residents = 331,726

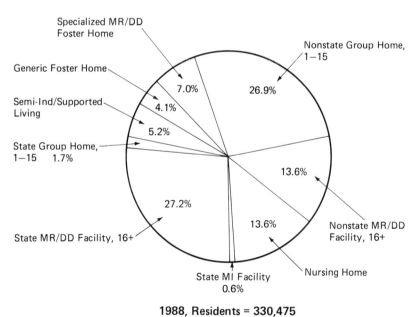

1988, Residents = 330,475

FIGURE 14.3. Distribution of residents among different residential options for persons with mental retardation and related conditions on June 30, 1977 and 1988. (MI, Mental Illness; MR/DD, mentally retarded/developmental disability.) (White, Lakin, & Bruininks, 1989)

facilities in upcoming years. In fact, residential services have been evolving and continue to evolve into an overwhelmingly adult system; and the more adults there are with mental retardation, the more demand there will be for residential services of one form or another. To exemplify the adult focus of residential services, as the overall placement rate decreased slightly between 1977 and 1988, and the rates of placements of children and youth into public and private mental retardation facilities decreased dramatically from 42.1 to 20.1/100,000 of the general population, the overall placement rates for all adults with mental retardation increased from about 77.8/100,000 in 1977 to 89.2/100,000 in 1988. In actual numbers, that represented an increase from about 156,600 to 220,300. Today an estimated 106,000 of these adults live in community-based residential settings with 15 or fewer other residents.

In terms of proportionally increased community presence, two groups in particular have seen dramatically improved opportunities in recent years: young people and people with severe cognitive impairments. With respect to young people, in 1977 there were 91,100 children and youth (birth to 21 years) in residential placements for persons with mental retardation; in 1982 there were 60,000 (Hill, Lakin, & Bruininks, 1984); and in 1986 there were 48,500 (the number of children and youth in state institutions decreased from about 54,000 in 1977 to 12,000 in 1987) (Taylor, Lakin, & Hill, 1989). These changes reflect growing tendencies for parents to provide a family life for their children at least until adulthood, particularly as they have had access to community schooling and other basic supports. In a growing number of states, these efforts are bring pursued more systematically under the concept of permanency planning. Permanency planning involves in order of priority (a) support of the natural family; (b) temporary out-of-home placement with family reunification; (c) if reunification is not in the child's best interest, parental release and adoption; (d) foster care; and (e) the least restrictive non-family placement with movement to a stable, permanent home as soon as possible (Taylor et al., 1989). In short, it is about assuring the same kinds of home and nurturing environments for children with mental retardation that we seek for the other children of our society.

In the last few years, there have also been rapidly increasing opportunities for people with the most severe cognitive limitations to live in natural communities. Although data from the 1987 National Medical Expenditure Survey show that 46.7% of the residents of large state and nonstate facilities (i.e., those with 16 or more residents) have profound mental retardation as opposed to only 13.6% of smaller facility residents (Lakin, Hill, Chen, & Stephens, 1989); the latter statistic reflects a substantial increase over previous years. Applying these estimates to state statistics on the total number of persons in small residential facilities in the United States yielded an estimated 16,000 persons with profound mental retardation living in community-based residential facilities in 1987.

This represents an increase of nearly 10,000 persons with profound mental retardation in community-based facilities between 1982 and 1987. Even though state institutions showed an increase in the proportion of residents with profound mental retardation (from 47% to 63%) during the 10-year period from 1977 to 1987, the total number of persons with profound degrees of mental retardation in state institutions actually decreased by over 11,000 from 71,100 to 59,800 (White, Lakin, Hill, Wright, & Bruininks, 1988). This numerical reduction is reflected in the increased community presence of people with profound mental retardation.

Findings and Issues of Relevance

The steady movement toward ensuring that people with mental retardation have a presence in the community has substantial momentum. Evidence of that momentum ranges from the vast majority of states and numerous federal agencies making formal commitments to continued reduction of institutional populations and to the closing of whole state institutions (Braddock, Hemp, Fujiura, Bachelder, & Mitchell, 1990; Lakin, Jaskulski et al., 1989); to the dramatically increasing amounts of applied research and demonstration focused on understanding and improving community living in general and more specifically for the increasing numbers of people with severe cognitive, functional, and behavioral limitations who live in the community. In addition to research focused on improving community living for persons with mental retardation, there is also a growing body of research that consistently documents that benefits accrue to people with mental retardation when they have opportunities for community living. Two particularly relevant examinations of this research have been (a) studies of changes in functional skills (i.e., adaptive behavior) among people living in institutional versus community settings and (b) studies of perspectives of families of persons with mental retardation regarding institutional and community placements.

Functional Skill Change

One generally accepted purpose of residential services is to provide people with an environment and appropriate support so as to facilitate the development of skills and to increase their independence. One method of assessing the differential achievement of such outcomes is with longitudinal measurement of changing skill levels through repeated adaptive behavior assessments. A review of 18 longitudinal and experimental–contrast group studies measuring the effects of deinstitutionalization on adaptive behavior over periods from 6 months to 6 years, concluded that residents of institutions consistently show less positive change in adaptive behavior than residents who moved to community settings (Larson & Lakin, 1989a). In all, 13 of the 18 studies noted statistically significant improvements associated with movement to community settings in either overall adaptive behavior or in basic self-help and domestic skills areas. Each of the five other studies showed at least some increase in favor of community living. The studies used 10 different assessment instruments, and a total of 1,358 subjects, persons who were for the most part diagnosed as having severe or profound mental retardation. They were conducted in 13 different states or regions from all over the United States. While the majority of the studies reviewed were not true experimental designs, they produced remarkably consistent evidence of improved outcomes favoring community living versus institutional living.

Parent Attitudes About Deinstitutionalization

Objective data on measurable developmental change are important, but the relative benefits of one type of home over another are not exclusively, nor perhaps even primarily, a matter of their ability to stimulate developmental change. How well a setting provides for all that might be sought from one's home (e.g., comfort, safety, autonomy, acceptance, status, etc.) is often somewhat subjective. Parents provide a particularly important perspective on how well the qualities they seek in long-term housing for their family member are available in the institutional and community-based settings in which their children, adults for the most part, are living. As debates about the merits of deinstitutionalization are waged across the country, many parents have been active participants, some as advocates of deinstitutionalization, others as adamant foes (Frohboese & Sales, 1980). But whatever their position, it must be appreciated that parents have a clear emotional interest in the relative quality of the out-of-home placements of their children, and they have unique perspectives on the extent to which different types of housing meet their children's needs. Therefore, parent perceptions of the satisfactoriness of institutional and community settings have been an interesting and valued source of outcome data.

A recent review of literature on this topic (Larson & Lakin, 1989b) identified 35 studies of parent attitudes about movement of their institutionalized children to community living arrangements, including 23 studies that reported statistical data. The review noted that across studies a very high proportion of parents with offspring currently living in institutions were satisfied with institutional living for their offspring (91.0% were satisfied and 74.6% were opposed to the prospect of movement to a community setting). However, parents whose offspring had been through the deinstitutionalization process and who were living in community settings at the time the parents were surveyed were overwhelmingly satisfied with the community setting (87.6% were satisfied) and reported much less retrospective satisfaction with institution settings (52.3% reported satisfaction) than parents interviewed while their child still resided in an institution. Four studies that surveyed parents both before and after deinstitutionalization showed a pattern of reversals from initial opposition to later high satisfaction with deinstitutionalization and with the specific community home of their son or daughter. In general then, there is an overwhelming tendency for parents to shift from opponents to advocates of community living once they have the opportunity to actually observe the experiences of their children in community living settings.

Challenges to Ensuring Access and Support

There are obviously many problems and issues in sustaining the general commitment to increase access to communities for persons with mental retardation. A few of the more notable of these follow.

Interstate Variability in Community Access

Although the general national trend is toward steadily increasing community access for people with mental retardation, an individual's access is often substantially influenced by his or her state of residence. For example in 1988, nationally, an average of 48.8% of persons residing in mental retardation facilities lived in homes with 15 or fewer people. However, the proportion of persons living in these relatively small settings varied enormously by state, from 14.2% in Mississippi to 86.6% in New Hampshire. In all, three states (Mississippi, Oklahoma and Texas) served fewer than 20% of the people with mental retardation in settings of 15 or fewer residents, while five states (Alaska, Arizona, Montana, New Hampshire and Rhode Island) served 80% or more persons in such settings (Lakin et al., 1990). Although residential services have been historically left largely to the discretion of states, statistics such as these raise questions about the extent to which significant federal inducements should be brought to bear on increasing congruence between articulated national goals regarding increased community living opportunities and the relative paucity of such opportunities in many states. It seems extremely likely that the 1990s will bring federal legislation that will substantially increase federal financial participation in all kinds of residential services, probably under Title XIX of Medicaid. But whether that increased federal role with respect to community living will come with an effort to reduce or limit federal financing of institutional services seems less certain.

Increasing Institutional and Total System Costs Affect Community Access

Access to community living arrangements is not solely a condition of preferability on the part of government agencies. Increased access to community settings and supports requires resources. Although, it has often been assumed that resources committed to institutions would be shifted to community settings with shifts in population, this assumption has been simplistic. In fact, from 1977 to 1988, as the average daily populations decreased from 151,532 to 91,582, the costs of operating these institutions increased from 2.46 billion dollars per year to 5.14 billion dollars per year (Braddock, Hemp, Fujiura, Bachelder, & Mitchell, 1989). Between 1977 and 1988, as the average daily population of institutions decreased by 40%, the per-resident real-dollar costs of institutional care increased by 75% and total institution expenditures were increased by over 20%. In only a few states has deinstitutionalization produced a "residential dividend" that can be applied to increasing or improving community residential opportunities. States are beginning to realize that such dividends can be produced only through institutional closure; otherwise, substantial fixed costs are merely spread over smaller numbers of residents. As a result, between 1977 and 1988, states closed or established plans to close 42 state institutions, but this represents only about 15% of state institutions operating on June 30, 1977. Achieving such outcomes has been made difficult by the many strong opponents of institution closures within the states (especially public employee unions, parents of residents, and local community groups). One potential factor of influence in this area will be whether the federal government will place financial restrictions on its participation in supporting inefficiencies in current practice and allow states increased flexibility to address such issues through the provision of certain Medicaid Title XIX reform proposals.

The shift from institutional to community-based settings has been, and apparently will continue to be, not only a shift in locus of services but also a shift from publicly to privately provided services. Since the shift from public to private management of residential services began, researchers have been particularly interested in comparing costs across facility types. The results of these studies, however, must be viewed with considerable caution. Many complex methodological problems are involved in such research, and these are compounded by the substantial variation among services provided in institutions and community-based settings. No national study has ever been structured so as to gather comprehensive cost data on a full set of comparable services for persons living in different types of facilities. However, six smaller studies have gathered generally comparable cost information for public institutions and small, community-based facilities (Ashbaugh & Allard, 1984; Bensberg & Smith, 1984; Campbell & Smith, 1989; Jones, Conroy, Feinstein, &

Lemanowicz, 1983; Minnesota Department of Public Welfare, 1979; Touche Ross & Co., 1980). In each of these studies, summarized in Table 14.1, the researchers tried to compare full "packages" of community services (residential care, day programs, case management, transportation, medical services, administration, and so forth).

One general conclusion derived from these relatively well-controlled studies would be that when comparable comprehensive services are included in the total computed program costs for residents of different types of staffed residential facilities, the total costs of these programs are fairly similar. Comprehensive community programs had costs that were from 72% (Campbell & Smith, 1989) to 92% (Jones et al., 1983) of total public institution program costs. The median finding was that the community-based programs were costing 86% of the institutional programs. Such differences are certainly significant, and for program cost estimation and policy analysis purposes, they are important. However, wage differentials between public and private facility staff alone generally account for that range of difference in cost. In addition, one might add that in only some instances were the private agencies' office administrative and training–technical assistance costs included. In short, we must expect, even with the closure of complete institutional programs, that resources needed to support development and enhancement of community-based programs will represent a major challenge for the rest of this century.

Attempts to find those new resources will meet with increased competition within the human services field. Quite likely, the remainder of this century will see heightened demands for community services for persons who are elderly, for persons who have mental illness, and for families, as well as for persons with mental retardation. This will add to the enormous problems of responding to the needs of as many as 60,000 people with mental retardation and related conditions currently on waiting lists for community residential services (Davis, 1987). Virtually all states currently claim a need for the new federal resources that a community-oriented Medicaid long-term care benefit would bring to their citizens with mental retardation (Lakin, Jaskulski et al., 1989). The ultimate question with respect to obtaining such a program is, given the huge waiting lists and growing total costs of our state instituions that house fewer and fewer people, whether and in what form Congress will try to meet the states' needs.

Shortages of Qualified Staff Could Affect Access to Community Service

A major challenge to providing increased access to community residential services in the last years of this century will be to recruit, train, and retain people who can provide direct-care services. No issue can be more important, because, as evolution toward less restrictive, better integrated

TABLE 14.1. Studies gathering comparable cost data on residents of public institutions and community-based facilities.

Study/Author (s)	Year	Residential programs compared	Types of costs included	Notes on costs included	General findings
Minnesota Department of Public Welfare	1979	Publc ICF-MR institutions and private community (ICF-MR) facilities in Minnesota	Residential, day programs, transportation, social services, (case management, family support, etc.), medical services	Cost of components calculated only for individuals in private facilities, presumed covered in institution per diem; institutional capital not included	Higher average annual costs in the state institution ($19,500 to $17,900 per year)
Touche Ross and Co.	1980	Beatrice State (ICF-MR) and community-based mental retardation (CBMR) programs (non-ICF-MR) in Nebraska	Residential, day program, support service (physical and speech therapy, transportation, etc.), social service (case management, social work), administration	Costs of components computed on a per-client average from budgets of six CBMR regions; Beatrice State cost components extracted from facility budget; medical costs for CBMR clients based on average of state Medicaid billings; institution capital not included	Average annual costs for persons in CBMR programs ($15,400) was less than in Beatrice State Hospital ($19,500)
Jones, Conroy, Feinstein, and Lemanowicz	1983	Pennhurst State (ICF-MR) and community residential facilities (CRFs) with average bed size of 3.2 clients in Pennsylvania	Residential, day programs, entitlements, medical costs, case management, other	Study based on a matched sample of 70 former and 70 current residents of Pennhurst; costs of components calculated for individuals in both CRFs and Pennhurst	Average annual costs for persons in CRFs ($40,300) was less than in Pennhurst State School ($44,200)

	Year	Facility	Components	Findings
Bensberg and Smith	1984	Public ICF-MR institutions and small (less than 15 res.) ICF-MR facilities in Texas	Residential (food, rent, utilities, phone, maintenance, staff), support services (day services, transportation)	Costs of components calculated only for individuals in small facilities, persumed covered in institution per diem; institution capital not included	Lower average annual costs in small ICF-MRs ($18,350 to $21,250) without including administrative costs in small facilities; costs higher in small facilities if agency administrative costs are included ($29,900)
Ashbaugh and Allard	1984	Pennhurst State (ICF-MR) institution and community living arrangements (CLAs) with three to six residents in Pennsylvania	Residential, day programs, case management, specialized support services, medical and transportation	Costs of components calculated for individuals in both CLA and Pennhurst	Average annual costs for persons in CLAs ($33,250) less than in Pennhurst ($44,900) or average for PA state institutions; wider range in client costs in CLAs ($7,200 to $92,200) than in Pennhurst ($36,400 to $76,250)
Cambell and Smith	1986	All large public institutions and all community facilities (1–8 res., 9–16 res.) in South Dakota	Residential, day programs, case management, administration, medical services, follow-along services for each individual; all other costs prorated to each individual in each type of facility	Actual costs computed for individuals in institutions and community settings, except for "other," which included all other costs for each category of facility (e.g., training, monitoring) equally apportioned to each resident of the facility type	Average annual institution costs of $30,536 were higher than $16,893 in community settings; controlling for four levels of resident service need (of nine total) with at least forty institution and 40 community residents, community costs averaged 71% of institution costs

ICF/MR, Intermediate Care Facility for the Mentally Retarded.

housing arrangements continues, we will by necessity see increased decentralization. At present, there are over 250,000 full-time equivalent direct-care positions in institutional and community-based residential settings. About 90,000 of these positions are in community-based facilities (Lakin, Hill et al., 1989), and by the year 2000, given current trends, the number of full-time equivalent positions in community-based facilities could increase to about 150,000. New direct-care roles will entail considerable greater autonomy and responsibility than typically experienced by direct-care staff of institutions. These increased responsibilities will be given primarily to paraprofessionals, that is, people without college degrees in a discipline relevant to their task (about 75% of all community direct-care staff according to Lakin & Bruininks, 1981). Because of this, the greater attention and resources given in recent years to training these individuals (e.g., as in the Developmental Disabilities Assistance and Bill of Rights Act Amendments of 1987) will need to be expanded even further in years to come. But the personnel issues in this area will be far more complex than just training. It will be necessary to recruit people who can acquire the needed skills, who will respect the people who are dependent on their assistance, and who can find satisfaction and value in their work. Once these individuals are hired and trained, it will be important to retain them so that their skills and familiarity with the individuals they serve can grow and continue to contribute to the well-being of people with mental retardation. Unfortunately, the near future will present enormous challenges in each of these areas.

In this past decade, there has been growing concern about personnel problems in residential services generally and especially in providing community-based residential services. Research has shown unacceptably high turnover rates (from 26% to 33% annually) in institutions (Lakin, Bruininks, Hill, & Hauber, 1982; Zaharia & Baumeister, 1979) but even higher rates (55% to 73% annually) in community-based residential settings (George & Baumeister, 1981; Lakin et al., 1982). Compounding the serious problem of extremely high turnover rates among existing employees is the increasing problem that recruitment represents, one that can be expected to worsen as we near the year 2000. Clearly, the low birth rates of the 1960s and 1970s will lead to labor shortages in the 1990s and beyond. The industries that will suffer most are those that pay the least, demand the most, and draw their personnel primarily from among young adults. Nothing better describes paraprofessional employment in residential services. These problems are only exacerbated by the fact that direct care has traditionally been a female-dominated industry, while young women of the 1990s are likely to continue the trend toward seeking employment outside the traditional occupations of women. Further adding to the challenges is the fact that foster-care programs, historically making up 15% to 25% of community residential placements, and usually among the best integrated and least costly alternatives, are being affected by the changing American family, which has led to fewer homes that are able or willing to meet current agency standards to provide foster care to children and adults with mental retardation. Indeed, there is stiff competition among child welfare, mental health, aging, and mental retardation service agencies for this limited pool of families willing and able to open up their homes.

These factors pose major challenges in the next few years. They will require changes in recruitment of staff, drawing much more heavily from nontraditional employment pools. They will also require much more attention to retaining staff. At present rates of growth in total employees and present rates of turnover, out of about 650,000 full-time equivalent direct-care positions filled for community residences nationally between the years 1990 and 2000, nearly 90% will be replacements for people who quit. Pay and benefits will need to be improved, but other forms of compensation will also need to be developed, including some innovative efforts to draw people to human services. Opportunities for advancement (i.e., career ladders) will need to be developed. In short, tremendous attention and effort will need to be given to recruiting, training, and retaining a work force of adequate size, skill, and experience as we move toward the end of this century.

The Limited Supply of Residential Services Requires Increased Attention to Family Support

There are many challenges to ensuring access to the out-of-home residential services needed by a minority of persons with mental retardation. But the single greatest challenge to the viability of the residential services system is to ensure that the demand for costly residential services is kept at a minimum. With up to 85% of individuals with mental retardation and related conditions living with their natural or adoptive families, policy makers have recently begun to acknowledge the importance of providing specific supports to those families. Therefore, even though this chapter focuses on residential services, it must attend, at least briefly, to those services that prevent or delay entry into the residential services system. The development of such services is one important challenge in supporting families to enable them to keep their children at home for as long as possible.

Family supports refer to a range of flexible forms of assistance that enhance a family's capacity to provide care at home (Bradley et al., 1990). In-home support services designed specifically for families were not begun in a substantial way until the 1980s (Bradley et al., 1990). Despite these late beginnings, by fiscal year 1988, 42 states and the District of Columbia offered a discrete family-support initiative, either cash subsidy, respite care services, or other family support (Braddock et al., 1990). Total expenditures on family support were $171 million in

FY 1988, and the family-support programs served an estimated 168,314 families nationwide (Braddock et al., 1990). One recent description of the types of support provided to families (Bradley et al., 1990) noted that 30 states provided at least one support service in four of eight categories including respite and child care, environmental adaptation, supportive services, in-home assistance, extraordinary and ordinary needs (e.g., transportation, special clothing), training for parents and family members, recreation, and systemic assistance (e.g., advocacy); 20 states provided most traditional developmental services such as occupational therapy, and behavior management; 23 states offered special case management services; and 22 states offered financial assistance through discretionary cash subsidies, allowances, vouchers, or other payment–reimbursement methods.

Although research on the effectiveness of family support services is limited, a few studies have examined this issue. For example, Zimmerman (1984) surveyed 38 Minnesota families who received a financial subsidy to enable them to care for a child with severe mental retardation at home. She found that 97% of the families regarded the Family Subsidy Program to be of great help in enabling them to care for their child at home. The specific areas in which most families found the program helpful were in purchasing special items for the child (95% of families surveyed), purchasing respite care and babysitting services (71%), and in providing support to care for the child's general needs (92%). In a controlled study, Meyers and Marcenko (1989) evaluated the impact of a cash subsidy program on 81 randomly selected families with children under age 18 who were diagnosed severely mentally retarded, severely multiply handicapped, or autistic from four counties in Michigan. The Impact on Family Scale was used to assess pretest–posttest changes associated with the provision of a $225 per month cash subsidy for 8 to 10 months. The results indicated that the amount of measured family stress was significantly lower after receiving the subsidy; the life satisfaction of parents increased significantly after receiving the subsidy; and the proportion of mothers who anticipated placing their child out of the home in the future declined significantly from 32% to 19%. While these studies provide some evidence that families find family support programs useful, further research is needed to address broader concerns about the best strategies to use when designing and implementing family support programs.

Bradley et al. (1990) presented a list of 14 characteristics that define comprehensive systems of family supports. Those conditions included (a) a legislative mandate to provide family support, (b) guiding principles for family-support systems articulated at the state level, (c) family-focused supports, (d) parental control, (e) parental oversight, (f) flexible funding, (g) provision of core services, (h) services brokerage approaches, (i) interagency collaboration, (j) inclusive eligibility, (k) statewide access, (l)

Medicaid policy for family support, (m) community-centered approach, and (n) active outreach. But their review of the family-support programs in each state in the United States revealed considerable variation, with states showing a range from having none of these characteristics to having all but two of them.

Clearly, meeting the demands for residential services in the 1990s and beyond will depend on minimizing the demand for these services and, conversely, on supporting families in their efforts to provide a place to live for their family members with mental retardation. Doing so will require attention to and nurturing of trends of tremendous relevance to the future of residential services including the following:

1. Families are keeping their children at home longer when they are properly supported.
2. Families are increasingly integrated into and vocal about decisions regarding their children, whatever their ages.
3. Families are becoming increasingly involved in and vocal about quality assurance in community-based residential services.

Attention to these trends for increased family support and involvement will be of great importance to the viability and quality of residential services for persons with mental retardation as we move toward the end of this century.

Prospects for the End of the Century

Projection of trends from 1977 to 1988 to the end of this century suggests a rather dramatic reorientation toward providing homes in the community for a very substantial majority of the people with mental retardation who received residential services. Continuation of current patterns of change would suggest that the total number of people with mental retardation receiving residential services could be expected to number about 290,000 people, to which would be added perhaps another 25,000 people from changes required in current use of nursing homes for persons with mental retardation under the Omnibus Budget Reconciliation Act of 1987 (Lakin et al., 1990). In short, the total size of the mental retardation residential care system by the end of the century appears likely to be around 315,000 people with only about 10% of the system's clients (31,500) still residing in state institutions. If trends maintain by the end of the century, large nonstate (private and local government) institutions (e.g., facilities serving 16 or more people) will house more people with mental retardation (about 39,000) than those directly operated by states. But the overwhelmingly most common placement will be the relatively small community settings of 15 or fewer residents, which could house as many as 245,000 people if the expected net reduction in nursing home placements is totally reflected in increased community placements. If changes in facility size continue at the same rates as they did from 1977 to 1988, about 135,000 of those people should be living in settings of six or fewer residents, with recent acceleration in trends (since 1982) suggesting that the number could be nearer to 150,000.

These statistics suggest the basic shape of residential service at the end of the century if all current trends continue in the same direction. The only fact of which we are absolutely certain, however, is that by the year 2000, the actual numerical distribution of people by residential placement will be different than projected here. How much we cannot say. Clearly, the development of a federal program through Medicaid reform is essential to the ability of states to continue the trends toward increased community access witnessed in the 1980s. Improving personnel policies and practices is essential to finding and keeping the staff, without whom increased community living opportunities will not be possible. Clearly, making difficult political decisions regarding the closure of the costly and inefficient state institutions currently operating at far below capacity is essential to moving essential funds with residents as they move from institutions to community settings. Introducing new efficiencies and continuing to move away from full-time supervised care for persons who do not need or benefit from "total care" also will be important. Continuing to increase support to families with youngsters and adult children at home to reduce overall demand for out-of-home placements will be important. In short, many potential factors within the residential care system will affect the rate at which increased opportunities for community living are made available to persons with mental retardation. There are many factors of relevance outside the system too, including the funds that our society and its economy will allocate to human services in general and the ability of the mental retardation systems to "compete" successfully for a sufficient share of the funds.

While the net effect of these and other factors can seem ominous, on another level, it seems not unlike other litanies of problems that for years have in the minds of some portended the end of steadily increasing community living opportunities for people with mental retardation. In two decades, this society's commitment to continue to expand these opportunities has always overcome the impediments to doing so. There is no historical foundation to think these opportunities will not be sustained in the decade leading to the year 2000. However, maintaining past momentum in the next several years may require much more systematic attention to problem solving at federal, state, local, and provider agency levels than ever before.

As more and more states are characterized as having most of the residential service recipients in community settings, greatly increased and often long overdue attention will be given to the quality of that experience. In the next sections of this chapter, we will review four important themes that relate much more directly to the quality of life for the people who are and will be living in the community settings, which by century's end will be by far the predominant residential experience for people with mental retardation.

Enhanced Growth and Development

Recent Trends

Good homes are environments in which household members experience opportunities to learn and develop their interests and skills. But good home environments also balance positive developmental experiences with other desired qualities of a "home": privacy, relaxation, individually determined activity (or inactivity), a place to bring friends, and so forth. Most of the last half of this century can be characterized as a struggle to incorporate into residential services efforts to enhance individual growth and development through "habilitation," "active treatment," and other facility-based training. Without doubt, the single act of greatest importance in ensuring that residential services in the United States were attentive to fostering personal growth and development on the part of people with mental retardation was the inclusion of an "active treatment" requirement in the federal Medicaid regulations governing services for persons with mental retardation (the Intermediate Care Facilities for the Mentally Retarded [ICF-MR] program). The active treatment requirement mandated regular participation in professionally developed and supervised activities, experiences, or therapies and an individual written plan of care that sets forth measurable goals or objectives stated in terms of desirable behavior and that prescribes an integrated program of activities, experiences, or therapies necessary for the individual to reach those goals or objectives. By 1982, those standards were formally governing the residential services provided to more than half (approximately 140,000) of the people living in residential settings for persons with mental retardation. They were also of substantial influence in other residential settings, as formal training within the residence became a standard aspect of residential care.

In the last few years, there has been some concern about the importance of the active treatment standard for persons with mental retardation. As the residential "facility" has been increasingly recognized in terms of its being a "home" to people living in it, there has been concern about whether the typical conditions of habilitation should be required of people who return home from a full day of vocational, educational, or other developmentally beneficial activity. Typical adults in our society undergo no equivalent of active treatment when they return home from a day of work. In recognition of this, recent efforts to enhance growth and development through residential services focus on enhancing people's interest and abilities to engage in and enjoy the typical activities of living in a community such as recreation–leisure activities, a trend exemplified in the 1988 revised ICF-MR regulations. Finding an appropriate balance between the requirements for developmental training and the right to a reasonably typical home life will probably become an issue of greater contention in upcoming years, particularly if Medicaid is reformed in ways that make federal reimbursements for residential services less directly linked to developmental training than under current ICF-MR regulations.

Findings and Issues

Throughout the last 40 years, it has been increasingly accepted that one's living arrangement should contribute to one's growth and development. Whether expressed as "habilation" or in less jargonistic ways, most professionals, policymakers, and consumers have come to see a major role for residential services in enhancing the personal development and community living skills of persons with mental retardation. Conversely, we have come to believe that certain environments can and do consistently have true or relative debilitating effects on their residents (Heal, 1988; Lakin, Bruininks, & Sigford, 1981). Deinstitutionalization has been a major product of that belief. As noted earlier, research has consistently and convincingly shown that adaptive behavior and functional living skills are more likely to be developed in community settings than in institutions (Larson & Lakin, 1989a). This finding is not particularly surprising, given what is known about learning among persons with mental retardation.

During this half century, expanding application of applied behavior analysis has dramatically changed the nature and amount of instruction provided to persons with mental retardation (Liberty, 1985). The effectiveness of these applications has been demonstrated in teaching an extremely wide range of skills directly relevant to personal growth and development (Martin, 1988; Snell, 1987; Wehman, 1981). But at least as important as the improvement in the technology of teaching have been changes in the focus of instruction. Increasingly, ideas concerning what should be taught to persons with mental retardation have become determined by analysis of what an individual needs to know in order to increase his or her level of independence and social participation. The instructional goals and activities developed through such analyses are sometimes said to be based on "the criterion of ultimate function" (Brown, Nietupski, & Hamre-Nietupski, 1976). According to this criterion, the curriculum of habilation (i.e., what is deliberately taught) should be based on analysis of both the capabilities and characteristics of the individual and of the specific skills required of him or her in the environments of present and probable future daily living. Methods and issues of selecting relevant behaviors as targets for instruction have been widely discussed (Falvey, 1986; Wilcox & Bellamy, 1982). In applying functional criteria to the planning of instructional programs, it is recognized that these programs for people with mental retardation should ultimately serve the same ends as those for normal people, that is, they should maximize the individual's ability to function independently and productively in the society into which he or she was born.

A related major change in efforts to effectively enhance the personal growth and development of persons with mental retardation has derived from increased attention given to the environment of instruction. This attention has broadened behavioral reinforcement theory applications to broader social learning or ecological applications. These have suggested that factors such as situation, setting, intent, natural reinforcement, and vicarious reinforcement are all important to learning and behavior. They have also suggested that learning is enhanced particularly for persons with limited ability to generalize, when the environment of instruction and of ultimate performance are as similar as possible, preferably identical (Gaylord-Ross & Holvoet, 1985). The relevance of these instructional principles to residential services is that, in terms of ultimately preparing people for community living, the best place for teaching needed community living skills is the community setting for which one is being prepared.

Despite their central role in promoting personal growth and development, relatively little attention has been given to providing community care personnel with the orientation and training needed for them to carry out their jobs well. The gap between current knowledge and daily practice is considerable, in part because of inadequate preparation of training materials and provision of effective training programs, and because the basic daily demands of household management may preclude much attention to systematic training; and in part because relatively little focus is placed on habilitation outcomes in living environments. Improving the response of community care providers, including foster parents, is a matter of orientation, training, and retention of effective staff. Little specific research on direct training has been conducted, and few specific standards for direct-care qualifications exist. Only recently has there been any effort to specifically study and identify the components of care provision to persons with mental retardation (Burchard & Thousand, 1988). Clearly, along with efforts to create home environments that foster personal growth and development of persons with mental retardation, better efforts are needed to support those homes with people who can help persons with mental retardation reach their full developmental potential, as well as their full potential to enjoy the opportunities to choose and participate in preferred activities that are enjoyed by people "at home" and in their communities.

Prospects for the End of the Century

The next decade will bring increased recognition of the importance of enhancing opportunities for community living and for developing community living skills. This recognition will be heightened by the continuing efforts to increase community living opportunities and capabilities of people with severe cognitive impairments. At the same time, there is likely to be considerably increased respect for people being "at home." This is likely to be manifested by greater concentration on recreation and leisure activities as the primary and proper domain of training and experience. Those advocating greater unstructured time and self-determined activity (and inactivity) will find others who argue that that is precisely what public institutions provided at the beginning of the half century. But it is likely that by century's end some degree of equilibrium and individualization will be reached. Home, for many more people with mental retardation, will be a place that approximates the cultural norm of providing a place of relative independence, privacy, relaxation, and a place where one engages in a balance of preferred activities and activities needed to maintain the home. But it will still be recognized that having a home also provides opportunities for people with mental retardation to continue learning to master the demands of the culture. In short, considerable focus on residence-based personal skill development is likely to remain in the future, but the focus of that learning is more likely to be individually determined and in service of an individual's own preferences, life-style, and areas of interest.

Fostering Typical Social Relationships

Recent Trends

Recent years have seen the publication of compelling arguments on the importance of social relationships in the lives of people with mental retardation and related conditions (O'Brien, 1987; Strully & Strully, 1985; Taylor, Biklin, & Knoll, 1987). Increasing attention is being given to support networks, a concept developed primarily in the mental health area in the mid-1970s (Bott, 1971; Guerin, 1976). Social networks are simply groups of people whose members provide reciprocal support and friendship. Fostering typical social relationships among persons with mental retardation involves facilitating both the development of social skills, and the establishment and maintenance of social networks. Social networks are increasingly being used to facilitate the involvement of typical peers and community members in planning for inclusion in school settings (Vandercook, York, & Forrest, 1989) and in community residential and work settings (Mount & Zwernik, 1988).

Current service systems are often not sufficiently responsive to the social needs of people with mental retardation. For instance, although it has been demonstrated that the deinstitutionalization process is associated with significantly improved social skills among those who move (D'Amico, Hannah, Milhouse, & Frohleich, 1978; Eastwood & Fisher, 1988; Horner, Stoner, & Ferguson, 1988; State of Wisconsin, 1986), improvements in social skills as measured by adaptive behavior assessments do not necessarily translate into positive changes in the number or the quality of social relationships. Qualitative and follow-up research studies document that physical integration of adults with handicaps in community settings does not guarantee that they will establish desired social and interpersonal relationships with typical community members (Bercovici, 1983; Bruininks, Thurlow, & Steffans, 1988; Bruininks, Thurlow, Lewis, & Larson, 1988). Limited community participation and social isolation are the themes common in the lives of far too many adolescents, young adults, and adults with handicaps—particularly for those who are in the residential service system (Bogdan & Taylor, 1987a; Calkins et al., 1985; Crapps, Langione, & Swaim, 1985). Some even suggest that people who have been deinstitutionalized appear to be as socially isolated in the community as they were when they were living in institutions (Bercovici, 1983). These findings point to the development of social relationships as the next major challenge in the field of developmental disabilities (Bogdan & Taylor, 1987a).

Findings and Issues of Relevance

The social networks of persons living in community settings typically include parents, staff members, peers with handicaps, and considerably less often, typical community members.

Family Members

Several studies have demonstrated that family members play an important role in the lives of people living in community settings. Researchers who have followed individuals through the deinstitutionalization process have noted that most (81% to 88%) persons living in community settings had contact with family members at least once a year, and many (30% to 44%) had monthly or more frequent contact with them (Eastwood, 1985; Feinstein, Lemanowicz, & Conroy, 1988). Other studies, however, have shown considerable variation in terms of both contacts and visits across community settings. For example, one recent study found that persons in foster care have fewer contacts with family members than those in group homes (Hill et al., 1989). As is typically found with variation within different residential facility categories, greater variation was found within the categories than between different facility categories. The importance of encouraging family contacts for adults living in community settings was further demonstrated in a recent cross-sectional follow-up study of postschool outcomes for students with moderate-to-severe mental retardation, which found that across time fewer former students lived at home (42% at 1 to 2 years vs. 26% at 7 to 10 years) (Thurlow, Bruininks, & Lange, 1989).

Several variables that influence social relationships between persons in residential settings and their family members have been identified. Parents of persons who had been deinstitutionalized frequently report that the move to the community had a positive impact on the relationship between the family, the person with mental retardation, and care providers (Bradley, Conroy, Covert, & Feinstein, 1986; Conroy, Lemanowicz, & Feinstein, 1987; Eastwood, 1985). Research also suggests that persons living in larger community facilities received fewer visits than those in smaller facilities (Feinstein et al., 1988). Finally, Stoneman and Crapps (1990) in a multiple-regression analysis of the factors predicting the frequency of family visitation, found that when variables such as having parents who are alive, the education level of the provider, and the age of the person were controlled, the level of involvement of the parents in the placement process and the encouragement of parents by the provider accounted for a significant amount of the variability in the frequency of visitation by family members. These findings suggest several policy interventions, such as focusing efforts on developing small facilities, involving parents in the placement process, and encouraging them to visit.

Typical Community Members

Unfortunately, relationships between persons in residential settings and typical community members are much less common than those with family members. It has been well documented that the most common friendships (between 43% and 85% of all friendships) for persons with mental retardation are ones established with other persons with mental retardation either from the residence or from the day program attended (Birenbaum & Seiffer, 1976; Hill et al., 1989; Lakin, Anderson, & Hill, 1988; Malin, 1982; O'Connor, 1976; Willer & Intagliata, 1984). Horner et al. (1988), in an analysis of the social networks of 67 people who had been deinstitutionalized, found that while average participants had 12.3 socially important people in their lives, 5.5 of them were paid providers, 2.4 were family, 2.0 were friends with or without disabilities, 1.9 were co-workers with or without disabilities, and only .45 were neighbors. Edgerton's classic study (1967) of former institution residents found the presence of a "benefactor" (a personal advocate and friend) to be key to an individual's success and integration in the community. However, Birenbaum and Seiffer (1976), in another study of deinstitutionalization, saw few examples of the benefactor relationships in the lives of the persons in supervised living arrangements that they studied. A fourth study found that only an average of 4.2% of best friends for people living in community residential settings were typical community members, and that 60% of the people in those settings did not have even one friend who was a typical community member (Hill et al., 1989). While instances of reciprocal relationships between people with mental retardation and other community members have been documented, these have typically been developed outside any direct or indirect program efforts to foster them (Bogdan & Taylor, 1987b). In general then research suggests limited success on the part of residential service providers to establish and maintain social relationships between the persons in these residential settings and members of the larger community.

The problem of social isolation of people with mental retardation, and the associated lack of skills in developing, accessing, or using interpersonal contacts, relationships, and networks, has many facets and contributing factors. Some work in the area of interpersonal relationships has focused on the exhibited deficiencies of individuals themselves in the primary areas of adaptive behavior and related social skills (Craig & McCarver, 1984; Gollay, Freedman, Wyngaarden, & Kurtz, 1978; Holman & Bruininks, 1985). The findings of such studies were supported in a recent study (Hill et al., 1989) that found that less severe retardation and greater adaptive behavior were associated with greater social integration. In work that looked at the nature of the residential setting itself, Willer and Intagliata (1980) found in a multiple-regression analysis that the social interaction of persons in community facilities depends both on the characteristics of the residents and on the characteristics of their residential environment. They found significantly increased social interactions among persons living in homes where practical skills were taught and where fewer residents lived after resident age and level of functioning were statistically controlled. Other research seems to suggest that social networks that include typical community members are more frequently evident among persons in foster care arrangements than among other types of community residential settings (Hill et al., 1989). In large measure it appears that persons in family–foster care are often included in the social networks of the families with which they live and that many relationships of persons with mental retardation tend to derive directly from the personal, social, or neighborhood associations of care providers. While small group facilities provide considerably better opportunities for social relationships with persons outside the facility than do large facilities, their residents are much less likely to benefit from existing interpersonal networks of their care providers than are residents in family–foster homes.

Another variable influencing the development of social relationships among persons with mental retardation is the extent to which community support systems provide opportunities for, and promote such development. Available studies report limited contact with typical community agencies and organizations (e.g., community education, social clubs, recreational resources) and few efforts by existing community resource agencies to reduce the social isolation of people with mental retardation (Bruininks & Lakin, 1985; Bruininks, Thurlow & Steffens, 1988; Certo, Schleien, & Hunter, 1983; Halpern, Close, & Nelson, 1986). Unfortunately, while there is a good deal of quantitative evidence that persons with mental retardation in community settings have limited social contacts outside the colleague and care-provider networks, qualitative studies focusing on nature of social relationships of persons with mental retardation have been few. Exceptions are represented in the early work of Edgerton (1967) and Edgerton and Bercovici (1976) and the recent work of Bogdan and Taylor (1987a, 1987b, 1989). Such qualitative approaches of participant observations and in-depth interviews are important to efforts to examine and promote interpersonal contacts and meaningful relationships between community respondents with mental retardation and their fellow citizens.

Prospects for the End of the Century

Several issues are important as we consider ways to improve the social relationships of persons in residential environments. Despite the focus of researchers and professionals on facilitating development of relationships with persons who do not have handicapping conditions, most people in residential environments view other persons with disabilities as their best friends. Like the rest of our society, persons with mental retardation tend to draw these friendships from residential surroundings and major day activity. Inadequate appreciation and valuing of these relationships has over the years separated people from key friends as they have moved to or within the community. Increasingly, selection of a home for persons with mental retardation includes careful appreciation of the person or persons that individual considers a friend and chooses to be with. That trend will surely continue as a part of the generally increasing respect for the personal preferences and right to maximum self-determination of citizens with mental retardation. While continuing to enhance the relationships with other community residents, it seems likely that there will be enhanced appreciation of the importance of relationships with peers with mental retardation, including those of the opposite sex.

Family Members

Respect for the importance and inherent rights of family relationships will continue to grow. Families not only are the most basic and enduring relationships people know but the emotional commitments to the well-being of members that are a part of the family bond are critical to people with mental retardation. The support and advocacy of an involved family member cannot be replaced by paid or volunteer surrogate advocates.

Efforts to sustain family involvement in the lives of persons with mental retardation in residential settings will be an increasing focus in years to come. Research is beginning to suggest ways of doing just that. Stoneman and Crapps (1990) found that the amount of involvement parents had in the deinstitutionalization process was the strongest predictor of their future involvement with their son or daughter. Other literature has provided clues about how to facilitate such involvement. The literature review on parent attitudes regarding deinstitutionalization by Larson and Lakin (1989b) summarized many suggestions made by families and recommendations addressed to those who work with families regarding family involvement in the community placement decision. Those suggestions include attending and responding to the perceptions, needs, and concerns of family members regarding the move; facilitating participation of the individual and family in decision making regarding placement (e.g., where, when, with whom); arranging opportunities for family members to learn about and visit potential community sites; and establishing and maintaining effective communication links between community providers and family members after placement. To the extent that such strategies improve family participation in the decision-making process, they promote ongoing social contacts between family members and persons who move to community settings from institutions.

Families who have raised their children in the era of increased publicly supported educational opportunities and who are used to community-based educational and other services can be expected to maintain a central role in the lives of children who grow up and move out. These ongoing relationships will bring new challenges and new opportunities to the residential care system. Ongoing family relationships will involve parents acting as case managers, parents securing housing on behalf of their sons or daughters with mental retardation, and other intensities of involvement that will be quite different from the passive acceptance of whatever services were offered in the past. These relationships not only will enhance the quality of advocacy for individuals with mental retardation but also will help sustain the quality and frequency of family relationships.

Typical Community Members

Social relationships with friends and neighbors are important to us all. Service providers will increasingly be expected to assist people with mental retardation to form friendships and become involved in community associations and organizations. Professional and popular literature has noted numerous successful efforts to establish friendships through community leisure/recreation programs and agencies (Putnam, Werder, & Schleien, 1985; Schleien & Meyer, 1988; Walker & Edinger, 1988), through casual contact with community members (Edgerton, 1967), and through participation in typical social institutions, like integrated school settings (Biklin, 1985) and churches (Taylor & Bogdan, 1989). However, despite evidence that social relationships develop more readily in community settings than in institutions, and despite evidence that relationships between persons with disabilities and nondisabled people tend to grow out of structured or existing relationships, there is much less information than is needed on successful methods of establishing social relationships between persons with mental retardation and others in communities. Future research is needed to address issues such as (a) how individual relationships are formed between people with mental retardation and community members; (b) how people with mental retardation can become effectively integrated with community associations and organizations; and (c) how service providers and families encourage or hinder the establishment and maintenance of supportive social relationships.

It seems important to look to the broader community for natural sources of relationships. There are obvious associations and organizations that should be explored. These include minimally (a) promoting continued use of the family social network once a child leaves home; (b) recognizing the value of friends and neighbors and taking them into consideration when contemplating a move; (c) involving persons with mental retardation in organizations that are typical sources of friendship (e.g., churches, recreation organizations, Boy or Girl Scouts, and other dedicated civic organizations); and (d) continued movement toward employment in typical integrated job settings. In exploring these areas, however, it is important to be sensitive to recommendations such as those made at the National Conference on Self-Determination (1989). There, self-advocates suggested that "friendships cannot be 'programmed.' . . . Training, demonstration, and research programs need to get people into settings where 'friendships can happen.' Then programmers need to develop natural ways of reinforcing those friendships" (p. 9). As we move toward the year 2000, one of the great challenges for providers of residential services will be to identify ways to provide opportunities for persons with mental retardation to meet and get to know typical community members.

Providing Opportunities for Valued Community Participation

Recent Trends

The phrase "providing opportunities for valued community participation" is used here to refer to both the quantity and the quality of participation by persons with mental retardation in the typical roles and activities of the community. As people with mental retardation have been increasingly provided with opportunities to live in communities, they have naturally or by design taken on many of the roles of the community (neighbor, shopper, bus rider, playground user, etc.). Increasingly, what is sought for people with mental retardation is that they have a valued identity in the community, that they are perceived to contribute to the community, that in short, they are seen as part of the community.

Being part of the community means using the resources and participating in the activities of the community. Much of the impetus for developing community-based residential facilities was derived from the logical presumption that such placements naturally led to increased participation in community activities and increased use of community resources. Normalization implies living in culturally typical housing; engaging in the productive activities associated with one's age in the settings in which those activities normally take place; participating in typical leisure, social/cultural, economic, and related roles of the culture; and having friends and associates who are valued in the society. These things increase the status and acceptance of persons with mental retardation. As such, cultural participation becomes an essential aspect of one of normalization's primary goals; "the establishment, enhancement, or defense of the social role(s) of a person or a group by the enhancement of people's social images and personal competencies" (Wolfensberger, 1983, p. 234).

Social images are increasingly being emphasized in providing housing for people with mental retardation. Greater attention is given to the way the house presents its residents to the local community. Not only is housing of typical size for a neighborhood increasingly sought but features that automatically identify the house and its residents as "different" are being removed. Ramps are made less conspicuous, and agency names are removed from vans. In many places, transport vans that present (and treat) the residential household as a group rather than individuals are being replaced by transportation that is typical for the neighborhood. Signs that pronounce a house to be a "facility" are disappearing, ranging from explicit facility identifiers to more implicit ones like numbered parking spaces.

Research Findings and Issues of Relevance

Community Resource Use

The community participation of persons living in community settings, when compared to the community participation of persons living in institutions is impressive (Conroy & Bradley, 1985; Felce, de Kock, & Repp, 1986; Hill & Bruininks, 1981; Horner et al., 1988; O'Neil, Brown, Gordon, Schonhorn, & Green, 1981). People in the community go to more movies, more restaurants, more stores, more sporting events. They go on more walks off the grounds of the facility or home and have more visits to friends away from the facility. They are more likely to participate in organized sports, to have friendships with nonhandicapped persons and to go places with their families. They are more likely to attend community churches. The list could go on.

Despite the personal, cultural, and habilitative values of participating in valued community roles, it has been noted that many individuals living in community settings participate in those communities less than might be expected or desired (Baker, Seltzer, & Seltzer, 1974; Bjaanes & Butler, 1974; Crapps et al., 1985; Hill, & Bruininks, 1981), although not necessarily less than persons who are not mentally retarded. In fact, a recent study of the use of community recreation and leisure resource use by 336 people in a nationally representative sample of people with mental retardation in settings of six and fewer residents compared a random sample of 100 adults in the general population and found the former to have slightly higher resource use than the latter (Hill et al., 1989). Indeed, in some studies participation in the institution and public environment of the community is quite high. Certainly, Intagliata, Willer, and Wicks's (1981) summary of the community engagements of 128 family care residents reflects a reasonably high level of community participation. Their data showed 93% of residents eating at a restaurant, 90% using a barber or beauty shop, 82% attending church, 86% attending parties, 75% using a park, 40% going swimming, 45% going to a zoo, 35% going camping, 20% attending a ball game, 22% going to a museum, 18% going to a library, and 4% going to a bar at least once over a 3-month period. A recent study of a nationally representative sample of 231 elderly persons with mental retardation in community facilities also showed a rate of community participation that seems reasonably high for persons who are elderly: 75% of sample members went to a grocery store at least once in a month, 85% went to a department store, 63% attended church, and 56% used a local park (Anderson, Lakin, Bruininks, & Hill, 1987).

Recreation/Leisure Participation

The importance of leisure, recreation, and other participatory activities in the community for engaging persons with mental retardation in social relationships and valued roles in the community settings has been noted for many years and by many people (Bell, Schoenrock, & Bensberg, 1981; Gollay et al., 1978; M. Seltzer, Sherwood, Seltzer, & Sherwood, 1981; Putnam et al., 1985). Program development demonstration and evaluation of concerted efforts at integrated recreation and leisure activities have occurred on a limited basis. For the most part, however, efforts at integration in recreation and leisure have focused on children and youth. Although these efforts have demonstrated direct social and physical benefits, they have not spread sufficiently to adult services.

One of the recurring findings in research on community resource–use and recreation–leisure participation is that the more severe the person's impairment, the less likely he or she is to engage in community activities (Bell et al., 1981; Dalgleish, 1983; Gollay et al., 1978; Hill, Rotegard, & Bruininks, 1983). Other findings suggest care-provider characteristics and attitudes are predictive of community engagement (Dalgleish, 1983; Intagliata et al., 1981). It is important to recognize that while opportunity is an important aspect of engagement in the community, given opportunities to participate in the community, people may choose different rates of participation or voluntarily reduce participation over time (Birenbaum & Re, 1979). Understanding the experiences of community engagement is greatly reduced by the near absence of objective qualitative studies of community living. Bercovici's (1983) qualitative studies of persons in group homes in the Los Angeles area suggested that isolation from other members of the community and restricted participation were common features of community living. Few of the many quantitative studies of community engagement have gathered data concerning the manner in which residents are presented to the community. That is, are they presented as individuals or as members of groups of persons with mental retardation, as being independent or as being directed or closely supervised? Such presentations are probably important in the status and experience derived from performance of otherwise culturally typical roles, although this issue has not been assessed systematically. There has also been limited attention to the engagement of persons with profound impairments and the nature of the adaptations and accommodations needed to increase or improve their participation.

Domestic Productivity

Participation in domestic activities among community facility residents is considerably lower than that of the general population (Hill et al., 1989), but it is considerably higher among people in community facilities than among those in institutions (Anderson et al., 1987; Horner et al., 1988). It also varies from facility to facility, with three factors clearly associated with differences: (a) severity of impairments of residents, (b) attitudes and length of service of care providers, and (c) type of facility. Persons who have been employed relatively long in group facilities or who are family care providers tend to engage residents in less domestic activity, and the severity of impairment reduces opportunities to participate actively in maintaining the household (Hill et al., 1989). This may suggest desires for efficiency that develop over time in employment or as part of providing care, whereas maintaining one's own household may lead to exclusion of persons from domestic tasks that might benefit them.

Engagement of people with severe and profound mental impairments in domestic tasks is a problem, but one that has been and can be remedied through staff training and response (Mansell, Jenkins, Felce, & de Kock, 1984).

Employment

Employment has been justifiably given special treatment elsewhere in this volume (see Chapter 15). Employment is one of the most explicitly valued and valuable activities for adults in our society. Any effort to increase the valued community participation of adults in residential settings must provide them with opportunities for employment, and those opportunities should to the maximum extent possible provide opportunity to perform those work roles in the manner and places where they are typically performed. People with mental retardation in residential settings enjoy such employment opportunities far less often than might be imagined, given the decade of focus on supported and competitive employment. According to the 1987 National Medical Expenditure Survey, only about 58% of all residents of community-based residences (15 and fewer residents) had any work they did for pay. For an estimated 85% of these individuals, the work took place in sheltered workshops. Put another way, only 9% of residents of community residential facilities worked for pay some place other than in sheltered workshops, and the paid job of some of these individuals was in the residential facility in which they lived (Lakin et al., 1989). Clearly, although there has been considerable improvement in the employment opportunities for people with mental retardation in general, and for some of those people in residential settings, much is left to be accomplished. Ultimately, providing opportunities for truly valued participation in community life will involve better opportunities to contribute to the community through work.

Prospects for the End of the Century

Three trends will have substantial influence on future opportunities for people with mental retardation to enjoy greater participation in valued ways in the community. The first is the increasing acceptance by community institutions and agencies of the rightful place of citizens with mental retardation as their clientele. Each year, greater numbers of public and private community organizations include people with mental retardation and other disabilities. This is to some extent a natural outcome of the increased presence of people with mental retardation within the catchment areas of those programs, to some extent a result of advocacy on the part of groups and individuals, and to some extent a natural outgrowth of our society's growing commitment to nondiscrimination. Along these lines, we must recognize that the passage by the U.S. Congress of the Americans With Disabilities Act will reinforce and further propel such change.

Another factor of likely importance to the participation of persons with mental retardation and related conditions will be the general aging of the society. Clearly, as the population as a whole ages, there will be increased efforts among community agencies to serve the aging population, including the relatively higher proportion of persons with physical and mental conditions within it. This could increase competition for resources and reduce opportunity for participation or it could produce greater opportunity for integration. One might expect, given current trends, that the latter will usually occur, but the former is by no means precluded. Continuation of the effective advocacy and demonstration of the 1980s clearly remains a key element to continued positive opportunities.

Finally, in the area of employment, demographic trends suggest that many new opportunities may be expected for people with mental retardation to participate in valued ways in their communities. The low birth rates of the 1960s and 1970s coupled with an aging work force are creating major labor shortages that will increase throughout this decade. The challenge to people providing training and other assistance to persons with mental retardation—particularly those with more severe impairments, who make up the bulk of the residential population—will be to demonstrate not only the ability to work, but the ability to do the job. If this can be accomplished, given the national commitment to assisting people with disabilities to find and maintain jobs; the Americans With Disabilities Act, which will prohibit employment discrimination against people who can do the job; and the labor shortage, which will mean that everyone who can do a job will be needed, the opportunities to enhance community participation of persons with mental retardation in residential settings seem very promising.

Permitting and Encouraging Increased Personal Autonomy

Recent Trends

Personal autonomy, including decision making, personal choice, self-advocacy, self-determination, and self-expression, is a right and expectation for most adults in America. The primary locus of expression of personal autonomy is one's home. But autonomy has only recently been recognized as an important goal for persons with mental retardation who are consumers of residential services. Personal autonomy has been identified as a key component of independent living for persons with severe disabilities (Budde & Bachelder, 1986). Self-determination, which includes the attitudes and abilities that lead people to define goals for themselves and to take the initiative to reach those goals (Ward, 1988), is one focus of self-advocacy efforts. Although personal autonomy is valued in our society and although it tends to be associated with community living, little is known about the association between it and facility type, how and why it appears greater in some than in others, how much it may vary as a result of care-provider and resident characteristics, and where and how it is fostered. The opportunity to develop and use skills required for personal autonomy has been identified as a significant need for persons with disabilities (Abery & Bruininks, 1990; Guess, Benson, & Siegel-Causey, 1985; National Conference on Self-Determination, 1989; Shevin & Klein, 1984).

Michael Kennedy, an effective advocate for people with disabilities and a 15-year veteran of state institution living, clearly expresses the importance of autonomy and the pride, responsibility, and freedom it brings:

The differences between my new living situation and my former living situations are numerous and immeasurable. I am now responsible for paying my own bills. Previously I had never been entrusted with responsibilities. It was always assumed I could not be responsible for myself because I was disabled. . . . Being responsible for my life led to having control over my life. I make decisions for myself. I have equal say in everything that happens regarding our house. I make all the decisions that directly affect me. In the institution and supported apartment, my decisions were all made for me, often without my consultation. I did not have real control of my life. . . . I did not control my choice of activity. . . . As a consumer, I would like to propose that parents and professionals give people the opportunity to make personal choices themselves. (Kennedy, 1989, p. 4).

As residential service providers continue to improve in their ability to provide and/or support homes for people with mental retardation, including increasing numbers of persons with severe and profound cognitive impairments, it seems clear that they must also strive to develop effective strategies to teach self-expression and choice making, and to create improved opportunities for expression of personal autonomy, choice and self-advocacy, and the important service of personal responsibility that derives from that expression.

Recent Findings and Issues of Relevance

Considerable research has focused on comparing different types of residential facilities in terms of the degree to which they facilitate and encourage personal autonomy. Community facilities have consistently been found to be superior to institutional facilities in attempting to grant autonomy to residents. On the *Characteristics of the Treatment Environment* (Silverstein, McLain, Hubbell, & Brownlee, 1977), community facilities have been found to be more likely to encourage residents to make their own decisions, to manage their own affairs, to maintain and improve their own living areas, and to be involved in decisions affecting them (Rotegard, Hill, & Bruininks, 1982). King, Raynes, and Tizard's (1971) study of residential facilities focused on four aspects of institutional versus individual orientation: "rigidity," "block treatment," "depersonalization," and "social distance," and concluded that small facilities tended to be more individually oriented than larger facilities. In G. B. Seltzer's (1981) study of 153 persons transferred from institutions to community facilities, he found functional skill gains and resident satisfaction associated with environmental normalization, training and responsibility for household tasks, access to community resources, and individual autonomy. However, importantly, as in all studies of community living, the general tendency toward greater autonomy, independence, and choice in the community by no means is uniformly or sufficiently available to all persons in community settings (Kishi, Teelucksingh, Zollers, Park-Lee, & Meyer, 1988).

Personal Autonomy Skill Development

Personal autonomy in choice making involves "the act of an individual's selection of a preferred alternative from among several familiar options" (Shevin & Klein, 1984) and requires skills in communication as well as skills in choice making. Researchers who have examined choice making among persons with severe and profound mental retardation have found that when presented with a situation in which individuals are free to make choices, the actual behavior observed often does not reflect the known preferences of the individuals (Shevin & Klein, 1984). A number of factors affecting this have been hypothesized. Mithaug and Hanawalt (1978) note ambiguities in situations where persons who are severely handicapped are given opportunities to choose, limited abilities to respond in an interpretable manner, and related development of task avoidance behaviors. Certainly the "acquiescence" that has long been evident in research on persons with mental retardation (Rosen, Floor, & Sizfein, 1974; Sigelman et al., 1981) is the most widely recognized evidence of the difficulty that persons with mental retardation have in expressing their personal independence and preferences. Among functionally oriented habilitation programs for persons with severe handicaps, being able to indicate preferences should be seen as a skill that is essential to the pursuit of independence. Still, there is very little evidence in literature that it has been the target of much intervention (Guess et al., 1985; Shevin & Klein, 1984). Limited research does exist that suggests that assertiveness training, and training for decision making among adults with mild or moderate mental retardation can successfully influence skills in the area of personal autonomy (Bregman, 1984; Tymchuk, Andron, & Rahbar, 1988), but they are only a beginning.

Systematic development of personal autonomy skills and orientations in residential settings may involve a range of activities including (a) direct instruction in choice making, assertiveness, decision making, and communicating preferences; (b) systematic integration of choice making, decision making, and self-expression throughout the individual's daily life; and (c) capitalizing on natural opportunities, as well as specific provision of opportunities to make and express choice and to experience the consequences of those choices. But, as Abery and Bruininks (1990) note:

Facilitating the development of self-determination skills and encouraging their use in multiple contexts is a complex task. It is affected by all aspects of the environment within which the individual functions, including: a) the personal characteristics of the learner (e.g., cognitive competencies, communication skills, etc.), b) characteristics of the home/family environment and other contexts within which the individual functions, and c) characteristics of the community within which the individual resides. (p. 13)

More demonstration is needed of effective methods for increasing skills and orientation toward autonomy, self-expression, and personal responsibility of people in residential settings, particularly people who have had little previous opportunity for such expression of individuality.

Communication

Communication abilities are obviously critical to increased self-determination, self-advocacy, and self-expression. Increasingly, these are stressed in instructional goals for persons with mental retardation, including persons with severe cognitive limitations. In recent years, increasing attention has been given to the potential use of augmentative or alternative communication interventions for persons with severe speech or language deficits. Augmentative communication systems use nonspeech methods such as sign language, graphic-based communication boards or wallets, or electronic communication aids to supplement verbal communication, and alternative communication systems use the same methods, alone or in combination, in place of spoken language. In the past, the inclusion of cognitive prerequisites in the decision rules regarding who shall receive augmentative communication training excluded many individuals with severe cognitive deficits from being candidates for such training (Reichle & Karlan, 1985; Romski & Sevcik, 1988). More recently, leading researchers in the area of augmentative communication have moved toward "a 'zero reject' model which allows [speech and language] professionals to provide services to all individuals with cognitive impairments, regardless of the degree of impairment" (Zangari, Kangas, & Lloyd, 1988, p. 62). Effective training strategies have now been developed to teach learners with severe handicaps the use of communication skills, such as requesting items and events, rejecting or protesting items and events, and indicating a choice from an array of two or more items, which are necessary for the exercise of personal autonomy and self-determination (Kangas & Lloyd, 1988; Keogh & Reichle, 1985; Orelove & Sobsey, 1987; Reichle & Keogh, 1986). Communication skills increasingly are seen as absolutely key to two main goals of residential services: increasing autonomy and increasing integration.

Environmental Support for Personal Autonomy

Environments that have provided few choices or ones in which the preferences of individuals were recognized and responded to by well-meaning parents or other caretakers without active participation by the person with disabilities have in many instances inhibited the expression of preference by individuals. Furthermore, even when people with disabilities do express choice, care providers are not always attentive to such expressions. For example, in a school setting for students with severe cognitive impairments, it was noted that only an average of 7% to 15% of student-initiated expressions of preferences or choice-making behaviors were responded to by teaching staff (Houghton, Bronicki, & Guess, 1987), hardly the recipe to stimulate the acquisition and maintenance of such behaviors. In a national study of 336 residents in 181 foster homes and small group home settings (Hill et al., 1989), more than one third of the staff members who claimed to know each particular resident well could not name a favorite food of the resident, hardly an indication of sensitivity to and fostering of choice. Whether such findings derive from a lack of sensitivity among staff, or inability to express personal preference among residents, they provide reason for concern about the attention given to expression of personal autonomy as an essential skill for the independence and integration of people with mental retardation.

Empowerment

Self-advocacy groups are an important exception to the general lack of attention to the expression of independence, preference, and self-determination by persons with mental retardation. According to a survey of 98 consumer self-advocacy groups operated in 35 states, the primary emphases of self-advocacy groups include self-advocacy (learning about rights and responsibilities); self-help (developing self-identity, worth, and confidence); group advocacy (collectively speaking for rights of the handicapped); and recreation (having a meaningful leisure time) (Browning, Thorin, & Rhoades, 1984). Although such groups tend to include persons with relatively mild cognitive limitations (in the Browning et al. study, 45% of the group members were diagnosed with mild, 42% with moderate, and 12% with severe mental retardation), self-advocacy has done much to promote the exercise of self-determination among persons with mental retardation and to develop the skills to act on those preferences. Self-advocacy is still quite limited in total participation and representation in all communities, with the estimated total membership in 1984 of only about 5,000 persons nationwide (Browning et al., 1984). Although memberships is growing rapidly and more and more materials are now available to assist in the organization of such groups and to teach the skills necessary to carry out its collective and individual purposes (Washington State People First, 1983), there is a need to continue to develop greater numbers of such programs. There is also a need to create environments where individuals are empowered as self-advocates to play critical roles in planning their own future, as well as in local, state, and federal policy making.

Prospects for the End of the Century

There is a growing recognition of the importance of personal autonomy for persons with mental retardation. This is being translated into increased attention to providing opportunities and skills required for attaining the maximum personal independence and self-expression. These trends will surely continue, fueled by increasing respect for the rights and responsibilities of people with mental retardation and by the expressed preferences of people with mental retardation and other disabling conditions. In a 1989 National Conference on Self-Determination, consumers articulated a number of recommendations relevant to the provision of housing and residential services, including increased efforts to (a) enable people with disabilities to determine their own futures; (b) support state and local self-advocacy organizations; (c) institute a program to reshape the attitudes of professionals who are currently working with persons with disabilities to value autonomy and choice; (d) include self-determination as a top priority in preservice and inservice training of professionals and paraprofessionals; (e) provide courses in self-assertion to persons with disabilities; (f) reinforce friendships between people with and without disabilities; and (g) facilitate the involvement of people with disabilities in their own program-planning sessions. Although there is a long way to go in incorporating these recommendations, evidence of appreciation and action is available and growing. Clearly, there exists nationwide an increased sensitivity to the acceptance and promotion of personal autonomy and self-expression for persons with mental retardation. Demonstrably effective means of doing so have been developed, and new training and technology-assisted methods continue to be developed. Further prompted by the Americans With Disabilities Act, and other recognitions of the rights of citizenship for persons with disabilities, increased forces in this areas can be expected throughout this next decade. Programs like Minnesota's Partners in Policymaking (Zirpoli, Hancox, Wieck, & Skarnulis, 1989), which provides high-quality training in policymaking and legislative processes at the local, state, and national level to parents and consumers, will be replicated. The self-advocacy movement will assuredly continue to grow throughout the decade. Increasingly, personal autonomy including personal choice, self-determination, self-advocacy, and self-expression will become a central expectation of residential services as we move toward the year 2000.

Conclusions

As the 21st century approaches, changes will continue in both the location and guiding principles of residential services for persons with mental retardation. We have noted that the continual shift from institution to community-based care will mean that by the year 2000 less than a quarter of persons with mental retardation in residential placements will be in facilities of 16 or more residents. But perhaps even more notable will be the growing acceptance that residential settings must be viewed first as the home of the people who live in them. The implications of these changes are revolutionary, and the challenges formidable. Financing residential services over the next decade will be tremendously challenging. Even with improved federal participation in funding community living, the vestiges of our institutional heritage will continue to drain inordinate resources for their dwindling populations. These economic pressures could be increased significantly by economic conditions that are presently unseen but could impact residential services substantially. In addition to the challenges of continuing deinstitutionalization, demographic pressures on the residential services system can be expected to increase demand (and probably the waiting lists) for community services, particularly as aging parents whose sons or daughters with disabilities have lived at home no longer can provide the care their children need. Community services may suffer shortages in staffing produced by a labor pool that is shrinking because of demographic shifts, particularly among the groups of young people who have traditionally staffed community services and among middle-age and older persons who now provide a disproportionate amount of foster–family care.

Much of the attention of advocates, policymakers, and service providers in the past 30 years has focused on the organization and financing of residential service models and related community service programs. The further refinement and expansion of community services and formal and informal supports for persons with mental retardation will continue in the 1990s. But the next decade will also be dominated by increased competition for investment in domestic programs of all types combined with growing public expectations for the development of information that supports the efficiency and effectiveness of service strategies. Increased competition for resources and expectations for accountability will impose pressures on our service programs, but these realities should also stimulate greater opportunities for flexibility and creativity in supporting the needs of persons with mental retardation and their families.

Many important challenges have been discussed throughout this chapter. These challenges are unlikely to reduce the clear national commitment to providing community living opportunities for people with mental retardation. It is clear, however, that the mere physical presence of people with mental retardation in our communities is not going to be in itself satisfactory. Goals for people with mental retardation increasingly will shift from ensuring a *place* in the community to ensuring a *part* in the community (Center on Human Policy, 1989). Having a role in the community means presence in the community, but it also includes personal growth and development in the community, relationships with others in the community, participation in respected aspects of community life, and the ability and opportunity to exercise personal choice, and to express and have respected one's preferences.

In this decade, greater numbers of "residential services systems" will be committed to assisting greater numbers of people with mental retardation to find a place in their communities. These commitments will be reflected as much more personalized approaches to residential services. It is not possible to predict exactly what these approaches will be or the extent to which they will be implemented, but we believe a number of new perspectives on residential services will become highly visible in this decade, including the following:

1. *Increased recognition of an individual's stake in his or her housing and the correspondingly increased involvement of consumers in selecting their own housing*: One's house dictates much of one's life; who one meets, how often one sees family and friends, what one is able to do in spare time, and even the safety with which one can live one's daily life. These are critically important aspects of life, and individuals have the right to have their home congruent with their desires in these areas.

2. *Increased recognition of personal preferences in the creation of a home*: Home is the environment where an individual can most be himself or herself. Home is where one does what one wants, wears what one wants, and eats what one wants. Home is where one's walls are painted a favorite color and the pictures on the walls are one's personal favorites. Increasingly, the personal touches of home will be encouraged and made available to people with mental retardation.

3. *Increased acceptance of affording people with mental retardation to the extent feasible, the same controls over their homes as generally enjoyed by others in the society*: People with mental retardation should have the opportunity to live with whom they choose. They should be able to expect honoring of their voice regarding who comes in and out of their home and for what purpose. They should enjoy the opportunity to entertain family and friends, including persons of the opposite sex. They

should be given opportunities to establish a long-term stake in their housing through purchase or long-term lease.

4. *Increased separation of the housing component of residential services from the residential supports needed by people living in their own homes*: The specific supports and instruction needed by people with mental retardation can be separated from their place of residence. This is a basic premise of the Medicaid Home and Community-Based Services Waiver alternative to institutional care, which offers supports such as case management, habilitative services, personal care and home health services, transportation, and other forms of assistance. Efforts to permit people with mental retardation to have their own homes will require targeting of support services to the specific needs of individuals.

5. *Increased participation of families and consumers in selecting and financing a home*: People with mental retardation and their families can enjoy the same sense of security and financial benefit from home ownership as others in the society. As the separation of residential and support components of residential services become more easily accomplished, more parents and consumers will bind together with developers and real estate brokers to purchase individual and cooperative housing for persons with mental retardation. This trend could also produce important financial dividends for the financing of programs, because housing equity will belong increasingly to consumers for supporting aspects of daily living.

6. *Increased participation by people with mental retardation in the neighborhoods in which they are living*. Finding a place in one's community means not only living in the community but also sharing in the activities and organizations of that community. There will be increased emphasis throughout this decade on people participating in the specific community in which they are living. This will include not only resource-consuming activities but also contributing activities. Passage of the Americans With Disabilities Act will foster such participation.

7. *Increased empowerment and promotion of the involvement of families in defining, authorizing, securing, and/or providing needed supports*: Parents who have raised their children at home and enjoyed the expanding benefits of free public education expect to be involved in the life of their child. Having raised their child to adulthood, they know him or her well and they know what he or she needs. The knowledge and sophistication of contemporary parents and their strong commitment to the well-being of their child increasingly will be brought together in a formal empowerment of parents to make service decisions regarding their child and to act as a broker in securing those services.

8. *Greater attention to the quality of life of people in residential settings*: Attention to quality of life in residential settings will bring added attention to the important aspects of social participation and contribution through employment, social relationships, and other considerations that

define quality of life for nondisabled members of the community. In turn, isolation experienced by many persons with mental retardation in our communities will be reduced. There will be growing public commitment to meaningful social integration, to improve access to technology, to support community participation and to provide economic opportunities to contribute to and benefit from economic activity.

9. *Increased emphasis on ensuring that services meet acceptable standards, and that programs provide information to evaluate their efficiency and effectiveness*: Increased expectations to account for public investment will accompany improvements in evaluation methodologies and growing competition for public resources. This emphasis on assessing the quality and return on public investment, if addressed creatively, will lessen the rigidity of current finance and organizational strategies in providing residential services and supports to individuals and families.

10. *Increased strategic attention to the recruitment, preparation, and retention of personnel in residential service programs*: Recruitment and retention of staff in times of chronic labor shortages, particularly among groups traditionally providing direct services will necessitate major and specific attention to personnel issues. In addition, continued growth in community services will mean increasing the numbers and responsibilities of paraprofessional staff. The majority of public and private investment gocs to the payment of salaries to personnel. Few accepted standards exist for training or experience for professional and paraprofessional personnel. In the next few years, increased attention will be given to all aspects of personnel management, including recruitment, training, compensation, implementation of standards and other areas relevant to the quality and stability of the work force.

Benjamin Friedman, economist and author of *Day of Reckoning* (Friedman, 1988), stated that "history runs in only one direction" (p. 87). The trends toward community living and more normal life-styles in residential services will continue in this decade and well into the next century. But designing and implementing strategic efforts to guide these trends will not be simple. The challenges ahead require continued change from centralization to decentralization, from an emphasis on agency to individual, from professional programs to paraprofessional and family supports, from limited, inefficient options to truly individualized, efficient, and productive approaches. Achieving the full measure of new directions discussed in this chapter will demand greater consensus among policymakers, consumers, providers, and others in matters of mission and purpose of residential services as well as policies of greater congruence with our mission and purpose. There is reason to believe that this will happen and that, although the future in residential services is not certain, the coming decade holds considerable promise for improving the quality of life for persons with mental retardation in residential settings.

Acknowledgment. Preparation of this chapter was supported in part by the National Institute on Disability and Rehabilitation Research (Cooperative Agreement No. H133B80050) and the Administration on Developmental Disabilities (Grant No. 90DD145/02).

References

Abery, B. H., & Bruininks, R. H. (1990). *Facilitating the self-determination of youth with disabilities*. Unpublished manuscript, University of Minnesota, Department of Educational Psychology, Minneapolis.

Amado, A. N., Lakin, K. C., & Menke, J. M. (1990). *1990 chartbook on services for people with developmental disabilities*. Minneapolis: University of Minnesota, Center for Residential and Community Services.

Anderson, D. J., Lakin, K. C., Bruininks, R. H., & Hill, B. K. (1987). *A national study of residential and support services for elderly people with mental retardation*. Minneapolis: University of Minnesota, Center for Residential and Community Services.

Ashbaugh, J., & Allard, M. A. (1984). *Comparative analysis of the cost of residential, day, and other programs within institutional and community settings*. Boston: Human Services Research Institute.

Baker, B. K., Seltzer, G. B., & Seltzer, M. M. (1974). *As close as possible: Community residences for retarded adults*. Boston: Little, Brown.

Bell, N. J., Schoenrock, C. J., & Bensberg, G. J. (1981). Change over time in the community: Findings of a longitudinal study. In R. H. Bruininks, C. E. Meyers, B. B. Sigford, & K. C. Lakin (Eds.), *Deinstitutionalization and community adjustment of mentally retarded people* (pp. 195–206). Washington, DC: American Association on Mental Deficiency.

Bensberg, G. J., & Smith, J. J. (1984). *Comparative costs of public residential and community residential facilities for the mentally retarded*. Lubbock: Texas Tech University, Research and Training Center in Mental Retardation.

Bercovici, S. M. (1983). *Barriers to normalization: The restrictive management of retarded persons*. Baltimore: University Park Press.

Biklen, D. (1985). *Achieving the complete school: Strategies for effective mainstreaming*. New York: Teachers College Press.

Birenbaum, A., & Re, M. A. (1979). Resettling mentally retarded adults in the community—Almost four years later. *American Journal of Mental Deficiency*, *83*, 323–329.

Birenbaum, A., & Seiffer, S. (1976). *Resettling retarded adults in a managed community*. New York: Praeger.

Bjaanes, A. T., & Butler, E. W. (1974). Environmental variation in community care facilities for mentally retarded persons. *American Journal of Mental Deficiency*, *78*, 429–439.

Bogdan, R., & Taylor, S. J. (1987a). The next wave. In S. J. Taylor, D. Biklen, & J. Knoll (Eds.), *Community integration for people with severe disabilities* (pp. 209–213). New York: Teachers College Press.

Bogdan, R., & Taylor, S. J. (1987b). Toward a sociology of acceptance: The other side of the study of deviance. *Social Policy*, *18*(2), 34–39.

Bogdan, R., & Taylor, S. J. (1989). Relationships with severely disabled people: The social construction of humanness. *Social Problems, 36*(2), 135–148.

Bott, E. (1971). *Family and social network.* New York: Free Press.

Braddock, D., Hemp, R., Fujiura, G., Bachelder, L., & Mitchell, D. (1989). *Public expenditures for mental retardation and developmental disabilities in the United States: State profile* (3rd ed.). Chicago: University of Illinois, University Affiliated Program in Developmental Disabilities.

Braddock, D., Hemp, R., Fujiura, G., Bachelder, L., & Mitchell, D. (1990). *The state of the states in developmental disabilities.* Baltimore, MD: Paul H. Brookes.

Bradley, V. J., Conroy, J. W., Covert, S. B., & Feinstein, C. S. (1986). *Community options: The New Hampshire choice.* Cambridge, MA: Human Services Research Institute.

Bradley, V. J., Knoll, J. A., Covert, S., Osuch, R., O'Connor, S., Agosta, J., & Blaney, B. (1990). *Family support services in the United States: An end of decade status report.* Cambridge, MA: Human Services Research Institute.

Bregman, S. (1984). Assertiveness training for mentally retarded adults. *Mental Retardation, 22,* 12–16.

Brown, L., Nietupski, J., & Hamre-Nietupski, S. (1976). The criterion of ultimate functioning and public school services for severely handicapped students. In L. Brown, N. Certo, & T. Crowner (Eds.), *Papers and programs related to public school services for secondary-age severely handicapped–students.* (Vol. VI, pp. 2–15). Madison, WI: Madison Metropolitan School District.

Browning, P., Thorin, E., & Rhoades, C. (1984). A national profile of self-help/self-advocacy groups of people with mental retardation. *Mental Retardation, 22,* 226–230.

Bruininks, R. H., & Lakin, K. C. (Eds.). (1985). *Living and learning in the least restrictive alternative.* Baltimore, MD: Paul H. Brookes.

Bruininks, R. H., Thurlow, M., Lewis, D., & Larson, N. W. (1988). *Post school outcomes for special education students one to eight years after high school.* Minneapolis: University of Minnesota, Institute on Community Integration.

Bruininks, R. H., Thurlow, M., & Steffans, K. (1988). *Follow-up of students after schooling and suburban special education district: Outcomes for people with moderate to severe handicaps.* Minneapolis: University of Minnesota, Institute on Community Integration.

Budde, J. F., & Bachelder, J. L. (1986). Independent living: The concept, model, and methodology. *Journal of the Association for Persons With Severe Handicaps, 11,* 240–245.

Burchard, S., & Thousand, J. (1988). Staff and manager competencies. In M. Janicki, M. Krauss, & M. Seltzer (Eds.), *Community residences for persons with developmental disabilities: Here to stay* (pp. 251–266). Baltimore, MD: Paul H. Brookes.

Calkins, C., Walker, H., Bacon-Prue, A., Gibson, B., Martinson, M., & Offner, R. (1985). *The learning adjustment process: Implications of a national profile of adult development.* Logan, UT: Utah State University, Developmental Center for Handicapped Persons.

Campbell, E. M., & Smith, G. A. (1989, March 20). *Predictors of service costs for people with developmental disabilities.* Paper presented at the Pacific Rim Conference on Quality of Life for Persons with Disabilities. Honolulu.

Center on Human Policy (1989). *From being in the community to being part of the community: The proceedings of a Leadership Institute for Persons With Developmental Disabilities.* Syracuse, NY: Syracuse University, Research and Training Center on Community Living.

Certo, N., Schleien, S., & Hunter, D. (1983). An ecological assessment inventory to facilitate community recreation participation by severely disabled individuals. *Therapeutic Recreation Journal, 17*(3), 29–38.

Conroy, J. W., & Bradley, V. J. (1985). *The Pennhurst longitudinal study: A report of five years of research and analysis.* Philadelphia: Temple University Developmental Disabilities Center.

Conroy, J. W., Lemanowicz, J. A., & Feinstein, C. S. (1987). *Pennhurst class members in CLA's: The views of families in 1986, and changes from 1985 to 1986.* Philadelphia: Temple University, Research & Quality Assurance Group.

Craig, E. M., & McCarver, R. (1984). Community placement and adjustment of deinstitutionalized clients: Issues and findings. In N. W. Bray & N. Ellis (Eds.), *International review of research in mental retardation* (pp. 91–122). New York: Academic Press.

Crapps, J., Langione, J., & Swaim, S. (1985). Quantity and quality of participation in community environments by mentally retarded adults. *Education and Training of the Mentally Retarded, 20,* 123–129.

Dalgleish, M. (1983). Assessments of residential environments for mentally retarded adults in Britain. *Mental Retardation, 21,* 275–281.

D'Amico, M. L., Hannah, M. A., Milhouse, J. A., & Froleich, A. K. (1978). *Evaluation of adaptive behavior: Institutional vs. community placements and treatment for the mentally retarded.* Stillwater: Oklahoma State University, National Clearinghouse of Rehabilitation Materials.

Davis, S. (1987). *National status report on waiting lists of people with mental retardation for community-based services.* Arlington, TX: Association for Retarded Citizens–United States.

Eastwood, E. A. (1985). *Community living study: Three reports of client development, family impact, and the cost of services among community-based and institutionalized persons with mental retardation.* Belchertown, MA: Belchertown State School.

Eastwood, E. A., & Fisher, G. A. (1988). Skill acquisition among matched samples of institutionalized and community-based persons with mental retardation. *American Journal on Mental Retardation, 93,* 75–83.

Edgerton, R. B. (1967). *The cloak of competence: Stigma in the lives of the mentally retarded.* Berkeley, CA: University of California.

Edgerton, R. B., & Bercovici, S. M. (1976). The cloak of competence: Years later. *American Journal of Mental Deficiency, 80*(5), 485–497.

Falvey, M. A. (1986). *Community-based curriculum: Instructional strategies for students with severe handicaps.* Baltimore, MD: Paul H. Brookes.

Feinstein, C. S., Lemanowicz, J. A., & Conroy, J. W. (1988). *A survey of family satisfaction with regional treatment centers and community services to persons with mental retardation in Minnesota, Welsch v. Gardebring class members.* Philadelphia: Conroy & Feinstein Associates.

Felce, D., de Kock, U., & Repp, A. C. (1986). An eco-behavioral analysis of small community-based houses and traditional large hospitals for severely and profoundly mentally handicapped adults. *Applied Research in Mental Retardation, 7,* 393–408.

Friedman, B. A. (1988). *Day of reckoning: The caregivers of American economic policy under Reagan and after.* New York: Random House.

Frohboese, R., & Sales, B. D. (1980). Parental opposition to deinstitutionalization: A challenge in need of attention and resolution. *Law and Human Behavior, 4,* 1–87.

Gaylord-Ross, R. J., & Holvoet, J. F. (1985). *Strategies for educating students with severe handicaps.* Boston: Little, Brown.

George, M. J., & Baumeister, A. A. (1981). Employee withdrawal and job satisfaction in community residential facilities for mentally retarded people. *American Journal of Mental Deficiency, 85,* 639–647.

Gollay, E., Freedman, R., Wyngaarden, M., & Kurtz, N. R. (1978). *Coming back: The community experiences of deinstitutionalized mentally retarded people.* Cambridge, MA: Abt Books.

Guerin, P. (1976). *Family therapy: Theory and practice.* New York: Gartner.

Guess, D., Benson, H. H., & Siegel-Causey, E. (1985). Concepts and issues related to choice-making and autonomy among persons with severe disabilities. *Journal of the Association for Persons With Severe Handicaps, 10*(2), 79–86.

Halpern, A. S., Close, D. W., & Nelson, D. J. (1986). *On my own: The impact of semi-independent living programs for adults with mental retardation.* Baltimore, MD: Paul H. Brookes.

Heal, L. W. (1988). Evaluating residential alternatives. In L. W. Heal, J. I. Haney, & A. R. Novak Amado (Eds.), *Integration of developmentally disabled individuals into the community* (2nd ed., pp. 211–225). Baltimore, MD: Paul H. Brookes.

Hill, B. K., & Bruininks, R. H. (1981). *Family, leisure, and social activities of mentally retarded people in residential facilities.* Minneapolis: University of Minnesota, Department of Educational Psychology.

Hill, B. K., Lakin, K. C., & Bruininks, R. H. (1984). Trends in residential services for people who are mentally retarded: 1977–1982. *Journal of the Association for Persons with Severe Handicaps, 9*(4), 243–250.

Hill, B. K., Lakin, K. C., Bruininks, R. H., Amado, A. N., Anderson, D. J., & Copher, J. I. (1989). *Living in the community: A comparative study of foster homes and small group homes for people with mental retardation* (Report No. 28). Minneapolis: University of Minnesota, Center for Residential and Community Services.

Hill, B. K., Rotegard, L. L., & Bruininks, R. H. (1983). Quality of life of mentally retarded people in residential care. *Social Work, 29*(3), 275–281.

Holman, J., & Bruininks, R. (1985). Assessing and training adaptive behaviors. In K. C. Lakin & R. Bruininks (Eds.), *Strategies for achieving community integration of developmentally disabled citizens* (pp. 73–104). Baltimore, MD: Paul H. Brookes.

Horner, R. H., Stoner, S. K., & Ferguson, D. L. (1988). *An activity-based analysis of deinstitutionalization: The effects of community re-entry on the lives of residents leaving Oregon's Fairview Training Center.* Eugene: University of Oregon, Specialized Training Program, Center on Human Development.

Houghton, J., Bronicki, G. J. B., & Guess, D. (1987). Opportunities to express preferences and make choices among students with severe disabilities in classroom settings. *Journal of the Association for Persons With Severe Handicaps*, *12*, 18–27.

Intagliata, J., Willer, B., & Wicks, N. (1981). Factors related to the quality of community adjustment in family care homes. In R. H. Bruininks, C. E. Meyers, B. B. Sigford, & K. C. Lakin (Eds.), *Deinstitutionalization and community adjustment of mentally retarded people* (pp. 217–232). Washington, DC: American Association on Mental Deficiency.

Jones, P., Conroy, J., Feinstein, C., & Lemanowicz, J. (1983). *A matched comparison study of cost-effectiveness: Institutionalized and deinstitutionalized clients*. Philadelphia: Temple University, Developmental Disabilities Center.

Kangas, K. A., & Lloyd, L. (1988). Early cognitive skills as prerequisites to augmentative and alternative communication use: What are we waiting for? *AAC Augmentative and Alternative Communication*, *4*, 211–221.

Kennedy, M. (1989, November). Out of my old life and into my new one. *Community Living for Adults*, pp. 3–4. Syracuse, NY: Syracuse University, Center on Human Policy.

Keogh, W., & Reichle, J. (1985). Communication intervention for the "difficult-to-teach" severely handicapped. In S. Warren & A. Rogers-Warren (Eds.), *Teaching functional language* (pp. 157–193). Baltimore: University Park Press.

King, R. D., Raynes, N. V., & Tizard, J. (1971). *Patterns of residential care: Sociological studies in institutions for handicapped children*. London: Routledge & Kegan Paul.

Kishi, G., Teelucksingh, B., Zollers, N., Park-Lee, S., & Mcyer, L. (1988). Daily decision-making in community residences: A social comparison of adults with and without mental retardation. *American Journal of Mental Retardation*, *92*(5), 430–435.

Lakin, K. C., Anderson, D. J., & Hill, B. K. (1988). *Community integration of older persons with mental retardation*. Minneapolis: University of Minnesota, Research and Training Center on Community Living.

Lakin, K. C., & Bruininks, R. H. (1981). *Occupational stability of direct-care staff of residential facilities for mentally retarded people* (Report No. 14). Minneapolis: University of Minnesota, Department of Psychoeducational Studies, Developmental Disabilities Project on Residential Services and Community Adjustment.

Lakin, K. C., Bruininks, R. H., Hill, B. K., & Hauber, F. A. (1982). Turnover of direct-care staff in a national sample of residential facilities for mentally retarded people. *American Journal of Mental Deficiency*, *87*, 64–72.

Lakin, K. C., Bruininks, R. H., & Sigford, B. B. (1981). Early perspectives on the community adjustment of mentally retarded people. In R. H. Bruininks, C. E. Meyers, B. B. Sigford, & K. C. Lakin (Eds.), *Deinstitutionalization and community adjustment of mentally retarded people* (pp. 28–50). Washington DC: American Association on Mental Deficiency.

Lakin, K. C., Hill, B. K., & Bruininks, R. H. (1985). *An analysis of Medicaid's Intermediate Care for the Mentally Retarded (ICF-MR) program*. Minneapolis: University of Minnesota, Center for Residential and Community Services.

Lakin, K. C., Hill, B. K., Chen, T. H., & Stephens, S. A. (1989). *Persons with mental retardation and related conditions in mental retardation facilities: Selected findings from the 1987 National Medicaid Expenditures Survey.* Minneapolis: University of Minnesota, Center for Residential and Community Services.

Lakin, K. C., Jaskulski, T. M., Hill, B. K., Bruininks, R. H., Menke, J. M., White, C. C., & Wright, E. A. (1989). *Medicaid services for persons with mental retardation and related conditions.* Minneapolis: University of Minnesota, Institute on Community Integration.

Lakin, K. C., White, C. C., Hill, B. K., Bruininks, R. H., & Wright, E. A. (1990). Longitudinal change and interstate variability in residential services for people with mental retardation. *Mental Retardation, 28*(6), 343–352.

Larson, S. A., & Lakin, K. C. (1989a). Deinstitutionalization of persons with mental retardation: Behavioral outcomes. *Journal of the Association for Persons With Severe Handicaps, 14,* 324–332.

Larson, S. A., & Lakin, K. C. (1989b). Parent attitudes about their daughter's or son's residential placement before and after deinstitutionalization. *Policy Research Brief, 1* (Whale No. 2). Minneapolis: University of Minnesota, Institute on Community Integration.

Liberty, K. (1985). Enhancing instruction for maintenance, generalization, and adaptation. In K. C. Lakin & R. H. Bruininks (Eds.), *Strategies for achieving community integration of developmentally disabled citizens* (pp. 29–71). Baltimore, MD: Paul H. Brookes.

Malin, N. A. (1982). Group homes for mentally handicapped adults: Residents' view on contacts and support. *British Journal of Mental Subnormality, 28,* 29–34.

Mansell, J., Jenkins, J., Felce, D., & de Kock, U. (1984). Measuring the activity of severely and profoundly mentally handicapped adults in ordinary housing. *Behavior Research and Therapy, 22,* 23–29.

Martin, J. E. (1988). Providing training in community and domestic skills. In L. W. Heal, J. I. Haney, & A. R. Novak Amado (Eds.). *Integration of developmentally disabled individuals into the community* (2nd ed., pp. 169–191). Baltimore, MD: Paul H. Brookes.

Meyers, J. C., & Marcenko, M. O. (1989). Impact of a cash subsidy program for families of children with severe developmental disabilities. *Mental Retardation, 27,* 383–387.

Minnesota Department of Welfare. (1979). *Residential care study.* St. Paul, MN: Author.

Mithaug, D. E., & Hanawalt, D. A. (1978). The validation of procedures to assess prevocational task perferences in retarded adults. *Journal of Applied Behavior Analysis, 11*(1), 153–162.

Mount, B., & Zwernik, K. (1988). *It's never too early, it's never too late: A booklet about personal futures planning* (Publication No. 421-88-109). St. Paul, MN: Metropolitan Council.

National Conference on Self-Determination (1989, January). *29+ Recommendations from the conference participants.* Minneapolis: University of Minnesota, Institute on Community Integration.

O'Brien, J. (1987). A guide to life style planning: Using *The Activities Catalog* to integrate services and natural support systems: In B. Wilcox & G. T. Bellamy (Eds.), *The activities catalog: A community programming guide for youth and adults with severe disabilities* (pp. 175–189). Baltimore, MD: Paul H. Brooks.

O'Connor, G. O. (1976). *Home is a good place: A national perspective on community residential facilities for developmentally disabled persons.* Washington, DC: American Association on Mental Deficiency.

O'Neil, J., Brown, M., Gordon, W., Schonhorn, R., & Green, E. (1981). Activity patterns of mentally retarded adults in institutions and communities— A longitudinal study. *Applied Research in Mental Retardation, 2,* 267–379.

Orelove, F. P., & Sobsey, D. (1987). *Educating children with multiple disabilities: A transdisciplinary approach.* Baltimore, MD: Paul H. Brookes.

Putnam, J. W., Werder, J. K., & Schleien, S. J. (1985). Leisure and recreation services for handicapped persons. In K. C. Lakin & R. H. Bruininks (Eds.), *Strategies for achieving community integration of developmentally disabled citizens* (pp. 253–274). Baltimore, MD: Paul H. Brookes.

Reichle, J., & Karlan, G. (1985). The selection of an augmentative system in communication intervention: A critique of decision rules. *Journal of the Association for Persons with Severe Handicaps, 10,* 146–156.

Reichle, J., & Keogh, W. (1986). Communication instruction for learners with severe handicaps: Some unresolved issues. In R. Horner, L. Meyer, & H. Fredericks (Eds.), *Education of learners with severe handicaps: Exemplary service strategies* (pp. 189–219). Baltimore, MD: Paul H. Brookes.

Romski, M. A., & Sevcik, R. A. (1988). Augmentative and alternative communication systems: Considerations for individuals with severe intellectual disabilities. *AAC Augmentative and Alternative Communication, 4,* 83–93.

Rosen, M., Floor, L., & Sizfein, L. (1974). Investigating the phenomenon of acquiescence in the mentally handicapped: I. Theoretical model test development and normative data. *British Journal of Mental Subnormality, 20,* 58–68.

Rotegard, L., Hill, B., & Bruininks, R. H. (1982). *Environmental characteristics of residential facilities for mentally retarded people.* Minneapolis: University of Minnesota, Center for Residential and Community Services.

Schleien, S. J., & Meyer, L. H. (1988). Community-based recreation for persons with severe developmental disabilities. In M. D. Powers (Ed.), *Expanding systems of service delivery for persons with developmental disabilities.* Baltimore, MD: Paul H. Brookes.

Seltzer, G. B. (1981). Community residential adjustment: The relationship among environments, performance and satisfaction. *American Journal of Mental Deficiency, 85,* 624–630.

Seltzer, M., Sherwood, C., Seltzer, G., & Sherwood, S. (1981). Community adaptation and the impact of deinstitutionalization. In R. H. Bruininks, C. E. Meyers, B. B. Sigford, & K. C. Lakin (Eds.), *Deinstitutionalization and community adjustment of mentally retarded persons* (pp. 82–88). Washington, DC: American Association on Mental Deficiency.

Shevin, M., & Klein, N. K. (1984). The importance of choice-making skills for students with severe disabilities. *Journal of the Association for Persons With Severe Handicaps, 9*(3), 159–166.

Sigelman, C. K., Schoenrock, C. J., Winer, J. L., Spanhel, C. L., Hromas, S. G., Martin, P. W., Budd, E. C., & Bensberg, G. J. (1981). Issues in interviewing mentally retarded persons: An empirical study. In R. H. Bruininks, C. E. Meyers, B. B. Sigford, & K. C. Lakin (Eds.), *Deinstitutionalization and community adjustment of mentally retarded persons* (pp. 114–129). Washington, DC: American Association on Mental Deficiency.

Silverstein, A. B., McLain, R. E., Hubbell, M., & Brownlee, L. (1977). Characteristics of the treatment environment: A factor-analytic study. *Educational and Psychological Measurement*, *37*, 367–371.

Snell, M. E. (1987). *Systematic instruction of persons with severe handicaps* (3rd ed.). Columbus, OH: Charles E. Merrill.

State of Wisconsin, Bureau of Evaluation, Division of Policy and Budget. (1986). *Evaluation of the community integration program*. Madison: Author.

Stoneman, Z., & Crapps, J. M. (1990). Mentally retarded individuals in family care homes: Relationships with the family of origin. *American Journal on Mental Retardation*, *94*, 420–430.

Strully, J., & Strully, C. (1985). Friendship and our children. *Journal of the Association for Persons with Severe Handicaps*, *10*(4), 224–227.

Taylor, S. J., & Bogdan, R. (1989). On accepting relationships between people with disabilities and nondisabled people: Toward understanding of acceptance. *Disability, Handicap and Society*, *4*(1), 21–36.

Taylor, S. J., Biklin, D., & Knoll, J. (1987). *Community integration of people with severe disabilities*. New York: Teachers College Press.

Taylor, S. J., Lakin, K. C., & Hill, B. K. (1989). Permanency planning for all children and youth: Policy and philosophy to govern out-of-home placement decisions. *Exceptional Children*, *55*(6), 541–549.

Thurlow, M. L., Bruininks, R. H., & Lange, C. M. (1989). *Assessing post-school outcomes for students with moderated to severe mental retardation* (Report No. 89-1). Minneapolis: University of Minnesota, Institute on Community Integration.

Touche Ross & Co. (1980). *Cost study of the community based mental retardation regions and the Beatrice State Developmental Center*. Kansas, MO: Author.

Tymchuk, A. J., Andron, L., & Rahbar, B. (1988). Effective decision-making/problem solving training with mothers who have mental retardation. *American Journal on Mental Retardation*, *92*, 510–516.

Vandercook, T., York, J., & Forrest, M. (1989). The McGill Action Planning System (MAPS): A strategy for building the vision. *Journal of the Association for Persons With Severe Handicaps*, *14*, 205–215.

Walker, P., & Edinger, B. (1988). The kid from cabin 17. *Camping Magazine*, *Fall*, 18–21.

Ward, M. J. (1988). The many facets of self-determination. *Transition Summary* (National Information Center for Children and Youth With Handicaps), *5*, 2–3.

Washington State People First. (1983). *The people first handbook*. Tacoma, WA: Author.

Wehman, P. (1981). *Competitive employment: New horizons for severely disabled individuals*. Baltimore, MD: Paul H. Brookes.

White, C. C., Lakin, K. C., & Bruininks, R. H. (1989). *Persons with mental retardation and related conditions in state-operated residential facilities: Year ending June 30, 1988 with longitudinal trends from 1950 to 1988* (Report No. 30). Minneapolis: University of Minnesota, Department of Educational Psychology.

White, C. C., Lakin, K. C., Hill, B. K., Wright, E. A., & Bruininks, R. H. (1988). *Persons with mental retardation in state-operated residential facilities: Year ending June 30, 1987 with longitudinal trends from 1950 to 1987* (Report

No. 26). Minneapolis: University of Minnesota, Department of Educational Psychology.

Wilcox, B., & Bellamy, G. T. (1982). *Design of high school programs for severely handicapped students*. Baltimore, MD: Paul H. Brookes.

Willer, B., & Intagliata, J. (1980). *Deinstitutionalization of mentally retarded persons in New York State*. Buffalo: State University of New York at Buffalo, Research Foundation.

Willer, B., & Intagliata, J. (1984). *Promises and realities for mentally retarded citizens: Life in the community*. Baltimore, MD: University Park Press.

Wolfensberger, W. (1983). Social role valorization: A proposed new term for the principle of normalization. *Mental Retardation, 21*(6), 234–239.

Zaharia, E. S., & Baumeister, A. A. (1979). Technician losses in public residential facilities. *American Journal of Mental Deficiency, 84*, 34–39.

Zangari, C., Kangas, K. A., & Lloyd, L. L. (1988). Augmentative and alternative communication: A field in transition. *AAC Augmentative and Alternative Communication, 4*, 60–65.

Zimmerman, S. L. (1984). The mental retardation family subsidy program: Its effects on families with a mentally handicapped child. *Family Relations, 33*(2), 105–118.

Zirpoli, T. J., Hancox, D., Wieck, C., & Skarnulis, E. R. (1989). Partners in policymaking: Empowering people. *Journal of the Association for Persons With Severe Handicaps, 14*, 163–167.

Part 4
Trends on Service and Policy Issues

15
Critical Issues in Planning Vocational Services in the 1990s

PAUL WEHMAN and WENDY PARENT

Efforts to predict the future are always difficult, even under the best of circumstances. In trying to assess what vocational opportunities will be available to people with mental retardation as this century closes, several difficulties come to mind. First, vocational programs depend heavily on the overall labor market and economy. As Stark and Goldsbury (1988) point out, one cannot analyze future trends for persons with disabilities out of the context of society as a whole. There is not a clear picture as of yet about how inflation, interest rates, or automation and mechanization will affect the labor force. We do know that there will probably continue for sometime to be a labor shortage in entry-level service occupations. Persons with mental retardation should be able to expand their growth into these positions.

A second difficulty in long-term assessments involves the availability of financial resources to fund social and rehabilitation programs for disadvantaged members of society. Who could have foreseen at the beginning of 1989 the crumbling of the Eastern European Communist bloc? Who, even now, knows the full implications of the transformation on the United States and other free-world economies, annual budgets, and reallocations of funds? It does seem possible, however, that domestic programs will suffer at the expense of the defense budget.

Yet a third difficulty, which cannot be ignored, is the continuing lack of coordination and strategic planning between the many agencies that are charged in some fashion with helping or advocating for individuals with disabilities. The conflicting intent of different pieces of legislation, laborious nature of regulatory procedures, and inability to gain compliance from under funded programs are major obstacles to reducing the unconsciousably high unemployment rate of persons with disabilities, which some have put as high as 66% (Harris Poll, 1986).

It is our purpose in this chapter to review those trends that we feel are here to stay and will not fade out with yesterday's news. We believe that some aspects of vocational progress in the 1980s, such as the move toward integrated employment or efforts to identify disabled youngsters (aged 18 to 21) as high-priority candidates for vocational services, will not be turned back but should continue to expand and be better defined. What follows is a review of several of these trends and needs, which we feel will characterize vocational services into the 1990s.

A total of 6 years have passed since the U.S. Department of Education established transition from school to work as a major federal initiative (Will, 1984). Since that time, significant research and scholarly activity have occurred, as have many state and federally funded model demonstration programs in the area of transition (Everson, 1988). Much of the impetus for this work has been stimulated because of the discouraging postsecondary employment outcome data that are associated with youngsters with disabilities after they leave school (e.g., Hasazi, Gordon, & Roe, 1985; Wehman, Kregel, & Seyfarth, 1985; see Chapter 2 in Wehman, Moon, Everson, Wood, & Barcus, 1988).

In lieu of the poor employment status attained by young adults with disabilities, Edgar (1987; 1988) has developed two highly provocative papers in which he seriously questions how justifiable secondary special education is. Edgar challenges the practices and philosophies of secondary special education and asks how transition can work in the present environment:

... analysis of data collected in recent follow-up studies of handicapped students who left school indicates that the transition process is incomplete: Few handicapped students move from school to independent living in communities. Secondary special education programs appear to have little impact on students' adjustment to community life. More than 30% of the students enrolled in secondary special education programs drop out. (Edgar, 1987, p. 555)

The Edgar papers (1987, 1988) are excellent because they are forcing educators and others to think critically about progress, or lack of it, which has been made to date. We have carefully reviewed the major concepts of these papers and, while agreeing that the outcomes are nowhere yet near what we wish to see, we fundamentally disagree with the ideas and thoughts for change. We believe that for the most part the field has in place many of the elements necessary for meaningful transition. These elements, however, simply have not yet been completely put together in most communities. Therefore, the purpose of the following sections is to review best practices in secondary special education and identify elements in transition that are necessary to effect positive postsecondary outcomes for young adults with disabilities.

Critical Elements in Meaningful Transition

Meaningful transition can be defined as postsecondary employment in real work once school is completed or toward the end of the school period. Transition also means moving toward postsecondary residential independence and individual competence in community living.

Transition is Community

In developing a sound conceptual framework for approaching the transition area, it is important to understand that school to adulthood activities must be planned in the context of the local community. Rural communities will implement transition differently from highly urban inner-city communities. The community will be influenced by the local economy, which will in turn influence the tax base of dollars from which schools and social service agencies can be funded. The status of postsecondary agencies, the educational level of parents of students with disabilities, and the availability of leadership and/or university personnel nearby are just some of the critical features that help to sharply influence whether meaningful transition can occur or not. As we have observed earlier (Wehman, Kregel, & Barcus, 1985), it is noteworthy that transition cannot be developed exclusively by the schools or vocational rehabilitation or any one agency alone. Transition is based heavily on the local community.

Transition is Individual Student Choice

Transition planning for adulthood requires major student input. What job(s) does the student want? Where does he wish to live? How does she wish to spend her free time? How does he wish to spend his money? What freedom does she have to change her mind? School curricular planning, individual educational rehabilitation plans, and above all, teacher and counselor attitudes do *not* currently reflect a major role for student choice. The solution seems to be the creation of a more formal mechanism to plan for meaningful and frequent input to postsecondary planning and outcomes. We believe that students and families must be educated in, first, what their options are; second, what they could be; and third, how they can exercise those options. The relationship between educator, student, and family must be educative and collegial, not supervisor–subordinate.

Transition is Shared Resources

There is not enough money, and almost certainly will never be enough, for one agency alone to provide for all of the promises that the transition initiative suggests. Furthermore, even if there were enough money, the very essence of effective transition requires *interagency* or cross-agency interaction. There are at least three ways for agencies to work together on behalf of transition-age youth (Wehman, et al., 1988). First, there can be *information sharing*, that is, vocational rehabilitation, special education, and adult community service programs simply communicate to each other about program alternatives. A second model, known as *responsibility transfer*, takes this one step further with their agencies contracting with each other or assigning responsibility from one agency to the other through a fee-for-service arrangement. Yet a third model is that of *interagency collaboration*. Within this model, all three agencies work together and share cash or in-kind resources for specific targeted outcomes, i.e., job placement of eight students with autism.

The shared resources approach seems to be a critical component distinguished between affective programs and those that are mediocre or fragmented. This model provides a structured way to sort out which students need what services, when the services will be delivered, and how programs will be funded.

Vocational Rehabilitation Counselors Need to Be in the Schools

For thousands of special education students, especially those with mild handicaps, rehabilitation counselors can play a major role in bridging the gap between school and work. However, the counselor needs to be physically present and available for teachers, guidance counselors, work-study coordinators, and administrators to see. At one time in the late 1960s and early 1970s, with the advent of the career education movement, rehabilitation counselors were frequently based in public schools. This practice was modified in many places when the new special education law (PL 94-142) was passed in 1976. Clearly, it would be advantageous to transition-age youngsters with disabilities if (a) rehabilitation counselors were based at special education programs and (b) sufficient numbers of counselors were available to handle what often turns out to be a crushing caseload. If, in fact, interagency collaboration and shared resources are critical elements toward the target of job placement, then the agency representatives absolutely must have physical proximity and regular contact with each other.

Business Linkage With School Programs

Although it has been commonly observed that business and industry linkage and communication are important in secondary education programs, amazingly, many schools have not actively courted the business community. It would appear, however, that a structured and formal linkage is absolutely essential for at least three reasons. First, local business representatives, if used appropriately, can be a major source of helping school officials determine the marketability of the special and vocational education curriculum. Members of the business community should be asked to assess how useful the school curriculum is in terms of vocational planning and outcomes. Second, businesses can be an excellent source of training sites in all types of occupations and industries. And, third, business is where students will work once leaving school, hence, the better business and schools understand each other, the more successful will a job placement become. Communication with employers about capacities and limitations of youngsters with disabilities is imperative. As we enter the 1990s, there is clearly a shortage of labor, especially in entry-level service occupations. Young adults with disabilities can prove to be a very effective source of labor, but educators must reach out to the business community.

Expanding Employment Opportunities

The effectiveness of even the best vocational education programs and transition plans is limited if employment opportunities are not available through adult rehabilitation services. Until the last decade, the vocational service option of choice has been placement into a sheltered workshop or day-activity program. The emphasis of these programs was on providing long-term evaluation, skills training, and work adjustment to prepare individuals for paid work in the community. The actual outcomes achieved, such as lack of movement out of the facility, long waiting lists for services, increased program costs, and lack of opportunities for integration, have prompted the development of alternative service options to better meet the employment needs of individuals with mental retardation (Bellamy, Rhodes, Bourbeau, & Mank, 1986; Wehman & Moon, 1988; Whitehead, 1979).

Numerous additional factors have influenced the movement away from segregated day programming to integrated employment services. These include (a) parent and consumer demands, (b) federal and state funding and policy initiatives, (c) supported employment demonstration project outcomes, and (d) labor market demands. Employment outcome data show that individuals with severe mental disabilities can work successfully in community businesses when they receive specialized training and ongoing support services (Hill, Wehman, Kregel, Banks, & Metzler, 1987; Wehman, Parent, Wood, Kregel, & Inge, 1989). The Rehabilitation Research and Training Center placed 21 individuals with measured IQ scores ranging from 24 to 39 into competitive jobs with reported cumulative earnings over $231,976.00 (Wehman, Hill, Wood, & Parent, 1987). Furthermore, these workers earned $2 in income for every public dollar spent on service delivery, which reflects a significant increase over their presupported employment status. The first-year annual cost for providing supported employment services is estimated at $5,784.00 as compared to $3,816.00 for sheltered workshops and $6,806.00 for day programs (Wehman, Shafer, Kregel, & Twardzik, 1989). Supported employment costs tend to be reduced over time, as indicated by 4-year projected cost comparisons of $5,963.00 for supported employment,

$16,137.00 for sheltered workshops, and $25,499.00 for adult day programs (Rehabilitation Research & Training Center Newsletter, 1986). Despite these outcomes, the number of individuals participating in integrated employment settings is small when compared to the numbers still being served in segregated programs (Kregel, Shafer, Wehman, & West, 1989).

Efforts to change vocational rehabilitation services for individuals with severe mental disabilities has created a great deal of controversy among parents, individuals with disabilities, teachers, facility staff, rehabilitation counselors, and administrators. Debates frequently occur over the permanency or stability of supported employment services and the appropriateness of the model for persons with severe disabilities. Additional issues include long-term funding, staff development, and strategies for implementation (Parent, Hill, & Wehman, 1989).

The value that persons with mental retardation can and should participate in real work in the community and the commitment to provide those services is essential for converting vocational services. Several factors will influence the degree and rate with which integrated employment opportunities are developed. First, existing dollars need to be reallocated and new monies targeted to fund supported employment services for qualified individuals currently in day programs, on waiting lists, and exiting special education programs. Second, direct service staff and program manager training workshops and resources must be made available for those facilities who are interested in changing their service-delivery system. Third, research on facility conversion projects needs to be conducted and disseminated on the federal, state, local, and program level to assist with policy development and implementation. Fourth, the criteria for program decision making must shift from professional opinion to feedback from the local business community and persons with severe disabilities who are the consumers of supported employment services (Parent & Hill, 1990).

Upgrading Quality of Vocational Personnel

The philosophical and programmatic changes in vocational services for persons with mental retardation have created a great demand for professionals who are qualified to provide those services (Renzaglia & Everson, 1990). The need for direct service staff to implement the variety of integrated employment models is great and will certainly continue to grow during the 1990s. It is estimated that approximately 4,000 direct-service personnel are needed to adequately staff the emerging supported employment programs nationwide (Kregel & Sale, 1988). In addition, numerous other professionals who are involved with providing vocational services for persons with mental retardation have been required to assume new responsibilities and to develop new skills. A shortage of qualified personnel as well as quality technical assistance and staff-development programs to meet existing training needs is one of the most frequently reported problems today (Wehman, 1989). To a great extent, the degree with which integrated employment services are implemented and the intended outcomes are achieved depends on the availability of quality staff to meet the demands for services.

Supported employment programs at the secondary and postsecondary levels are staffed by professionals, known as employment specialists, job coaches, or job trainers, who are responsible for completing all of the activities essential for placing and maintaining individuals with severe disabilities into integrated employment situations (Wehman & Melia, 1985). Direct-service staff functioning in the role of employment specialist must be skilled at communicating with employers, analyzing jobs in the community, making a job–consumer match, providing behavioral skills training, collecting data, systematically increasing independent work performance, coordinating interagency services, and communicating with parents and other agency representatives. Skill training is most often provided through inservice training workshops and one-to-one mentoring by an experienced employment specialist. More recently, university preservice programs have begun to emerge with curriculums designed to train supported employment professionals. Unfortunately, the need for trained staff far exceeds the training opportunities that are currently available. The implications of this shortage are that inadequately trained staff are providing services that can adversely effect the quality and success of the employment outcomes.

Training workshops must also be developed to meet the needs of other professionals who play a critical role in the delivery of supported employment services. Vocational rehabilitation counselors, special and vocational education teachers, case managers, and rehabilitation facility staff and managers are being expected to provide integrated employment services for those persons who have traditionally been excluded from participation in real employment opportunities. Rehabilitation counselors must be skilled at assessing individual training and support needs, arranging long-term funding and support services, and evaluating the quality of services provided by supported employment vendors. Teachers need to be skilled at providing systematic instruction in community-based settings, communicating with adult service agencies, and coordinating transition services from school to work (Renzaglia, 1986). Case managers may be called on to solve problems and to coordinate support services focusing on keeping an individual with mental retardation employed, quite unlike traditional case-management services. Facility managers and staff must be skilled at providing community-based employment training while maintaining the operations of the facility during the conversion period.

University training programs have been slow to develop curriculums that will prepare professionals with the competencies required to effectively meet the employment needs of persons with mental retardation (Kregel & Sale, 1988). In-service workshops designed to provide specific skill training for different professional groups are rapidly emerging; however, research suggests that personnel training and technical assistance are still critically needed (Renzaglia & Everson, 1990).

Although preservice and in-service training programs increased dramatically during the 1980s, the predicted growth of supported employment programs, the high rates of job turnover among direct-service staff, and the reported training needs of existing personnel indicates that meeting the demand for qualified service providers will continue to be a major problem of the future. Several factors can be expected to influence how well these training needs are actually met in the 1990s. One is the amount of federal funds that are allocated for the development of personnel preparation programs to meet long-term staffing and staff development needs (Wehman, 1989). Second is the degree to which universities modify their curriculums to include programs in the areas of supported employment and courses in the rehabilitation counselor and vocational education preparation programs (Kregel & Sale, 1988; Renzaglia, 1986). Third is the acceptance of paraprofessional training as an additional option and the development of community college degree programs to prepare supported employment personnel (Karan & Knight, 1986). Fourth is the extent with which workshops and technical assistance programs designed to meet the individualized needs of each group of professionals involved in the delivery of supported employment services are developed and made available.

It can be assumed that the success of future staff development efforts will in many ways be contingent on the value placed on integrated employment and the employment specialists who provide those services. Continued lack of recognition that supported employment specialists are professionals with unique and important skills will undoubtedly perpetuate low salaries, high turnover rates, and poor service quality. Equally important for achieving the goals of having well-trained personnel and quality service provision are the collection of training needs assessment data, the delivery of unduplicated and relevant training workshops, and the evaluation of training outcomes for program effectiveness.

Toward Integrated Employment Opportunities

As mentioned earlier, vocational services for individuals with developmental disabilities have primarily included segregated placement in a day-activity, work-activity, or sheltered workshop program. These programs typically offered large numbers of persons with disabilities with the opportunity to socialize with paid staff or other persons with a disability. Community participation and interactions with nonhandicapped persons were rare or nonexistent for the majority of the individuals served by these programs. Supported employment has opened the doors to new opportunities for integration for those persons previously excluded from participation in real work settings. One distinguishing feature of supported employment is the training of relevant job skills and work-related behaviors directly at the job site by an employment specialist (Wehman & Kregel, 1985; Wehman & Melia, 1985). In addition, the employment specialist is responsible for identifying the valued social interactions that occur at the work place and for training the employee to participate appropriately with co-workers, supervisors, and the public (Chadsey-Rusch, 1986; Moon, Goodall, Barcus, & Brooke, 1986).

Interestingly, research has shown that employees with mental retardation *do* participate in the social interactions and activities that are available during work with the same frequency as their co-workers (Parent, Kregel, Twardzik, & Metzler, 1990). The advantages of participating in these socially integrated employment situations are the same for persons with mental retardation as for their nonhandicapped co-workers. These include opportunities for the development of friendships, the establishment of support networks, access to the community, and personal enjoyment. Perhaps most important is the status associated with working in integrated employment settings that changes perceptions of persons with severe disabilities to one of being valued and productive members of society.

Today, more than 20,000 individuals with severe disabilities are successfully working in integrated jobs because of the supported employment services they have received (Wehman, Kregel, & Shafer, 1989). Data collected for the 1,081 individuals participating in Virginia's supported employment programs suggest that more than half of these employees work in settings where integration with nonhandicapped persons occurs on a daily basis (Wehman, 1989). Similar observations are reported by other supported employment programs nationwide. The current emphasis in the field of supported employment has shifted from whether we can successfully place individuals into integrated employment to how can we enhance the quality of the integration that workers with severe disabilities are experiencing.

The major factor limiting professional activities directed toward improving integration is the lack of consensus on what integration actually is. Federal regulations define integration as a work site that has no more than eight individuals with a disability employed (*Federal Register*, August 14, 1987). The optimum number for integration provokes controversy among professionals who feel that eight is either too small or large or too restrictive for all settings. Additional research is needed to determine the best numbers that define physical integration. While numbers are important for programmatic decisions, experience has shown that integration cannot be defined exclusive of other factors. Too often, individuals are placed into a job that meets federal regulations but lacks opportunities for social integration. For example, suppose all of the nonhandicapped individuals employed by the company work on a different shift, in a separate geographical location, or take their break at a different time from the worker with a disability who is employed in the same position. This job would be considered integrated because only one worker with a disability is employed by the company, however, the availability and quality of that integration would be questionable.

A second important factor that must be considered in any definition of integration is the individuality of each job setting. Variations in the opportunities for integration and the manner in which co-workers participate in those opportunities are going to be found across job types and individual businesses. Any definition must be comprehensive to include the multiple factors that constitute an integrated employment situation and flexible enough to apply across a variety of job settings.

It is clearly evident that the integrated employment opportunities for persons with mental retardation have increased dramatically in recent years. Future research and demonstration efforts will continue to focus on the parameters that define integration and the best strategies for ensuring quality physical and social integration. It is expected that products will soon be developed that are aimed at assisting practitioners with assessing integration on the job site both to make placement decisions and to monitor employee participation for job retention (Parent, Kregel, Twardzik, & Metzler, 1990). An important focus of the integration research over the next few years will be on improving strategies to facilitate the match between individual choice for social integration and actual level of participation. This is essential for delivery of quality integrated employment services that meet the individualized needs of persons with mental retardation.

Persons With Mental Disabilities Need to Have Vocational Choices

We all have vocational choices. In how many cases, when we choose to stop working, can we quit one job and move on to another? If we choose to select a different job and have the necessary qualifications, we can change fields. How many individuals with disabilities, especially severe disabilities, can say the same? As one reviews the type of services available, it is clear that sheltered workshops, which number 5,700 in the United States, are the principle choice for many persons with mental and physical disabilities. Within these workshops the main choices usually are

(a) sheltered/benchwork employment for very poor pay; (b) limited job placement with no support and follow-along; and (c) occasionally, sheltered enclave arrangements in the community.

It is clear to us that clients need to have two types of choices:

1. The choice to perform work in a variety of vocational settings and/or arrangements (i.e., with support in a real job; opportunity to work on a mobile work crew)
2. The choice to perform work in a variety of different vocational fields (i.e., technology, food service, clerical)

These are opportunities that historically have not been available and that very much need to be in place for students who leave school to enter the world of work for the first time as well as for those who are older and may want to change their career.

Individuals with disabilities must perform their job at a similar level of proficiency as their nonhandicapped counterparts. Maintaining disabled persons on the payroll because of their disability is not constructive over the long run for those persons or for other disabled individuals who seek employment. In our experiences of using a supported work approach to competitive employment (Wehman & Kregel, 1985), it is clear that initial client training by the job coach or on-site staff person is a major factor in persuading the employer of the individual's commitment to employment. This approach is also a reflection of how serious the client and staff person feel about employment.

Those professionals actively involved in job placement may be faced with the issue of whether to maintain a client in a job that is not being performed well. An employment specialist who is closely involved with the client and the job site often knows before the employer does the level of progress and adjustment being made by the client. This progress or lack of it may signal the need for movement to a more appropriate job. Such communication and partnership with the employer can only serve to tighten the relationship and respect the employer will have for the client and trainer.

Training Must Reflect Local Market Needs: The Role of Business

As noted in the previous section, working with business and industry will enhance employment prospects for those with disabilities. Surveys of local businesses and industry should reveal potential appropriate jobs for persons with disabilities. General screening techniques such as checking classified advertisements and contacting employment agencies and chambers of commerce should reveal not only types of jobs available but also what jobs are most often available. Further contact by phone or in person with specific employers gives one an even better idea about the types of job skills required and the rate of turnover on a particular job. This kind of information must be incorporated into school and community agency vocational training programs in terms of the types of jobs adolescents and young adults with handicaps are trained to enter. For example, a school in a community where there is always a need for farm laborers does its students a disservice by training all the mentally retarded students in a year-round food service vocational training program. On the other hand, training someone to be a farm laborer will be in vain unless the specific methods used on local farms are trained in real work settings.

One way to ensure that training reflects labor market needs is to establish a business advisory board that provides continued input into your training program (Wehman & Barcus, 1985). This board can also help with public relations and educational efforts between agencies and employers. Another method involves assigning a staff person to regularly assess the community for jobs and to work with businesses in formulating cooperatively sponsored training programs.

Long-Term Funding

Vocational rehabilitation services for persons with severe disabilities have changed from a time-limited approach to one that recognizes that successful employment can mean employment with ongoing support. The realities of this service system require that financial resources are available and directed to supporting integrated employment of people with severe disabilities. Vocational rehabilitation monies are available to fund the initial time-limited services as with traditional employment services. However, no funding source has been assigned the financial or service responsibility for providing long-term support. This lack of a permanent, long-term funding base has been reported to be the greatest obstacle limiting implementation of supported employment services (Moon & Stern, 1988; Wehman, 1989).

The need for support in the workplace is not unique to persons with severe disabilities. If the reader considers his or her own job, it is quite likely that a variety of supports can be identified. For example, a friend to provide transportation when the automobile needs repair, a co-worker to explain office procedures, or an employee-assistance program to assist with personal problems. A nonhandicapped employee may not use all of the supports that are available or may not need them all of the time, but job retention and satisfaction tends to be enhanced by the fact that supports do exist. Employees with a severe disability will require assistance from a trained professional or advocate to access the available supports or to identify and develop additional supports that may be needed. Examples of long-term supports for persons with severe developmental disabilities might include such services as the following:

On-site training, retraining, or supervision available for employee, employer and co-workers as needed
Problem solving for job success
Regular contact and communication with the employee, employer, family, or home provider
Checks at least twice monthly on work performance at job site, including contact with supervisors or co-workers
Coordination of other services that effect employment including transportation
Off-site and after-work assistance including support groups
Counseling
Reassessment of an employee with regard to career advancement when needed for whatever reasons
Employee assistance with management of medical needs and services
Employment specialists serving as a backup to natural supports
Continual job modification and adaptation of equipment
Technology assistance as needed

The type and intensity of the supports required for job retention will vary for each individual and over time. It is important that services are proactive and tailored to meet the individual needs of each person regardless of the severity of their disability. This requires a flexible and adaptive system both in terms of funding and service provision.

The greatest challenge of providing ongoing supports is identifying the long-term funds to pay for them. Many states have established and successfully implemented diverse and creative funding patterns (Wehman, Kregel, et al., 1989). However, these funding options often are based on temporary or unpredictable resources. Several strategies can be used to increase the availability of long-term funds. First, existing noncategorical funding should be expanded to include supported employment. Second, new dollars need to be prioritized for supported employment "start-up" and follow along funds. Third, individuals with severe disabilities and their advocates must demand services and encourage disability groups to act together. Fourth, private and nontraditional sources for ongoing support, such as business and industry, need to be pursued. Fifth, data collection and evaluation efforts should be designed to measure effects, efficiency, and costs of providing long-term supports for policy decisions and resource allocation.

Conclusion

The 1980s has witnessed a great deal of progress in the development of innovative vocational services for individuals with mental retardation. As a result, increasing numbers of individuals with significant disabilities are working in competitive employment situations and earning substantial wages alongside persons who are not handicapped. Critical elements which make these outcomes possible include: interagency transition planning, expansion of employment opportunities, availability of qualified personnel, focus on integration, vocational choices, community and business involvement, and long-term funding resources. Continued high unemployment rates and inconsistent service implementation suggest that these elements may not yet be available or may not be systematically coordinated in all communities. Although it is difficult to predict future employment opportunities, it is anticipated that the progress and growth of the last decade will continue throughout the 1990s. A vision of flexible long-term support and support services for improving the employment outcomes of individuals with mental retardation is as follows.

All individuals, regardless of disability, receive the amount and kind of supports needed.

Support services are those that are required for individuals to be successfully integrated in employment.

Decisions about appropriate services are made as close as possible to the individual and are custom tailored for each person.

Basic principles include equity, access, duration, continuity, consumer directed, and individualization.

Services are oriented toward career development, not merely job retention.

Natural supports are encouraged. There are an infinite number of "models" of supported employment programs.

People with different disabilities receive different forms of individualized ongoing support, as needed.

Long-term services are proactive, not merely reactive.

Long-term support means forever, if needed, without gaps.

Individuals should not be able to tell when time-limited services change to follow-along or long-term support.

References

Bellamy, G. T., Rhodes, L. E., Bourbeau, P. E., & Mank, D. M. (1986). Mental retardation services in sheltered workshops and day activity programs: Consumer benefits and policy alternatives. In F. R. Rusch (Ed.), *Competitive employment issues and strategies* (pp. 257–271). Baltimore, MD: Paul Brookes.

Chadsey-Rusch, J. (1986). Identifying and teaching valued social behavior. In F. R. Rusch (Ed.), *Competitive employment issues and strategies* (pp. 273–287). Baltimore, MD: Paul Brookes.

Edgar, E. (1987). Secondary programs in special education: Are many of them justifiable? *Exceptional Children, 53*(6), 555–561.

Edgar, E. (1988). Transition from school to community. *Teaching Exceptional Children, 20,* 73–75.

Everson, J. M. (1988). An analysis of federal and state policy on transition from school to adult life for youth with disabilities. In P. Wehman & M. S. Moon (Eds.), *Vocational rehabilitation and supported employment* (pp. 67–78). Baltimore, MD: Paul Brookes.

Federal Register. (1987, August 14). Final regulations. Vol. 52(157), pp. 30546–30552. Washington, DC: Government Printing Office.

Harris Poll. (1986, February). *A survey of the unemployment of persons with disabilities.* Washington, DC.

Hasazi, S. B., Gordon, L. R., & Roe, L. A. (1985). Factor associated with the employment status of handicapped youth exiting high school from 1979–1983. *Exceptional Children, 51*(6), 455–569.

Hill, M. L., Wehman, P. H., Kregel, J., Banks, P. D., & Metzler, H. M. D. (1987). Employment outcomes of people with moderate and severe disabilities: An eight year longitudinal analysis of supported competitive employment. *The Journal of the Association for Persons With Severe Handicaps, 12*(3), 182–189.

Karan, O. C., & Knight, C. B. (1986). Training demands of the future. In W. E. Kiernan & J. A. Stark (Eds.), *Pathways to employment for adults with developmental disabilities* (pp. 253–269). Baltimore, MD: Paul Brookes.

Kregel, J., & Sale, P. (1988). Preservice preparation of supported employment professionals. In P. Wehman & M. S. Moon (Eds.), *Vocational rehabilitation and supported employment* (pp. 129–143). Baltimore, MD: Paul Brookes.

Kregel, J., Shafer, M. S., Wehman, P., & West, M. (1989). Policy and program development in supported employment: Current strategies to promote statewide systems change. In P. Wehman, J. Kregel, M. S. Shafer (Eds.), *Emerging trends in the national supported employment initiative. An analysis of twenty-seven states* (pp. 15–45). Richmond, VA: Virginia Commonwealth University, Rehabilitation Research and Training Center.

Moon, M. S., Goodall, P., Barcus, M., & Brooke, V. (1986). *The supported work model of competitive employment for citizens with severe handicaps: A guide for job trainers* (2nd ed.). Richmond, VA: VCU, RRTC.

Moon, M. S., & Stern, J. (1988). Long-term funding. In M. Barcus, S. Griffin, D. Mank, L. Rhodes, & M. S. Moon (Eds.), *Supported employment implementation issues* (pp. 101–120). Richmond: VCU, RRTC.

Parent, W. S., & Hill, M. L. (1990). Converting adult day care to supported employment: Economic and human resource considerations. In F. R. Rusch (Ed.), *Supported employment: Models, methods, and issues* (pp. 317–336). Sycamore, IL: Sycamore.

Parent, W. S., Hill, M. L., & Wehman, P. (1989). From sheltered to supported employment outcomes: Challenges for rehabilitation facilities. *Journal of Rehabilitation, 55*(4), 51–57.

Parent, W. S., Kregel, J., Twardzik, G., & Metzler, H. M. D. (1990). Social integration in the work place: An analysis of the interaction activities of workers with mental retardation and their co-workers. In J. Kregel, P. Wehman, & M. Shafer (Eds.), *Supported employment for persons with severe disabilities: From research to practice* (pp. 171–195, Vol. 3). Richmond, VA: VCU, RRTC.

Rehabilitation Research and Training Center Newsletter. (1986). From research to practice: The supported work model of competitive employment. VCU, RRTC, *3*(2).

Renzaglia, A. (1986). Preparing personnel to support and guide emerging contemporary service alternatives. In F. R. Rusch (Ed.), *Competitive employment issues and strategies* (pp. 303–316). Baltimore, MD: Paul Brookes.

Renzaglia, A., & Everson, J. M. (1990). Preparing personnel for supported employment. In F. R. Rusch (Ed.), *Supported employment: Models, methods, and issues* (pp. 395–408). Sycamore, IL: Sycamore.

Stark, J., & Goldsbury, T. (1988). Analysis of labor and economics: Needs for the next decade. *Mental Retardation, 26*(6), 363–368.

Wehman, P. (1989). Supported employment: Current strategies to promote statewide systems change. In P. Wehman, J. Kregel, & M. S. Shafer (Eds.), *Emerging trends in the national supported employment initiative: An analysis of twenty-seven states* (pp. 1–14). Richmond, VA: VCU, RRTC.

Wehman, P., & Barcus, M. (1985). Unemployment among handicapped youth: What is the role of the public schools? *Career Development for Exceptional Individuals, 8*(2), 90–101.

Wehman P., Hill, J. M., Wood, W., & Parent, W. (1987). A report on competitive employment histories of persons labeled severely mentally retarded. *Journal of the Association for Persons With Severe Handicaps, 12*(1), 11–17.

Wehman, P., & Kregel, J. (1985). A supported work approach to competitive employment of individuals with moderate and severe handicaps. *The Journal of the Association for Persons With Severe Handicaps, 10*(1), 3–11.

Wehman, P., Kregel, J., & Barcus, J. M. (1985). From school to work: A vocational transition model for handicapped students. *Exceptional Children, 52*(1), 25–37.

Wehman, P., Kregel, J., & Seyfarth, J. (1985). Employment outlook for young adults with mental retardation. *Rehabilitation Counseling Bulletin, 29*(2), 91–99.

Wehman, P., Kregel, J., & Shafer, M. S. (1989). *Emerging trends in the national supported employment initiative: A preliminary analysis of twenty-seven states*. Richmond, VA: VCU, RRTC.

Wehman, P., & Melia, R. (1985). The job coach: Function in transitional and supported employment. *American Rehabilitation, 53*(3), 23–28.

Wehman, P., & Moon, M. S. (1988). *Vocational rehabilitation and supported employment*. Baltimore, MD: Paul Brookes.

Wehman, P., Moon, M. S., Everson, J. M., Wood, W., & Barcus, J. M. (1988). *Transition from school to work: New challenges for youth with severe disabilities*. Baltimore, MD: Paul Brookes.

Wehman, P., Parent, W., Wood, W., Kregel, J., & Inge, K. J. (1989). The supported work model of competitive employment: Illustrations of competencies in workers with severe and profound handicaps. In P. Wehman &

J. Kregel (Eds.), *Supported employment for persons with disabilities focus on excellence* (pp. 19–52). New York: Human Sciences Press.

Wehman, P., Shafer, M. S., Kregel, J., & Twardzik, G. (1989). Supported employment implementation: II. Service delivery characteristics associated with program development and cost. In P. Wehman, J. Kregel, & M. S. Shafer (Eds.), *Emerging trends in the national supported employment initiative: A preliminary analysis of twenty-seven states* (pp. 75–96). Richmond, VA: VCU, RRTC.

Whitehead, C. W. (1979). Sheltered workshops in the decade ahead: Work and wages, or welfare. In G. T. Bellamy, G. O'Conner, & O. C. Karan (Eds.), *Vocational rehabilitation of severely handicapped persons* (pp. 66–92). Baltimore, MD: University Park Press.

Will, M. C. (1984). *Supported employment for adults with severe disabilities: An OSERS program initiative*. Washington, DC: U.S. Department of Education.

16
A Brief Look at Technology and Mental Retardation in the 21st Century

GREGG C. VANDERHEIDEN

Technology will have an impact on persons with mental retardation in the 21st century in many ways. These will include medical technology, therapeutic–educational technologies, assistive technologies, and technology in the community. The use of technology in medicine is more properly addressed within the total context of medical impact on mental retardation and is therefore not addressed in this chapter. That leaves three major types of interaction between technology and persons with mental retardation.

1. Technologies in therapy and education
2. Assistive technologies
3. Standard technologies in the workplace, community, and home

The purpose of this discussion is to provide a brief overview of some of the roles technology can play in the lives of persons with mental retardation in the future as well as some of the issues surrounding its use. Throughout the discussion, it should be remembered that technology as it relates to mental retardation is a two-edged sword. The rapid advances in technology will provide us with new tools to help individuals with mental retardation to develop and maintain their skills. However, technology also has the potential for creating an ever more complex and fast-paced world, which could pose new difficulties for persons with mental retardation. Advancing technology may also displace many low-skill workers, creating further difficulties. Whether technology will result in a net gain or a net loss for persons with mental retardation will be a function of our ability to predict and forecast the technological trends, our ability to capitalize on technological advancements to develop better assistive devices, and our ability to increase the awareness of standard product manufacturers so that they can create a world that is technologically gentler and easier.

Technology in Therapy and Education

Therapy and education are combined here because it is often difficult to determine where one ends and the other begins. Basically, technology is used in both of these areas in a similar way. In both cases, the technology is used on a temporary basis to develop or enhance some skill or ability. Once the individual develops the skill or ability, the technology is no longer used (except perhaps periodically, to maintain the skill). This is in contrast to technology used as an assistive device (see following), when the individual would continue using the technology over time (as we would use a pair of glasses or a hearing aid).

Therapy and education technologies are also similar in that they generally are used in the context of a broader intervention program. That is, they are not themselves the total therapeutic or educational activity, but rather are tools or components within a broader therapy or education program.

In this area, advancing technologies will provide teachers and therapists with increasingly more powerful and easy-to-program therapy–education aids. One area of advancement will be programming, where simpler and more English-like languages will allow teachers and therapists to create their own tools (programs) rather than having to rely exclusively on commercial software. A taste of this phenomenon can be seen in the HyperCard™ environment on the Apple Macintosh™. Special tools are being developed using the HyperCard system that are enabling teachers to easily assemble custom therapy or educational materials. For example, one program allows teachers to make up custom talking books (K. Barnes, personal communication, 1990). Using a standard blank "book," teachers are able to create their own talking books with little or no programming experience. Pictures that they would like to use in the story can be put into the book using a scanner (a copier-like attachment to the computer, which causes images to be copied onto the screen where they can easily be positioned and "pasted" into the book). The teachers can then type any text they wish to go along with the pictures. Clicking the mouse or pointing to a touch screen with the finger will cause the text to be read. Using this or similar tools, it is also possible to easily assemble a scene, where touching the various elements on the screen will cause them to speak or move. For higher level individuals, it is also possible to have text with "hot" words. That is, touching any of the "hot" words will cause that word to be read aloud. The students can first try to read the sentence, and, when they find a word that they cannot read, touch the word to have it spoken aloud. The feature could also be programmed to spell and repeat the word, if so desired. Although most of these tools use synthetic speech, it is also possible to use high-fidelity digitally recorded speech to provide very distinct pronunciations for the words. Speech synthesis is progressing so rapidly, however, that by the year 2000 it should be possible to use synthetic speech that is as clear and articulate as human speech, particularly when diphone concatenation techniques are used.

Another area of advancing technology is that of animation and sound. Although previous technological aids tended to be rather stereotypic and simple, advances in graphic animation and sound can provide the therapist with flexible tools that are much more interesting. It is also possible to create increasingly realistic visual representations and actions (complete with real-life sounds) to make these simulated experiences much more concrete. Using these tools, it will be possible to create more realistic situations for the individual while still maintaining control over the level of complexity of the task. For example, two-dimensional static pictures of objects are harder for individuals with retardation to recognize than the objects themselves. With technologies available today, it is possible to create three-dimensional animated displays of an object or objects. In fact, Toshiba has developed a three-dimensional home video camera. With these technologies, actual scenes and objects could be presented to the individual, as reduced or life-size representations. The complexity or simplicity of the objects and actions could also be easily controlled to meet the requirements of the individual and the subject being taught or the therapy being conducted.

Assistive Technologies

Assistive technologies are those technologies that an individual keeps and uses as a tool or an extension of their abilities. While educational and therapeutic technologies are only used for a short period of time, assistive technologies would be used by the person on a long-term or permanent basis. For persons with a physical disability, an example of an assistive technology functioning as a tool is a wheelchair or a reacher. Examples of assistive technologies that function as extensions are braces, splints, hearing aids, and glasses. For persons with mental retardation, the assistive devices will fall into these two basic categories. For the purpose of this discussion I will categorize these two uses as (a) extensions/enhancers and (b) companions/tools.

Extending/Enhancing Aids

Enhancing/extending aids are designed to help strengthen the skills that an individual already has. Common examples of enhancing aids for other types of impairments are glasses (visual impairment), hearing aids (hearing impairment), or braces (physical impairment). In each case the aids enhance the individual's residual abilities. An enhancing or orthotic aid for an individual with mental retardation could take a variety of forms, including such things as a memory or reminder aid, a prompter, or an assister in problem solving.

A reminder aid could be something as simple as a variation on the pocket calendar, which could store appointments and cue the individual when the appointments were imminent. They can also provide storage for phone numbers and other memoranda. Although today the entry of such information is usually by push-button, by the year 2000, speech recognition and synthesis should also be emerging as common components of these pocket notebook aids. As a mass-market device, the cost should also be quite low.

A prompting device would assist an individual in stepping through a sequence of activities. If properly done, the prompting device can act as a checklist reinforcer for individuals who can mostly do the activities themselves. It could also function as a more active prompting mechanism for those who have difficulty with sequenced activities.

Problem-solving devices are similar to prompting devices, except that they have more sophisticated algorithms, capable of helping individuals solve more generalized problems than the "canned" or stereotypic prompting routines.

Enhancing aids can also take the form of simple, single-function aids such as calculators or automatic checkbooks. By the year 2000, we will have very powerful computers that will run on batteries the size of watch batteries and fit in our pockets. As a result, it will be possible to implement fairly sophisticated enhancement routines at relatively low hardware cost. The biggest challenge in this area, and the greatest barrier to our progress, will be in our own understanding of mental retardation and ways that we can facilitate cognitive processing and daily living skills.

Companion/Tool Technologies

Companion/tool technologies are those that not only extend or enhance the individual's cognitive abilities but also augment the user's cognitive abilities with a second separate cognitive entity. Aids that incorporate artificial intelligence techniques to the point that they begin to take on the characteristics of an intelligent entity themselves could be very helpful to an individual with mental retardation and would fall into this category. One example of such a device is a hypothetical device I will call the "Companion."

The Companion consists of a small device approximately the size of a large wallet. It has four or five large buttons on it, which are brightly and distinctly colored and have symbols on them. One of the buttons stands for "Help." Two other buttons stand for "Yes" and "No." Another button is a request button. The Companion has voice output and speech recognition. It has an artificial intelligence system programmed within it, which is specifically designed to facilitate problem-solving and crisis resolution. In addition, the Companion acts as a reminder and monitor system for the individual. The Companion has a built-in Loran system, which allows it to keep track of its exact position using signals from navigation satellites. Finally, the Companion has a cellular communication system similar to a cellular telephone, allowing it to put the individual into instant contact with a crisis line in case of an emergency that cannot be easily handled by the Companion.

In daily use, the Companion would work something like this. Certain regular activities would be programmed into the system. The Companion could wake the individual up in the morning and then periodically ask the individual questions, which could help cue or prompt them through their morning routine, or it could operate as a check for individuals who do pretty well at progressing through their morning routines on their own. While of some benefit in the routine operations, the Companion would really be much more useful in helping to remember the breaks in routine. This would include days when the individual is *not* supposed to go someplace they normally go (because of a special appointment, a holiday, etc.), as well as unusual things they must do or places they must go (doctor's appointments, etc.). Because the system always knows its physical location, it can automatically check the individual's progress and determine when the individual is not making suitable progress toward the programmed goal. For example, if the individual has a doctor's appointment, the Companion would remind them in time for them to get to the doctor's office. If the time for the appointment was drawing near and the individual had not made progress toward the doctor's office, the Companion would provide additional reminders to the individual, help them problem solve the situation, or put them in contact with someone who could help.

As the day progressed, the individual would be able to request information or assistance from the Companion by pressing the "Request" button. The Companion would respond by talking to the individual and running through a list of functions to see what it was that the individual wanted. Because of the speech-recognition capability of the Companion, the individual could also simply respond to the initial questions of the Companion by saying what it was that they wanted. Some of the functions that the Companion could provide include providing time of day, providing directions, checking appointments, providing telephone numbers, providing addresses, and assisting in problem situations.

For example, Tim falls asleep on the bus on his way home from work and rides past his normal stop. When he wakes up, he looks out the window, and finds himself in a totally strange part of town. He panics, gets off the bus, and begins walking aimlessly about the streets, becoming more alarmed as he goes. The Companion, recognizing that he is in an area that he has never been to before and that is not on his agenda, beeps and asks him if he is okay, and if he knows where he is going. Using speech or the yes/no buttons, Tim answers the Companion's questions until the Companion is fairly certain that he does or does not know where he is headed. If the Companion determines that he has a problem, it will go into crisis–problem-resolution mode, figure out what the problem is, and attempt to help him.

The Companion starts by asking Tim questions to try to determine what type of problem exists. It then runs through a number of problem-solving strategies to try to help Tim to solve the problem himself. (While doing this, it will function in an enhancement mode.) If this does not work, then Tim might be advised to seek help from those around him (depending on the environment and situation).

Finally, if the Companion is unable to help Tim to solve the problem himself or with the assistance of those around him, the Companion would use its wireless phone-like capability to contact a central, shared "Help" facility. This central facility is manned 24 hours per day by individuals trained to provide assistance and problem solving to people who have Companions. Because the central facility has a basic file on each individual, as soon as the Companion contacts the central facility, background information on Tim is instantly displayed on the operator's screen, along with any information that the Companion has been able to glean through its processes, including the individual's current location. At this point, Tim is in direct voice and visual contact with the operator, who is able to talk to him in a fashion appropriate to his abilities, determine what the problem is, and help him to resolve the problem.

Tim does not have to wait until the Companion detects a problem if he is in trouble. Tim can signal directly that he has a problem by pushing the Help button. Tim can also skip the Companion's assisted self-resolution phase and go directly to the call to the central operator by pressing the Help button more than once.

Although Tim's Companion doesn't have it yet, a new model of the Companion has just come out on the market which also has a built-in reading capability. This new model of the Companion has a small window, like the viewfinder on a camera. Using the new model, if Tim saw some writing on a sign or paper that he could not read, he would be able to just look through the viewfinder, aim it at the text, and push a button. The Companion would take an electronic "picture" and then read the text aloud to Tim. This technique is also helpful in the way-finding strategies, because the Companion would also know what the sign said, and could provide some assistance, if it was a familiar type. For example, if Tim were near a bus stop, the bus numbers could be noted and used to help Tim get on the right bus. Similarly, when a bus approached, Tim could just aim the viewfinder at the word written on the bus and the Companion could confirm whether this was the proper bus for Tim to board. This reading capability would also have a certain therapeutic value to Tim, because it would display the picture of the text and then highlight the words one at a time as it spoke them. In this way, the Companion could facilitate Tim's learning and recognizing common or familiar printed words. It would also be possible for the Companion to transmit the digitized picture back to the central operator, in the event of an emergency or problem solving. As a result, the operator would be able to "see" the problem more clearly, by simply asking Tim to "take pictures" of what the operator was interested in.

The purpose of the Companion would, of course, be to allow individuals with mental retardation to live more independently. If the Companion could enable an individual to live safely in a less supervised or more independent fashion, the cost savings would very quickly cover the cost of the Companion. Even a moderate shift in the independent living status can be a savings of $10,000 or more per year. The cost of the Companion would be kept reasonable because of its widespread application with elderly individuals, where it could help allow them to live safely outside of nursing homes for longer periods of time, and in nursing homes, allow greater degrees of freedom while still allowing maintenance of supervision to whatever level is desired.

Technologies such as the Companion are easily within our reach. The Loran (a navigational system that determines latitude and longitude from remote radio signals), cellular telephones, miniature cameras, voice synthesizers, and microprocessors all exist and are in use today. The artificial intelligence and expert system routines that would be needed for the problem-solving systems in a Companion-class device exist but not in the sophistication required for this application. However, steady progress is being made in these areas, and the computing power necessary to support these capabilities is advancing rapidly and will easily outstrip our ability to apply it effectively. What we do not have is knowledge of how to best use these technologies, how to provide useful prompting to help a client figure out a problem rather than thinking for them, how to identify problems without visual context, and so on. These are the critical missing components, and are necessary to transform an engineer's toy into a viable tool for persons with retardation.

Technology in the Workplace, Community, and Home

Everyday technology in the world about us will probably have the most significant impact on persons with mental retardation and on their ability to live and work independently.

As mentioned previously, the rapid advances in technology are leading to technification of our daily lives. Most of us now do our banking with an automated teller machine. Soon we will be increasingly sending our mail via electronic mail or fax. As electronic shopping technology advances, we will soon find it faster and cheaper to do at least some of our shopping electronically. Even when we do go shopping, we may find ourselves using cash less and less, and cash cards more. (For example, we would slip our card into a slot at the grocer's counter, and then punch a secret number into a keypad, after which, the money for the purchases would be directly subtracted from our account, similar to writing a check but faster.)

The increasing use of technology has the potential for making our community more technical and more difficult for persons with mild-to-moderate mental retardation to survive in. In the workplace, we are seeing an even faster incorporation of various technologies. As computers and robotics reduce the number of low-skill jobs, replacing them with jobs involving at least some use of technology, increasing pressure is put on those with mental retardation. In fact, if the community and workplace became significantly more complex, our functional definitions of mental retardation and the percentage of the population categorized as functionally retarded may need to be expanded to account for the greater numbers of individuals who have difficulty living and working independently.

On the other hand, technology also has the capability to make complex things simpler. For example, driving a car in the early days meant not only adjusting the accelerator but also the spark advance, double-clutching to shift gears, and so on. Technology has now made driving much simpler by providing us with automatic transmissions, power steering, automatic choke, and spark advance. Similarly, early televisions used to require that we master not only the volume and channel controls but also the horizontal hold, the vertical hold, the brightness, contrast, and fine tuning, to get a clear picture as we changed channels. Advancing technology has automated most or all of these functions, so that with most televisions it is unnecessary (and often impossible) to find the controls for horizontal hold, vertical hold, contrast or fine tuning. You simply change channels and adjust the volume. In like fashion, advancing technology can act to simplify other aspects of the world about us. Advances in both artificial intelligence and speech synthesis and recognition are making it possible to interact with machines in a more natural fashion. In place of complicated bus route maps, it will soon be possible to push a button on a bus stop sign, announce your destination, and have the electronics in the sign tell you the proper bus to take and the time that it will arrive at that particular bus stop. More intelligent signs could tell you if a bus is running late, or if you are at the wrong bus stop. In the latter case, it might also direct you to the correct bus stop if it is nearby. Automated teller machines already use a prompting strategy to assist people in stepping through the sequence of actions necessary to withdraw or deposit money.

Realizing the Potential of Technical Advances

To take advantage of any potential that technological advances may have for creating a simpler world, it is very important that we determine how this might be possible and communicate this to the right people. First, we must define what makes a device easier or more difficult for a person with mental retardation to handle. This is not always as easy as it may seem. We must then communicate these "design guidelines" to the manufacturers of consumer products and business–information systems. Manufacturers are in fact interested in identifying and incorporating these improvements into their products. This is primarily because products that are simpler and take fewer cognitive skills to operate are easier to operate for everyone. In addition, these design changes can help reduce fatigue and result in fewer errors. These techniques will also increase the usability of their products by the ever growing elderly population. By 2050, it is estimated that over one third of the population will be over 55 years of age (Office of Technology Assessment, 1985). Again, the greatest barrier to realization of this potential will be our own understanding of how to design things so that they require fewer cognitive skills, and in our effectiveness at communicating these to the actual design teams who are creating the devices that will constitute our world tomorrow.

Ethical Issues in the use of Artificial Intelligence

Artificial intelligence holds great potential for applications with people having cognitive impairments. However, its application must be carefully implemented to preserve the independence and freedom of these people.

If we were able to provide a person with mental retardation with an artificial brain that could think for them, would we have provided the person with new intelligence or would we have provided the artificial brain with a human body? Although artificial intelligence today is nowhere near the thinking or creative capacity of the human mind, we should be mindful that advances in this area are being made at a previously inconceivable rate. The power of our computers is increasing faster than any other technology we know of. It is in fact increasing by a factor of 10 every 4 years. In addition, the cost for equivalent computing power is going down by a factor of 10 every 5 years (Huray, 1990).

To get some conception of these numbers, let's draw a parallel with the automotive industry. In 1965, for $10,000 you could buy a Cadillac that went 120 mph. If automobiles were progressing at the same rate that computers are progressing, in 1990 you'd be able to buy either a $10,000 Cadillac that went the speed of light, or a Cadillac that went 120 mph for 10 cents. By the Year 2000, the car would travel 316 times the speed of light, or you'd be able to buy ten 120-mph cars for a penny (Huray, 1990). (316 times the speed of light is equivalent to traveling around the world 2,370 times in 1 second.) Computers and computing technologies are therefore advancing at a rate that is inconceivable by ordinary technology standards, and the potential of artificial intelligence will increase along with it.

This is a tremendous and rapidly advancing resource that we can tap to benefit those with mental retardation. We must, however, take great care in how we do this. If we attempt to make cognitive prostheses (an artificial brain for the person), we run the danger of thinking for the individual instead of facilitating his or her thinking and decision-making processes. For this reason, I think that we must focus our attention on "companion" classes of assistive technologies. These technologies constitute an approach that involves the use of artificial intelligence to stand alongside a person with mental retardation or other cognitive impairment, accompany them through their lives, and provide assistance to them in the same manner as a human companion or guardian might. It should be programmed to facilitate the natural thinking and problem-solving capabilities of individuals, thus maximizing their inherent cognitive abilities. In addition, its companion or guardian function can allow individuals to move about more freely than would otherwise be possible while still maintaining a link back to assistance should they need it.

With advancing artificial intelligence programming, the "companion" device may in fact be superior to a human companion or guardian with respect to the individual's independence. Human companions and guardians are susceptible to imposing their own points of view as well as their own wants and needs on the people in their care. The "companion" device could be programmed to offer assistance or reminder services on any level deemed appropriate for the given individual. The individual would therefore be left to make their own decisions based on the input from the "companion" or others in their environment.

Summary

Currently, technology can address only a small portion of the problems faced by individuals with mental retardation. In general, it is much easier to apply technology to meet individual's needs in the area of physical or sensory disability. This will probably continue well into the next century. However, advancing technologies are slowly beginning to provide us with tools that are powerful enough to better address some of the needs of persons with cognitive disabilities. Currently, the use of technology in therapy and education represents the bulk of the application of technology with persons with mental retardation. This role will continue and will expand. In addition, we should see increasing applications of technology as assistive devices to either enhance the person's cognitive skills, or to act as a "companion," which can facilitate independent living. One of the most important ways, however, that technology will affect persons with mental retardation is through its incorporation into the community around us. Depending on our skill and ability at advising product designers, this increased use of technology in the community can be either a negative or a positive factor in the ability of persons with mental retardation to live and work more independently. In all of these areas, however, our progress will be limited most, not by the limitations in technology, but by the limitations in our understanding of what technology could do for this population and, exactly how we should go about doing it.

References

Huray, P. G. (1990). The US information science initiative. Proceedings of the fifth annual national symposium on information technologies. Columbia, SC: University Printing, University of South Carolina.

Office of Technology Assessment. (1985, June). Technology and aging in America (U.S. Congress, OTA-BA-264). Washington, DC: U.S. Government Printing Office.

17
Beyond Benevolence: Legal Protection for Persons With Special Needs

STANLEY S. HERR

In the space of a mere two decades, a legal revolution has broken over the once-quiet field of mental retardation. Where change was formerly sought by appeals to virtue, beneficence, patriotism, or even shrill xenophobia, there is now an insistent call for new legislation, rules, and judicial decisions. Where medical superintendents were once the authors of legislative programs of isolation, there is now a broad constituency for integration.

This chapter offers an overview of these new realities, and dynamic legal and political forces. It focuses on the identification of 10 significant legal trends affecting persons with special needs. It then concludes with speculations on the prospects of realizing the international human rights of those persons. The term *persons with special needs* refers to persons with mental retardation, other developmental disabilities, other disabilities, and other infirmities associated with age. As a shorthand, this term will also be used interchangeably with the term *persons*, both for convenience and to emphasize the essential equality under law due all persons, disabled and nondisabled alike.

The New Realities

From Charity to Rights

Until the 1970s, services and aid for persons with special needs were commonly viewed as matters of charity rather than of right. Out of the almshouses and poorhouses of the past emerged the institutions and the workshops that survived into the 20th century. Concepts of rights, individual liberty, and due process were alien to those environments. Philanthropists, not lawyers, "Boards of Charities," not judges, exerted influence in this pre-civil rights era (Rothman & Rothman, 1984).

Appeals to rights were attempts to undo this legacy of powerlessness and prejudice. Some of these appeals were grounded in natural or human rights. The Declaration on the General and Special Rights of Mentally Retarded Persons, promulgated by the International League of Societies for the Mentally Handicapped (ILSMH), in Jerusalem, exemplified this approach (ILSMH, 1968). The so-called Jerusalem Declaration formed the basis for the United Nation's (U.N.'s) Declaration on the Rights of Mentally Retarded Persons, which proclaimed, among other rights, the right to medical care, physical therapy, and the education, training, rehabilitation, and guidance needed to develop the individual's potential (U.N., 1971). Although one commentator has criticized this approach as extending rights to persons with mental retardation that are not extended to other persons (Kass, 1988), this assertion is false. Comparable international declarations for disabled persons generally (U.N., 1975) and international covenants for children (U.N., 1989) adopt a similar approach to human rights, reaffirming and elaborating the principles contained in the Universal Declaration of Human Rights (1948).

Courts in the United States have also looked to the 1971 U.N. Declaration as a parallel support to a constitutionally grounded right to habilitation (*Wyatt v. Stickney*, 1972). Through the courts and legislatures, the rights strategy has emerged as a dominant form of social change discourse in the United States. Several reasons account for this influence. Appeals to humanity and fellow feeling have failed in the past to remedy gross indignities against persons with mental retardation. The themes of equal justice and legal protection have a powerful resonance in the American legal and popular culture. Notable early successes in judicial and legislative arenas encouraged subsequent efforts. Finally, the development of advocacy systems has lowered the barriers to access to lawyers, courts, and legislatures that traditionally confronted persons with special needs.

The rights strategy captured international attention. It has led to the overhaul of guardianship, special education, and commitment laws in many countries (Israel Special Education Law, 1988). It has also spurred new laws in developing countries, and antidiscrimination and community care laws in industrialized countries. As acknowledged by a position paper of the International League of Societies for Persons With Mental Handicap, advocacy is now internationally recognized as a basic support service to protect the rights articulated under law and to ensure appropriate access to needed services and facilities (Herr & Schuster-Herr, 1984). This emphasis on the implementation of rights is also reflected in the International League's theme for its Tenth World Congress, "Turning Rights Into Realities" (ILSPMH, 1990).

From Neglect to Protection

In the past, the lives, liberties, and pursuit of happiness of persons with special needs could be trampled with little or no legal recourse. Involuntary sterilization was upheld by a unanimous U.S. Supreme Court out of a misplaced fear that the public would otherwise be swamped by "incompetents" (*Buck v. Bell*, 1927). Infants with Down syndrome were denied life-saving medical treatment, and learned panels of experts opined that parents of such infants could not be "second-guessed" (Kennedy Foundation, 1971). Persons suspected of the taint of mental retardation could be segregated for life, put to institutional peonage, and their ancient commitment orders were never reversed (*In the Matter of Turner*, 1984). Under that legal regime of laissez-faire, neglect and abuse were rampant.

If discovered, such cases would today evoke protest and petitions for legal protection. Now, the reproductive choices of persons with disabilities are vigorously defended, even against their parent's preferences (*E. (Mrs.) v. Eve*, 1986), and the physical health and well-being of children with Down syndrome trump the life-denying wishes of their guardians (*Guardianship of Becker*, 1981). Institutions retain residents who are able to live in relative freedom at their legal peril (*Clark v. Cohen*, 1986; *O'Conner v. Donaldson*, 1975). Legal protection is common-place rather than a rarity in the disability field.

From Silence to Assertion

Advocacy by and for persons with mental retardation has had transform-ing effects. In the past, they were mischaracterized as permanent chil-dren, "holy innocents," or "social menaces." Even their organizational champions stressed their being "retarded children"; while pioneering works of legal scholarship focused on those labeled as "the silent clients" (Mickenberg, 1979). And in silence or wailing inside barren institutional dayrooms, many did suffer without legal redress.

The self-advocacy movement has changed many of those expectations and stereotypes. In Connecticut, a self-advocate was an effective lobbyist for a State constitutional amendment protecting persons with physical or mental disabilities from discrimination and segregation (Connecticut, 1984). In Pennsylvania, two former residents of Pennhurst provided effective and moving testimony on why they had preferred to live in the community (Ferleger & Boyd, 1979; *Halderman v. Pennhurst State School and Hospital*, 1977). By lobbying Congress, the disability-rights move-ment has addressed the nation with increasing sophistication and firmness in demanding an end to discrimination (Americans With Disabilities Act, 1990). Strikingly, it has done so through a wide array of spokespersons—disabled and nondisabled, physically and mentally challenged alike—to make the point that 43 million Americans with disabilities and their family and friends are a constituency that will be heard and heeded.

Trends in Legal Protection

This section analyzes some of the legal milestones in protecting the legal rights of persons with special needs. The focus is on the apex of the judicial system—the U.S. Supreme Court—and Congress as its vital check and balance. This emphasis reflects the supremacy of federal law, and the reverberations that decisions of the Court and Congress have on the Executive Branch and the States. Although Congress has proven a reliable champion of disability rights, changes in the composition of the Supreme Court may lead to an erosion of judicially declared rights by the year 2000. However, one promising trend is the increasing dynamism of state courts and the vigilance of state-level coalitions of advocates in pressing their own legislatures to defend the rights of persons with disabilities. For those readers interested in comprehensive treatises or in reporters of the torrent of new cases and bills, additional references are noted (Brakel, Parry, & Weiner, 1985; *Mental and Physical Disability Law Reporter*).

Valuing the Lives of Devalued Persons

One of the more contentious issues of the 1980s was the legal regulation of so-called Baby Doe cases. Out of the turmoil of anguished medical decision making of doctors who advised against treatment for a handicapped newborn and parents who acquiesced in that nontreatment decision came a barrage of federal rules, a Supreme Court decision, and a political consensus embodied in federal laws.

The debate began with the much-publicized Johns Hopkins Hospital case when parents of an infant with Down syndrome and intestinal atresia refused to authorize surgery. In the postmortem discussion that followed, leading ethicists failed to identify a potential role for the courts in saving the lives of such infants, arguing that it would be wrong to "second-guess" the parents (Kennedy Foundation, 1971). But when a similar case arose in April 1982, which became known as the Bloomington Baby Doe incident, the legal and political climate had changed. Then, the President and the U.S. Department of Health and Human Services (U.S. DHHS, 1982) reminded federally assisted health-care providers of the need to protect infants with handicaps from discrimination under Section 504 of the Rehabilitation Act (1973). Ultimately, federal rules were adopted to require the posting of informational notices, access to records, and action by state child-protective service agencies to prevent "unlawful medical neglect" of infants with handicaps (U.S. DHHS, Final Rules, 1985). But these rules proved anything but final, because the Supreme Court invalidated them in 1986 on the grounds that when treatment was withheld it was the result of a parent's failure to give consent not the discriminatory action of heath-care providers (*Bowen v. American Hospital*

Association, 1986). This plurality opinion by the Court also criticized DHHS for attempting to "commandeer state agencies" and its child-protection workers as "the foot soldiers in a federal crusade" (*Bowen*, 1986, p. 642). The dissenters opined, correctly, that handicapped newborns were entitled to some federal legal protection, and that the DHHS Secretary had authority to regulate in this field.

Congress had already provided that authority through the Child Abuse Amendments of 1984. By tying regulations to grants to state child-protective services agencies, Congress knew that agencies in accepting those grants could not protest that new duties were imposed against their wills. Furthermore, well-crafted compromise language by organizations of pediatricians and disability-rights activists ensured a high level of agreement on cases requiring outside intervention. Each state's protective agency must investigate complaints and apply legal remedies for medical neglect, defined as the withholding of medically indicated treatment in the face of life-threatening conditions. The only exceptions permitted for withholding treatment are extraordinary cases of (a) a chronically and irreversible comatose infant, (b) the futility of such treatment in merely prolonging dying, and (c) the virtual futility of treatment in terms of the infant's survival coupled with the inhumanity of the treatment itself. Thus, as the year 2000 approaches, there is fundamental consensus on the goals, if not the procedures for saving the lives of infants heretofore devalued.

Guaranteeing the Right to an Education

The right to a free, appropriate, publicly supported education is the clearest legal success story in the disability field. Federal courts first articulated the equal protection basis of that right and the due process underpinnings for the child's opportunity to be heard to challenge a classification or placement decision (*Mills v. Board of Education*, 1972; *P.A.R.C. v. Pennsylvania*, 1972). Congress fully embraced those rationales and due process hearing remedies in the Education for All Handicapped Children Act of 1975 (PL 94-142). This public law ensured every handicapped child of a free appropriate public education consisting of individualized instruction and related services according to an "individualized education program" (IEP). As a result of this legal activity, children with handicaps could no longer be excluded from their schooling or relegated to substandard custodial program. Their educational needs had to be clearly identified, and an annual infusion (now $2 billion) in federal funds helped to subsidize some of those needs.

For the year 2000, the law's target should shift from access to success. *Rowley v. Hendrick Hudson School Board of Education* (1982) confirms the propriety of Congressional action to open schoolhouse doors to children with disabilities. In *Honig v. Doe* (1988), the Supreme Court again defined access rights for such pupils, even those whose behavioral problems might otherwise expose them to disciplinary sanctions. Thus, a handicapped pupil is entitled to the protection of PL 94-142 in these circumstances, cannot be suspended for more than 10 days in drastic cases and can only be reassigned to a different education setting after notice and an opportunity to be heard. Although these precedents vigorously support rights of access to education, activism at state and local levels is needed to ensure that pupils receive effective instruction and placement in the least restrictive educational environment. Future contests loom on the extent to which local districts must provide effective, integrated education.

Defining Rights to Habilitation

The courts have lent considerable impetus and legal validation to the movement for habilitation rights. Initially, the landmark decree in *Wyatt v. Stickney* (1972) declared a constitutional right to habilitation enforceable through a set of minimum standards detailing staffing, program planning, and individual rights norms. In *Wyatt v. Aderholt* (1974), this right was affirmed and the role of an activist federal judiciary was broadly endorsed. Subsequent lower court decisions relied on the *Wyatt* precedent, as well as rationales of rights to "protection from harm" and to "training," to upgrade habilitation and to foster deinstitutionalization. With this legal leverage, lawyers for class-action plaintiffs were able to negotiate consent decrees closing large institutions (*Halderman v. Pennhurst State School and Hospital*, 1985; *Michigan Association for Retarded Citizens v. Smith*, 1979). In a similar case, the Willowbrook decree resulted in a 5,300-bed institution being drastically reduced to a facility 1/20th the size and then actually closed (*N.Y. State Association for Retarded Children v. Carey*, 1975).

Although the *Pennhurst* case (1981, 1984) also led to an institution's closing, the Supreme Court questioned the legal grounds for court-supervised deinstitutionalization. In 1981, the justices rejected the Developmentally Disabled Assistance and Bill of Rights Act as a basis for comprehensive relief when Congress had given the states an ambiguous command (*Pennhurst State School and Hospital v. Halderman*, 1981). Three years later, the Court overturned federally implemented state law as a grounds for an enforceable right to habilitation (*Pennhurst State School and Hospital v. Halderman*, 1984). Before the constitutional claims relied on by the trial court could be tested by the Supreme Court, the parties negotiated a consent decree closing Pennhurst and transferring its remaining residents.

Ironically, an initially little-noticed case of an individual resident of Pennhurst produced the clearest Supreme Court declaration on the rights of institutionalized persons. *Youngberg v. Romeo* (1982) held that such individuals had a constitutional right to training to live in safety and free from undue restraints. The case is also significant in recognizing that a mental retardation professional's judgments are presumptively due judicial respect if they are within accepted professional standards.

Post-*Romeo* judgments have led to mixed results. Some courts have limited relief to the development and implementation of internal standards of institutional care (*Society of Good Will to Retarded Children v. Cuomo*, 1984). Other circuit courts of appeal have upheld orders requiring least restrictive placements in the community (*Clark v. Cohen*, 1986; *Thomas S. v. Murrow*, 1986). A recent appellate decision ordered individual plans for transferring plaintiff class members to more normal settings in the community and identified other violations of accepted professional standards relating to drugs, restraint, and habilitation (*Thomas S. v. Flaherty*, 1990). Advocates have also turned to state courts for enforcement of their state rights to community-based habilitation. In a notable decision of the Pennsylvania Supreme Court, a young adult with mental retardation was held entitled to normalization and a placement to avoid institutionalization, on the basis of a legislatively created "right to live a life as close as possible to that which is typical for the general population" (*In re Schmidt*, 1981, p. 636).

Increasingly, the advocates' attention has focused on state legislatures for the creation, financing, and implementation of a wide panoply of habilitation rights. These rights include rights to broadly defined habilitation, medical care, freedom from coerced nonemergency treatments, and individual dignity. As a result of the advocates' labors, a majority of states now recognize the right to habilitation, with the principle of normalization reflected in the growth of family-sized community living arrangements.

Exploring Least Restrictive Alternatives to Guardianship

Guardianship is another legal area that is undergoing rapid change. Legislative rather than court-created reform characterizes this field. Court cases have, however, highlighted the dangers of rubber-stamped orders, lack of legal representation for the alleged disabled persons, and perfunctory evaluations (*Michigan Association for Retarded Citizens v. Wayne County Probate Judge*, 1977). Judicial opinions also have limited the powers of natural or appointed guardians to withhold medical treatment (*Guardianship of Becker*, 1981) or nutrition and hydration (*Cruzan v. Missouri*, 1990). Similarly, a guardian's decision-making powers can be limited in cases of nonconsensual sterilization (*Wentzel v. Montgomery County Hospital*, 1982; *E. v. Eve*, 1986).

Thorough revision of the concept and practice of guardianship is underway in many countries. In Sweden, guardianship is now largely confined to the protection of substantial financial interests. Instead, the law provides for the appointment of a *"godman"* ("goodman") to offer personal advocacy for individuals with mental handicaps. In Austria, guardianship has been replaced by a network of personal support services. Recently, New Zealand and West Germany have passed reform laws on guardianship that emphasize principles of necessity before any restriction can be imposed and the least restrictive alternative. Thus, under the German Guardianship Law (1990), a guardianship court may not appoint a *"betreuer"* ("guardian") if the individual with a disability can handle her own affairs independently or with the support of a third person or a social services agency. New Zealand law also requires the welfare guardian to tutor their wards "to encourage that person to develop and exercise such capacity as that person has to understand the nature and foresee the consequences of decisions relating to the personal care and welfare of that person, and to communicate such decisions" (New Zealand Protection of Personal Property Rights Act, 1988, § 18[3]). Similarly, some Australian states require the guardian to consult with the represented person in making decisions, to assist that person to become capable of self-care, and to serve only if no other means less restrictive of the person's freedom of action and decision is possible (Victorian Guardianship and Administration Board Act, 1986).

Where traditional guardianship continues to exist, it is likely to be challenged in the future on several fronts. With new forms of social support, advocacy services, and helping arrangements, fewer people will require guardians. With concern for enhancing the autonomy and self-determination of persons, the restrictive and civil-rights–nullifying features of total guardianship will fall under stiffer criticism. And with heightened procedural safeguards, and more vigorous advocacy, fewer persons with handicaps will be subjected to any form of guardianship. The advocates' careful consideration of alternatives to guardianship can also help to avoid excessive protection and undue restriction of rights. By the year 2000, plenary guardianship may become a relic of the paternalistic past, displaced by more individually tailored supports.

Safeguarding Equality Rights in the Community

The right to live in the community is the keystone to many fundamental political, social, and human rights. The U.N. Declaration on the Rights of Disabled Persons (adopted December 9, 1975) enunciates this principle and provides a useful benchmark from which to assess national laws. Article 9 declares that disabled persons, defined expansively to include persons functionally limited in their physical or mental capabilities, have the right to live with their families or with foster parents and to participate in all social, creative, or recreational activities. Although this formulation seems to have primary application to children and young adults, Article 9 recognizes the principle of normalization and a need for group homes and other specialized living arrangements for older persons as well. Thus, the U.N. Declaration further states: "If the stay of a disabled person in a specialized establishment is indispensable, the environment and living conditions therein shall be as close as possible to those of the normal life of a person of his or her age" (U.N., 1975, art. 9).

In 1975, when the U.N. adopted, and the U.S. Government voted for, this resolution 3447, those rights were honored more in rhetoric than in reality. By the year 2000, however, most U.S. states and localities will have real resources, supports, and rights to ensure community living. Many jurisdictions have already achieved the legal basis for community-based care. In the previously discussed *Halderman v. Pennhurst State School and Hospital* (1977, 1985) case, the Commonwealth of Pennsylvania agreed in 1985, after a protracted legal battle, to close that not atypical institution for the mentally retarded. In its stead, they guaranteed the availability of decent community-living arrangements. Through this act of vision and statesmanship, those authorities have demonstrated that all persons with mental retardation can benefit from services in community-based group homes, foster homes, other sheltered and independent-living arrangements.

This is not an isolated case. In New York, beginning in 1972, a persistent band of consumer activists and their legal warriors came to bury Willowbrook, not to praise it. The consent decree they initially negotiated called for phasing down that 5,300-bed monstrosity. But the lawyers eventually realized that even a 250-bed facility can be a disaster. Learning from this implementation experience, the parties modified the consent decree to close Willowbrook completely. Similarly, at Detroit's Plymouth Center, the Michigan Association for Retarded Citizens found that even shiny new institutions were dead-ends for clients subject to abuse and segregation. And so the court and the parties jointly sounded "taps" for Plymouth in 1983 and instead fully implemented a right to community-living arrangements (*Michigan Association for Retarded Citizens v. Smith*, 1979). The same outcome resulted at Maryland's Henryton Center, under the aegis of a case called *Bauer v. Hughes* (1984). On a crisp autumn day in 1984, the last of the residents of Henryton moved out of that institution to join the rest of us in a world of vicissitudes and triumphs.

By the year 2000, the litany of such class-action cases could be even more extensive. Already half of Nebraska is institution free in the field of mental retardation. Litigation at Rhode Island's Ladd School (*Iasimone v. Garrahy*, 1982) led Governor Edward DiPrete to make that state the first to eliminate mental retardation institutions completely.

If attaining the goals of community reintegration and equal rights is to be accelerated, the field of mental retardation will need more than reliance on the judiciary to safeguard client interests. *City of Cleburne v. Cleburne Living Center* (1985) shows the limits of the Supreme Court's solicitude for the mentally handicapped. By a six to three margin, the Court held that persons with mental retardation were not sufficiently disadvantaged as a group to merit heightened scrutiny of allegedly discriminatory governmental classifications. However, in applying the customary rational relationship test to a zoning ordinance, the justices engaged in a searching examination of a decision to exclude a group home and ruled that the ordinance was discriminatory as applied. The reality of the heightened scrutiny employed by the justices suggests that advocates can still use the judiciary to undo irrational prejudice that threatens to exclude persons with disability from neighborhood living.

In the wake of the *Cleburne* (1985) decision (and the ever more conservative composition of the Supreme Court), advocates will increasingly turn to Congress and state legislatures for codes that will spare potential group home residents from gauntlets of delay and discrimination. Recently, those efforts have resulted in the Fair Housing Amendments Act (1988) and the Americans With Disabilities Act (1990). These federal laws offer potent tools for safeguarding access to nondiscriminatory housing opportunities. Other long-term legislative advocacy efforts could redirect the Medicaid legislation to place greater emphasis on community-living supports and eventually to the avoidance of institutionalization altogether. With enactment of such a law, the right to live in the community would not hinge on the judicial class to which one might belong or the region in which one might be fortunate to live.

Combatting Neglect and Abuse

The most basic form of legal protection is to ensure the physical and psychological integrity of every person from abuse, neglect, or degrading treatment. The U.N. Declaration on the Rights of Mentally Retarded Persons (1971) proclaims this "right to protection from exploitation, abuse and degrading treatment" (art. 6). These are wide words and persons with mental retardation must look to national laws and to vigilant advocates for their interpretation and enforcement.

In the United States, this pursuit of protection from harm has been a significant element of the advocacy agenda. It is a recurrent motif in the institutional litigation (*Youngberg v. Romeo*, 1982; *N.Y. State Association for Retarded Children v. Carey*, 1975) and the legislative purposes of statutes creating systems of advocacy. As a result, protection and advocacy (P&A) systems now exist in the 50 states and the District of Columbia to represent and otherwise advocate for clients whose rights are in jeopardy (Developmentally Disabled Assistance and Bill of Rights Act, 1975). The federal Attorney General also has the right to sue on behalf of persons with disabilities who are subject to patterns of discrimination (Americans With Disabilities Act, 1990) or a pattern or practice of denials of federal rights in institutions (Civil Rights of Institutionalized Persons Act, 1980). Private attorneys may also recover attorney's fees as an incentive to vindicating civil rights (Civil Rights Attorney's Fees Awards Act of 1976).

Protection and advocacy systems have a special mission to make their services accessible to vulnerable and abused individuals. To ensure that institutionalized clients have meaningful access to legal protection, they have successfully litigated the right to visit those clients and to take other measures for outreach and the monitoring of potential rights violations (*Developmental Disabilities Advocacy Center v. Melton*, 1982; *Mississippi P&A System v. Cotten*, 1989). In the coming decade, these programs must also be geared to protect clients from abuse or neglect in community settings in which the majority of persons with special needs live. Eternal vigilance remains the price of not only liberty but freedom from harm.

Sparing Offenders With Mental Retardation From Execution

The United States is one of the few Western nations that exacts capital punishment. Regrettably, persons with mental retardation are not constitutionally relieved from this harsh sanction. The American Association on Mental Retardation and other disability organizations had urged the Supreme Court that "all mentally retarded people, regardless of their degree of retardation, have substantial cognitive and behavioral disabilities that reduce their level of blameworthiness for a capital offense" (AAMR, 1989, p. 30). The Supreme Court, however, held that mental retardation must only be considered as a mitigating factor, and that the Eighth Amendment (barring cruel and unusual punishment) does not preclude "the execution of any mentally retarded person of Penry's ability convicted of a capital offense simply by virtue of their mental retardation alone" (*Penry v. Lynaugh*, 1989, 109 S. Ct. 2934, 2958).

In support of its decision, the Court asserted a lack of consensus on barring the death penalty as a punishment for persons with mental retardation. It claimed that only Georgia had barred such executions (Georgia Code, 1988). This conclusion overlooked the enactment of a similar statute in Maryland precluding any person with mental retardation from being sentenced to death (Md. Code, 1989), the lack of any death penalty in 14 states, and the consistent opinion polling data that Americans (even in those states that have the highest rates of execution) do not believe offenders with mental retardation should be subject to the death penalty.

Drawing on this popular support, advocates for persons with mental retardation and foes of capital punishment have launched a multistate campaign to narrow or abolish the death penalty. In Kentucky (1990) and Tennessee (1990), state legislatures followed the lead of Georgia and Maryland in precluding the death penalty for persons with mental retardation. Other states are likely to follow in this decade leading to the year 2000.

As such statutes became more common, there are predictable consequences. More capital cases are likely to raise the issue of the offender's retardation or borderline mental retardation. There will be growing need for forensic experts capable of making the critical diagnostic assessments. Finally, as the costs of trying such cases and the inevitable multitiered appeals of convictions escalate and as the lack of deterrence of the death penalty can be statistically demonstrated, political pressure will mount for its outright abolition. Additionally, the number of nations that impose the death penalty will shrink, and the United States will not long wish to remain in the company of Iraq and South Africa as one of the handful of countries using this barbaric punishment.

Representing the Medical Choices of Adults Who Are Incompetent

The doctrine of informed consent requires that, before an individual can be subject to medical treatment, his or her consent must be knowing, voluntary, and competent. Some competent individuals with mental retardation have suffered from prejudice and discrimination when their informed consent to treatment has not been honored. A different set of difficulties arises when the individual lacks the cognitive or communicative abilities to provide or withhold consent. In such routine cases, this problem can be resolved through the consent obtained from the natural guardian of a minor, or the appointment of a temporary or limited guardian to exercise medical decision making. Many states also authorize such proxy decision making through durable powers of attorney, so-called living wills, or other mechanisms for providing substituted consent. For example, in the absence of either a durable power of attorney or a judicially appointed representative, Maryland permits certain family members to give substitute consent for the medical or dental treatment of a disabled individual (Md. Code Health-General, 1990).

In precedent-setting opinions, the courts have developed standards and procedures to be applied if life-sustaining treatment is to be withheld from a person who is severely incompetent. For example, the Massachusetts Supreme Judicial Court ordered that chemotherapy could be withheld from a 67-year-old man with profound mental retardation on the basis of the limited life extension possible and his fears arising from the likely unexplainable side-effects (*Superintendent of Belchertown v. Saikewicz*, 1977). In such cases, the court adopted a substituted judgment test to be based on the known interests and preferences of the patient, rather than his best interests. It further ruled that the ultimate decision lay with the judiciary, and not an ethics committee. However, a subsequent Massachusetts decision clarified that a doctor could end life-prolonging care on the doctor's initiative subject to legal liability for any wrongs committed (*In re Springs*, 1980).

The U.S. Supreme Court has recently addressed some of these complex legal, moral and political decisions. By a narrow five-to-four margin, the Court held that a young woman rendered incompetent by an accident cannot be denied life-saving hydration and nutrition (*Cruzan v. Director, Missouri Dept. of Health*, 1990). With little difficulty, the justices acknowledged that competent persons have a constitutional right to decline life-saving hydration and nutrition based on their liberty interest to refuse unwanted medical treatment. However, the majority opinion held that, as a matter of constitutional law, a state could require proof by clear and convincing evidence of the patient's own wishes when life-sustaining treatment was at stake. This procedural safeguard means that a surrogate decision maker may act to cause the patient's death only if "the action of the surrogate conforms as best it may to the wishes expressed by the patient while competent" (*Cruzan*, p. 4920). The Court reasoned that the state is entitled to erect strict safeguards against potential abuses by surrogates, or the lack of diligent, adversarial fact-finding in the trial courts entrusted with such matters. Courts and the states, therefore, need not defer to family decision making when some form of substitute judgment must be obtained.

The *Cruzan* (1990) opinion has broad implications for the future. It rejects so-called quality of life judgments as a basis for rationing medical treatment, upholding a state's right to "properly decline to make judgments about the 'quality' of life that a particular individual may enjoy, and simply assert an unqualified interest in the preservation of human life to be weighed against the constitutionally protected interests of the individual" (*Cruzan*, 1990, p. 4921). Although Cruzan's situation differs from that of individuals with developmental disabilities who have never experienced a period of competence, they will also be affected by the legal principles in *Cruzan* that allow states broad latitude to regulate medical decision making for incompetent persons. In the wake of this decision, it is likely that many states will comprehensively review their laws and policies in such matters. As part of that review, advocates should ensure that the predicament raised by *Saikewicz*-type situations is also resolved through legislative reforms. The most significant issues to be answered will be the qualifications of a substitute decision maker, the forum in which controversies will be resolved, the triggering event for judicial review, and the procedural safeguards and substantive standards of review to be imposed. For competent individuals, counseling is essential to ensure that some advance direction is provided to doctors and proxy decision makers when the individual can no longer articulate his or her wishes at the twilight of life.

Expanding Zones of Personal Autonomy

One of the revolutionary developments in the field of mental retardation is the expansion of the choices offered to clients and their families. No longer are the options limited to large institutions and sheltered workshops. No longer are the protective options restricted to plenary guardianship or no protection at all. To cope will new choices and to the possibilities of integration and full participation in society, many clients desire training in the exercise of their rights to self-determination. To avoid state-imposed stigma, legal systems must be subject to searching scrutiny as to its modes of assessing and recognizing various competencies. A positive emphasis on support systems of self-advocacy and personal advocacy is also essential if individuals are to acquire or regain particular competencies to vote, to associate with others in common cause, to use the services of the medical and legal professions, and to otherwise enjoy the normal benefits of community and social life to the extent of the individual's interests and capacities.

To accomplish these goals, consumers, professionals, and advocates must reexamine the rationale and necessity for limitations—legal as well as de facto—on client choices. Vague and unnecessary prohibitions on marriage by persons with mental disabilities will not likely survive that reexamination. Similarly, involuntary or nonconsensual sterilization of a nontherapeutic nature will also face invalidation by progressive courts (*E. (Mrs.) v. Eve*, 1986). In *Eve*, the Supreme Court of Canada held that the parens patriae jurisdiction (the court's protective power) does not permit a person with a mental handicap to be required to submit to a nontherapeutic sterilization authorized by the court at the behalf of a parent, next-of-kin, a facility administrator, or other third party. This decision upholds the principle that some rights are so personal to the individual affected that only that individual can decide to forfeit them. This principle is consistent with the emphasis on personally expressed wishes evident in the US Supreme Court's *Cruzan* (1990) opinion. This legal trend and advances in habilitation underscore the need to assist individuals with a disability to learn the skills to participate in, and to gain self-determination over, a wide spectrum of personal decision making. As legal barriers to full citizenship fall, the individual will need support and community acceptance to enjoy its benefits.

Eradicating Discrimination on the Basis of Handicap

A global movement is building to minimize, if not eradicate, discrimination based on handicap. Under the New South Wales Anti-Discrimination Act (1977), this Australian state has provided a system to reduce discrimination through a mechanism for complaints, enforcement remedies, and sanctions. In 1990, France enacted a similar law that would impose fines and even criminal sanctions for discrimination against handicapped persons in public accommodations and other public services. The International League of Societies for Persons With Mental Handicap has identified discrimination in everyday life in laws such as immigration laws barring the entry of such persons and in attempts to legalize the termination of the lives of severely impaired newborns as resulting in the mentally handicapped being "amongst the most discriminated against in the world of disability" (Lachwitz, 1990). Based on the prevalence and persistence of this experience, the International League has urged all nations to adopt antidiscrimination laws covering persons with disability.

A new law in the United States has stimulated calls for such legislation. Sweeping in its coverage and historic in its mission, the Americans With Disabilities Act (1990) (ADA) aims at nothing less than "a clear and comprehensive national mandate for the elimination of discrimination against individuals with disabilities" (Sec. 12101 [b] [l]). Persons with mental retardation are squarely within the Act's definition of disability because such persons likely possess a physical or mental impairment that substantially limits a major life activity, a record of such impairment, or are regarded as having such an impairment. Thus, the statutory definition covers individuals who are presently disabled, were formerly disabled, or are erroneously regarded by others as being disabled. One of the key concepts undergirding the Act's duties and remedies is that of "reasonable accommodation." In the employment context, this concept requires affirmative action. Existing facilities must therefore be made readily accessible to individuals with disabilities, while job restructuring, modified work schedules, reassignment, and other appropriate adjustments must be made to permit such individuals to be a part of the work force. These employment requirements become effective in July 1992 for larger employers with 25 or more employees and by July 1994 for employers with between 15 to 24 employees. Other specific antidiscrimination measures ensure access to public accommodations, state and local government activities, transportation, and telecommunications networks. In essence, ADA is a Magna Charta for all Americans with disabilities, and a civil rights affirmation that walls of exclusion must come down.

The future impact of ADA for persons with special needs will depend on the vigor of their advocates in noting complaints and demanding proactive implementation of its provisions. The Act contains a wide array of remedies, including court orders to stop discrimination, back pay orders, complaints to the Equal Employment Opportunity Commission, and complaints to the Attorney General (who is empowered to obtain money damages, penalties, and injunctions). Perhaps most significantly, in ensuring active enforcement, the law also permits private lawsuits and awards attorney's fees to prevailing plaintiffs.

With these tools, by the year 2000, many discriminatory barriers likely will fall. In planning and carrying out their operations, government agencies, employers, and others who serve the public will be obliged to reconsider, and desist from, potentially discriminatory and prejudicial actions against persons with mental retardation and other disabilities. One thing is certain: The disability-rights movement will have an active role to the second millennium and beyond.

Lurching Toward Jerusalem: The Future of Law for Persons With Special Needs

In the Jerusalem Congress of 1968, the International League of Societies for the Mentally Handicapped (as it was then known) proclaimed a new vision of human rights and full integration. In the Declaration of General and Special Rights of the Mentally Retarded, it boldly demanded equal treatment and equal rights. From its first article, the Declaration adopted an unambiguous egalitarian model: "The mentally retarded person has the same basic rights as other citizens of the same country and the same age (International League of Societies for the Mentally Handicapped, 1968, art. 1)." Realization of that egalitarian model and the elevation of the human services and the material conditions of life available to all members of society remain the universal goals of advocates.

Prejudice, poverty, war, and greed continue to hinder attainment of these goals. Prejudice—born of fear and lack of knowledge of the real possibilities of persons with mental retardation—are still reflected in timid constructions of human rights. Thus, the U.N. Declaration on the Rights of Mentally Retarded Persons (1971), largely modeled after the Jerusalem Declaration, waffled in its article 1 when it referred to persons with mental retardation having, "to the maximum degree of feasibility," the same rights as other human beings. It also added the caveat "whenever possible" to the rights to family and community living, noting that institutions might provide out-of-home care in "surroundings and other circumstances as close as possible to those of normal life" (art. 4). But only 4 years later, the U.N. took an unambiguous stance in declaring that disabled persons have "the same fundamental rights as their fellow-citizens of the same age, which implies first and foremost the right to enjoy a decent life, as normal and full as possible" (U.N., 1975, art. 3). But as long as the peoples of the world are troubled by homelessness, abject poverty, war and the threat of war, and domination by totalitarian states, these fundamental rights are in jeopardy.

By the year 2000, the challenge will be to extend the blessings of a decent, normal, and full life to all citizens with special needs. Inevitably, this leads to another challenge: minimizing the disparity in legal treatment of persons with mental retardation from persons with all other disabilities. To this end, few, if any, laws should single out persons with mental retardation for unique treatment. In general, they should have the same means to claim their rights and assert their interests as others do. Since article 11 of the U.N. Declaration on the Rights of Disabled Persons requires that disabled persons "shall be able to avail themselves of qualified legal aid when such aid proves indispensable for the protection of their persons and property" (1975, art.11), then persons with mental retardation must equally be assured of qualified and effective advocacy assistance. That assistance should include training those persons to better understand, and advocate for, their own rights. Self-advocates will then be able to evaluate and accept or reject professional advice with greater confidence.

By the year 2000, advocates will have become more sensitive to gradations of competency, more skilled in tutoring self-advocates, and more zealous in their defense of the zones in which clients make their own choices without undue risk. With additional supports for more independent living, the growth-inspiring options of family and community living, and advocates more attuned to client choices, the year 2000 will not become an Orwellian 1984. Instead, through the collaboration of persons with disabilities, legislators, disability professionals and advocates, the dream of equal rights and justice proclaimed in Jerusalem can improve the quality of choices to persons with special needs throughout the world. Beyond benevolence lies a universe of rights and options waiting to be claimed.

Acknowledgment. This chapter is dedicated to Gunnar and Rosemary Dybwad, whose pioneering and lifelong leadership for persons with special needs have inspired worldwide progress. This research was, in part, sponsored by the International Disability Exchanges and Studies (IDEAS) project, which is operated by the World Institute on Disability, in collaboration with Rehabilitation International and with funding from the U.S. Institute on Disability and Rehabilitation Research. The author also acknowledges with gratitude the assistance and insights that Professor Gunnar Dybwad generously contributed to this chapter.

As a Senior Fulbright Scholar in 1990–1991, the author also benefitted from the warm hospitality of the Tel Aviv University Shapell School of Social Work and the Hebrew University of Jerusalem Faculty of Law.

References

American Association on Mental Retardation et al., brief of amici curiae, Penry v. Lynaugh, 109 S.Ct. 2934 (1989).

Americans With Disabilities Act of 1990, Public Law No. 101–336, 42 U.S.C. §§ 12101–12231 (enacted July 26, 1990).

Bauer v. Hughes, Civ. No. 22871 (Md. Cir. Ct. Anne Arundel Co., May 16, 1984).

Bowen v. American Hospital Ass'n, 476 U.S. 610 (1986).

Brakel, S., Parry J., & Weiner, B. (1985). *The mentally disabled and the law* (3rd ed.). Chicago: American Bar Foundation.

Buck v. Bell, 274 U.S. 200 (1927).

Child Abuse Amendments of 1984, 42 U.S.C. §§ 5106a(b)(10), 5106g(10) (Supp. 1990).

City of Cleburne v. Cleburne Living Center, 473 U.S. 432 (1985).

Civil Rights Attorney's Fees Awards Act of 1976, 42 U.S.C. § 1988 (1981).

Civil Rights of Institutionalized Persons Act of 1980, 42 U.S.C. §§ 1997–1997j (1981).

Clark v. Cohen, 794 F.2d 79 (3d Cir. 1986).

Connecticut Gen. Stat. Ann. Const. Art. 21, (enacted 1984) (Supp. 1986).

Cruzan v. Director, Missouri Dept. of Health, 110 S. Ct. 2841 (U.S. Sup. Ct. June 25, 1990).

Developmental Disabilities Advocacy Center v. Melton, 689 F.2d 281 (1st Cir. 1982).

Developmentally Disabled Assistance and Bill of Rights Act of 1975, 42 U.S.C §§ 6041–6043 (Supp. 1990).

E. (Mrs.) v. Eve, (1986) 2 S.C.R. 388.

Fair Housing Amendments Act of 1988, Public Law No. 100–430, 42 U.S.C. § 3602 and scattered sections (Supp. 1990).

Ferleger, D., & Boyd P. (1979). Anti-institutionalization: The promise of the *Pennhurst* case. *Stanford Law Review*, *31*(4), 717–752.

Georgia Code Ann. § 17-7-131(j) (enacted 1988) (Supp. 1989).

German Guardianship Law. (1990).

Guardianship of Becker, No. 101981 (Cal. Super. Ct., Santa Clara Co., August 7, 1981), *aff'd* 188 Cal. Rptr. 781, 139 Cal. App. 3d 407 (1st Dist. 1983).

Halderman v. Pennhurst State School and Hospital, 446 F. Supp. 1925 (E.D. Pa. 1977).

Halderman v. Pennhurst State School and Hospital, No. 74–1345. Final settlement agreement (E.D. Pa. April 5, 1985).

Herr, S., & Schuster-Herr, R. (1984). *Advocacy and mental handicap.* Approved and adopted as an official position paper of the International League of Societies for Persons with Mental Handicap [ILSPMH]. Brussels: ILSPMH.

Honig v. Doe, 108 S. Ct. 592 (1988).

Iasimone v. Garrahy, No. 77-0727 (D.R.I. April 29, 1982).

In re Schmidt, 494 Pa. 86, 429 A.2d 631 (1981).

In re Springs, 405 N.E.2d 115 (Mass. 1980).

In the Matter of Charles Turner, Md. Board of Public Works (May 1984).

International League of Societies for the Mentally Handicapped. (1968, October 24). Declaration of General and Special Rights of Mentally Retarded Persons, adopted in Jerusalem.

International League of Societies for Persons with Mental Handicap. (1990, August 5–10). *Turning rights into realities: 10th World Congress*, program brochure. Paris.

Israel Special Education Law. (1988), Statutes of the State of Israel (No. 1256), p. 114.

Kass, L. R. (1988). Citizens with mental retardation and the local community. In L. Kane, P. Brown & J. Cohen (Eds.), *The Legal Rights of Citizens with Mental Retardation*, pp. 7–23.

Kennedy Foundation. (1971). *Who should survive?* [Documentary film]. Washington: Joseph P. Kennedy, Jr. Foundation.

Kentucky Session Law (1990), S.B. No. 172 (to be codified at Ky. Rev. Stat. Ch. 532).

Lachwitz, K. (1990, August 5–10). *ILSMH seminar on rights and advocacy: Key issues paper*. Paper presented at the 10th World Congress of ILSMH. Paris.

Md. Code Art. 27, § 412 (enacted May 1989) (Supp. 1990).

Md. Code Health-General, § 20–107 (1990).

Mental and physical disability law reporter (published 6 times a year). Washington, DC: American Bar Association.

Michigan Association for Retarded Citizens v. Smith, 475 F. Supp. 990 (E.D. Mich. 1979).

Michigan Association for Retarded Citizens v. Wayne County Probate Judge, 79 Mich. App. 487 (1977).

Mickenberg, N. (1979). The silent clients: Legal and ethical considerations in representing severely and profoundly retarded individuals. *Stanford Law Review*, *31*(4), 625–636.

Mills v. Board of Education of the District of Columbia, 348 F. Supp. 866 (D.D.C. 1972).

Mississippi Protection and Advocacy System v. Cotten, No. J87-0503(L) (S.D. Miss. Aug. 7, 1989).

New South Wales Anti-Discrimination Act. (1977).

New York State Association for Retarded Children v. Carey, 393 F. Supp. 715 (E.D. N.Y. 1975).

New Zealand Protection of Personal Property Rights Act. (1988), No. 4.

O'Conner v. Donaldson, 422 U.S. 563 (1975).

Pennhurst State School and Hospital v. Halderman, 451 U.S. 1 (1981) [Pennhurst I].

Pennhurst State School and Hospital v. Halderman, 465 U.S. 89 (1984) [Pennhurst II].

Penry v. Lynaugh, 109 S. Ct. 2934 (1989).

Pennsylvania Association for Retarded Children v. Pennsylvania, 343 F. Supp. 279 (E.D. Pa. 1972).

Rothman, D. J., & Rothman, S. M. (1984). *The Willowbrook wars: A decade of struggle for social justice*. New York: Harper & Row.

Rowley v. Hendrick Hudson School Board of Education, 458 U.S. 176 (1982).

Section 504 of the Rehabilitation Act of 1973, 29 U.S.C. § 794 (Supp. 1990).

Society for Good Will to Retarded Children v. Cuomo, 737 F.2d 239 (2d Cir. 1984).

Superintendent of Belchertown v. Saikewicz, 370 N.E.2d 417 (Mass. 1977).

Tennessee Session Law (1990), S.B. No. 1851 (to be codified at Tenn. Code Ann. tit. 39, ch. 13).

Thomas S. v. Flaherty, No. 89-1006 (4th Cir. May 2, 1990), *cert. denied*, 111 S. Ct. 373 (1990).

Thomas S. v. Morrow, 781 F.2d 367, *cert. denied sub nom.*, Childress v. Thomas S., 479 U.S. 869 (1986).

U.N. Convention on the Rights of the Child. (1989, December 5). G.A. Res. 44/25, U.N. Doc. 89-31648.

U.N. Declaration on the Rights of Disabled Persons. (1975). G.A. Res. 3447, 30 U.N. GAOR, Supp. (No. 34) 88–89, U.N. Doc. A/10034.

U.N. Declaration on the Rights of Mentally Retarded Persons. (1971). G.A. Res. 2856, 26 U.N. GAOR Supp. (No. 29) 93–94, U.N. Doc. A/8429.

U.N. Universal Declaration of Human Rights. (1948). G.A. Res. 217, U.N. Doc. A/810.

U.S. D.H.H.S. (1982). Notice to health-care providers, May 18, 1982, 47 Fed. Reg. 26027.

U.S. D.H.H.S. (1985). Final rules on procedures relating to health care for handicapped infants, January 12, 1984, 45 C.F.R. § 84.55.

Victorian Guardianship and Administration Board Act. (1986). §§ 22, 28(2).

Wentzel v. Montgomery County Hospital, 293 Md. 685 (1982).

Wyatt v. Aderholt, 503 F.2d 1305 (5th Cir. 1974).

Wyatt v. Stickney, 344 F. Supp. 387 (M.D. Ala. 1972).

Youngberg v. Romeo, 457 U.S. 307 (1982).

18
Staffing Issues in the Early 21st Century: Labor Supply, Program Models, and Technology

James F. Gardner and Michael Chapman

The community-based service programs that arose in the period from 1965 to 1980 were derivatives of the institutional models. Training and habilitation programs moved from the institution to smaller, more normalized community-based settings. Half-way homes and group homes were designed as mini-components of the larger facilities. Alternative living units, supervised apartments, and co-resident living arrangements were logical extensions of the continuum toward smaller community-based programs.

Several factors influenced the design of community service programs. There was an adequate labor force to staff the new programs. In addition, prevailing wages were sufficient to attract needed labor. Finally, the staffing patterns and management models were based on programs and experiences from institutional settings.

The issues of manpower availability, staffing, and training can be considered within the context of a human service labor market (Beauregard & Indik, 1979). Numerous studies have explored the relationship between labor supply and labor demand, productivity, and satisfaction (Levitan et al., 1972). Lester Thurow (1975) has challenged the neoclassical economic supply–demand interpretation by noting that organizations do not employ on the basis of projected productivity in relation to wage rates but rather on the cost of training the worker to perform the job. The quality of the labor force, the impact of education on productivity, and the role of social policy and public spending in human services have been examined (Boulding, 1967; Thurow, 1970).

The staffing models and training methods that emerge in the new century will reflect the intersection of three interdependent variables. The first variable is the labor supply. The second variable is the range of program models that defines employment responsibilities and the corresponding wage. The third variable is the use of available teaching and training technologies. The three variables will provide the basis for a relevant analysis of staffing issues for both the traditional range of community and institutional programs as well as the newly emerging supportive service programs.

Labor supply refers to the availability and characteristics of personnel to fill positions in programs serving people with developmental disabilities in the next century. The qualitative and quantitative characteristics of the labor supply will influence the direction and intensity of new program design and development. Service providers will consider the availability of needed personnel as they develop new program models.

Future program models will determine the expected performance level and compensation for human service workers. Residential and vocational program staff can be considered as "habilitation and training" staff or "care" staff. The former description assumes competencies related to teaching and habilitation, while the latter anticipates an entry-level human service job. Program models will be influenced by public sector policy priorities, funding, and if confronted by an insufficient or under-prepared labor force, the commitment to staff development and training.

The third variable, the use of available teaching and training technology, refers to the ability of state developmental disabilities agencies and provider organizations to adapt new technology. Training technologies might increase employee performance and responsibility so that program models continue to develop despite a contracting labor pool.

Recent Staffing Patterns

In 1962, the President's Panel on Mental Retardation (1962) report stated:

Society's special responsibility to persons with extraordinary needs is (1) to permit and actually foster the development of their maximum capacity and thus bring them as close to the main stream of independence and "normalcy" as possible; and (2) to provide some accommodation or adjustment in our society for those disabilities which cannot be overcome (p. 13).

The following year, Congress passed PL 88-164, which authorized the development of mental retardation research centers, university-affiliated facilities, and community mental health centers. That year also marked the peak in the number of persons residing in institutions. In the following years, the number of community-based programs increased dramatically and the number of persons residing in institutions for individuals with developmental disabilities decreased 57% between fiscal year 1967 and 1987, from 228,500 to 97,533 (White, Lakin, Hill, Wright, & Bruininks, 1988).

The development of alternatives to the institution has resulted in a proliferation of small, typically 15 beds or less, community-based alternative living arrangements. Between 1967 and 1985, alternative living arrangements have increased from approximately 22,000 to over 100,000

(Bruininks, Hill, Lakin, & White, 1985). During the last 10 years, community beds increased from 16.3% to 41.3% of the total number of individuals served (Lakin, Hill, White, & Wright, 1987).

The increase in community placements resulted in the need for additional qualified staff. Unfortunately, many of the concerns expressed during the 1960s continue to exist throughout the community-based network. Programs remain underfunded and understaffed. The shortage of qualified personnel persisted through the 1980s (Benson, 1979; Smull, 1989).

For the adult service system, there is a significant lack of professional staff to adequately meet the needs of individuals with developmental disabilities (Richardson, West, & Fifield, 1985). Occupational therapists, physical therapists, speech pathologists, psychologists, and other allied health professionals who are qualified and trained in developmental disabilities are not present in many communities. Many specialists do not want to work the hours required or needed by residential providers. In addition, physicians lack adequate training in developmental disabilities and have little experience working with nonmedical staff to address the health needs of individuals with developmental disabilities (Willer, Ross, & Intagliata, 1980). Physicians are often not prepared to participate in an interdisciplinary planning process (Garrard, 1982; Powers & Healy, 1982).

The terms *direct-care workers* and *paraprofessionals* usually describe those individuals involved in the day-to-day responsibility for and contact with individuals with developmental disabilities. These individuals are typically high school graduates with little or no formal preservice training in developmental disabilities. Over 78% of all personnel who come in contact with individuals with developmental disabilities are direct-care workers (Schalock, 1983). The responsibilities of the direct-care worker includes such tasks as data collection, mealtime supervision, activity of daily living training, participation on the interdisciplinary team, and individualized program development and implementation. Community programs are currently confronted with shortages of underprepared direct-care workers and high turnover rates (Richardson, West, & Fifield, 1985).

This growing scarcity of qualified entry-level staff and the increase in the number of geographically decentralized residential and vocational programs challenges the validity of the current staffing and management models (Smull, 1989).

Future Staffing Patterns

Demographics

Between 1990 and 2000, the 50-year and older age group will grow by 18.5%, while the number of people under the age of 50 will increase by 3.5%. The number of people over 75 will increase by 26% (Ostroff, 1989). The American population will continue to age in the new century. By 2030, the baby boom generation of 77 million people will be senior citizens. For the first time in history, the average American will have more living parents than children (Beck, 1989).

The greying of the population will be accompanied by a changing face of American youth. By the year 2010, more than one third of American children will be African American, Hispanic, or Asian. In seven states, they will represent 50% or more of the youth population—Hawaii (80%); New Mexico (77%); California (57%); Texas (57%); New York (53%); Florida (53%); and Louisiana (50%) (Ostroff, 1989).

In the absence of a radical policy change, the number of legal and illegal immigrants will also continue to rise. Projections of past trends indicate that at least 450,000 legal and 200,000 illegal immigrants will enter the United States each year during the next decade. Both the Hispanic and Asian populations are expected to double to 30 million and 10 million by the year 2000 (Johnston & Packer, 1987). These changes will be reflected in the population with developmental disabilities entering the service system and in the labor force providing services.

The Labor Supply

During the period 1968 to 1988, the American labor force swelled by about 50% (Johnston & Packer, 1987). The average age and experience of the new workers shifted downward. Faced with the increase in cheap new labor, American business increased hiring rather than investing in labor-saving methods and machinery.

The change in the work force in the last decade will be dramatic. The work force will grow slowly and become older, more female, and more disadvantaged. The labor force, which expanded at an annual rate of 2.9% in the 1970s will grow at a projected rate of 1% in the 1990s. The average age of the work force will increase from 36 in 1987 to 39 in the year 2000. Young workers in the age range 16 to 24 will decrease by 2 million or about 8% (Cetron, Rocha, & Luckins, 1988; Johnston & Packer, 1987).

Two thirds of the new workers between 1987 and the year 2000 will be women, and two thirds of all employable women will hold jobs by 2000. That number should increase to 75% in the next decade. Immigrants will constitute the largest share in the increase in the work force since the

First World War. During the period 1987 to 2000, about 15% of new workers will be native white men as compared to 47% in that category in 1987 (Cetron et al., 1988; Johnston & Packer, 1987). In total, minorities, women, and immigrants will represent more than 83% of the new workers though they make up only 50% in the late 1980s (Johnston & Packer, 1987, p. 93).

The changing nature of the work force will present challenges to the field of developmental disabilities. Employees will constitute a much more heterogeneous work group with more varied cultural and linguistic differences. In-service and on-the-job training programs will become more complex. Provision of culturally normative habilitation programs will become more challenging as the heterogeneity of both individuals with developmental disabilities and employees increases. University Affiliated Programs will be challenged to recruit a wide range of cultural and ethnic minorities as short- and long-term trainees.

The Growth of the Service Economy

There is much greater agreement about the direction of the economy than about the rate of growth (Cappo, 1990; Cetron & Davies, 1989). Although less than 50% of the national income came from service industries in 1950, the figure reached 66% in 1985 and will be close to 75% by 2020 (Stewart, 1989). In terms of employment rather than income, only 5% of the jobs in the year 2000 will be in manufacturing, food production, or industrial goods production. Approximately 95% of the jobs will be in the service and information processing sectors (Cain & Taber, 1987).

Recent and projected growth in the service industry indicate that newly emerging jobs in professional, technical, and sales fields require the greatest education and skill level. Following an analysis of job opportunities in the service sector and areas of greatest growth, Hugh B. Stewart (1989) concludes, "With half of all the demand for workers coming in areas requiring high skills, but with only 25 percent of the candidates being college graduates, the competition for highly qualified people could be extraordinarily vigorous" (p. 312).

Another analysis of the service industry concludes that the largest growth occupations of the 1990s are bottom-level service jobs—janitors, nurses' aides and orderlies, sales clerks, waiters and waitresses. Without new skills and education, minorities will dominate such jobs as other workers with the education and technical skill reach for the narrower band of better service sector jobs (Norton, 1984).

The increased competition for skilled labor in the service economy may pose some difficulties for organizations serving people with developmental disabilities that are unable to provide attractive wages or challenging work. Jobs in the field of developmental disabilities may not be located in that "narrower band of better service sector jobs."

The labor market for young workers will become more competitive. Organizations that have traditionally found young workers at lower wages will face the choice of raising wages, searching for employees further down in the labor queue, substituting technology for labor, or all three.

The Changing Structure of Work

The decline in the growth of the labor force coupled with the advances in technology will place a larger emphasis on productivity. The United States sustained a rising standard of living throughout the 1970s and early 1980s by increasing the number of people at work and by borrowing from abroad. Both of these phenomena will reach their limit at the end of the century (Johnston & Packer, 1987; Stewart, 1989).

The key to economic growth in the last decade will be to increase the productivity of the service sector in which the productivity per worker declined .02% over the last 15 years (Johnston & Packer, 1987). Several authors (Johnston & Packer, 1987; Stewart 1989) have noted that the key to such growth will be more competition and productivity in traditionally noncompetitive sectors such as education, health care, and government service.

The emphasis on productivity and the decrease in the traditional work force may cause health and human service organizations to shift attention to technologies and systems that improve efficiency and reduce expenses. The technology that will automate factories in the year 2000 will be available for the automated nursing home and the computerized Intermediate Care Facility for the Mentally Retarded (ICF/MR) (Cain & Taber, 1987; Johnston & Packer, 1987). Advanced robots linked with artificial intelligence that are capable of assisting people with basic self-help and daily living skills will be considered adaptive extensions of individual capacity (Johnston & Packer, 1987; Stewart, 1989). Technology, guided by values, can enhance the independence, productivity, and integration of people with developmental disabilities. Technology driven by efficiency and cost savings alone will further the process of dehumanization in human services.

The increases in productivity through the use of new technology mean that the quality of work life will improve. Isaac Asimov (1984) writes that "the dull, the boring, the repetitive, the mind-stultifying work will begin to disappear from the job market" (p. 26). Futurist Caroline Bird (1984) also writes, "Dull, demeaning jobs will go unfilled because no one will be willing to do them at the wage they're worth in competition with other goods and services. It's happening already" (p. 135). The changing structure of work in a service economy suggests that, because of the alternative employment possibilities, only the less qualified, experienced, and trained will opt for entry-level jobs in the field of developmental disabilities.

Program Models

There are three distinct possibilities for future program development: maintaining the status quo, the rebirth of institutionalization, and expansion of community programs.

Maintaining the status quo involves no changes in the current service system. The issues that community agencies face today are projected into the future. Patterns of underfunding, understaffing, and high turnover rates will persist into the next decade. For most states, the waiting list for services is growing (Smull, Sachs, Cahn, & Feder, 1988). States are unable to meet the demand for services. In addition, the majority of individuals with developmental disabilities remain in their parents' home and as these parents become older (Black, Cohn, Smull, & Crites, 1985), the demand for community-based services will increase. During the past two decades, the solution to the problem was to reduce the size of the institutions, while building the capacity of the community to meet the needs of individuals with developmental disabilities. In effect, the large institutions were downsized, and many areas of the community have become saturated with group homes and smaller three-person alternative living units. Smull and Bellamy (1991) state:

The needs to improve the quality of community programs, expand services to accommodate individuals on waiting lists, and reduce the size of institutions constitute a set of mutually reinforcing pressures on available resources. Yesterday's solutions have become today's crisis. (p. 508)

To maintain the status quo into the next decade may place unbearable pressures on the service system. To do so is to jeopardize continued community placements for individuals with developmental disabilities.

There is the possibility of a return to the institution as the focus of service. Many states are struggling to build the community's capacity to meet the needs of individuals with developmental disabilities and to eliminate waiting list for services. At the same time, many states are spending significant amounts of moneys on institutional care to comply with the evolving active treatment regulations imposed by the Health Care Finance Administration (HCFA). The threatened loss of federal financial participation has forced many states to continue their support for institutional care. Coupled with a shrinking labor pool in entry-level positions in the community for direct care and professional staff, and the increasing demand for services, the institutional census in some states may begin to rise.

Community expansion involves developing new residential options. Residential services are designed to provide individuals with developmental disabilities a place to live and to become a part of community life. The service system, however, has failed to develop innovative, cost-effective residential options for individuals in need of levels of care different from that provided by a group home or alternative living unit (Bruininks et al., 1985). As a result, if the individual does not fit into an existing community "slot" or "bed," the individual goes unserved or underserved.

Future community expansion will require new conceptual frames to replace the continuum of care. Smull (1989) calls for a paradigm shift away from community-based residential living units to community-based networks of support. The focus is on building natural support systems in the community.

Building natural support systems begins with the individual with developmental disabilities. In contrast to the existing service system, a support system begins by asking individuals where they want to live, who they want to live with (if anyone), how they want to spend their day, and who they wish to spend their time with. Neighbors and friends are untapped resources. They offer a resource, either paid or as volunteers, that could meet the needs of individuals with developmental disabilities. Maximizing these opportunities could lead to a reduction in full-time agency staff. A few programs have begun to develop informal community support systems relying on family members, friends, or neighbors that replace the paid agency staff (Rusch & Hughes, 1988).

The program models that emerge in the next century will be influenced by the availability of the number and quality of workers. The dominant models will also influence the development of labor markets. The strategies for preservice and in-service training programs will be very different for staff residing in a centralized institution, employees in a decentralized community based system, and for volunteers and friends in an informal support network.

The future development of support service models, of informal helping networks, and of volunteers represents more than an evolutionary trend in the field of developmental disabilities. Rather, the debate over informal support systems, the use of peers and volunteers, and the role of the voluntary association is part of the ongoing dialogue about the role of government in American society.

Continued indications of the contraction of the welfare state suggest an increasing role for the voluntary organization. Strengthening the role of the voluntary sector is also advanced as a means for recapturing the lost sense of community and preventing the advances of federal and state bureaucracy. Reflecting John Dewey's and Mary Follett's early 20th-century faith in neighborhood groups to provide social services, Berger and Neuhaus (1977) argue for a greater use of the mediating structures of neighborhood, family, church, and voluntary association, which provide some distance between the individual's private life and the megastructures of public life.

In contrast, Kramer (1981) argues that supporters of empowerment treat all forms of volunteerism the same in countering excessive government size. There are considerable differences, he notes, between volunteers as unpaid staff and peer self-help; between mutual aid, neighborhood, and community-based service agencies; and between forms of citizen participation and the institutional structures of family and church. Volunteers, argues Kramer, "are no substitute for necessary services best delivered by professionals and other types of paid staff" (1981, p. 284).

Economics, politics, demographics, and performance standards for human service systems will influence the evolution of program models. However, the scarcity of qualified labor will increase the concern for the quality of services and will result in a reevaluation of management models for decentralized scattered site programs.

Continued development of community-based options with an emphasis on social integration might reflect organic organizational characteristics, as displayed in Table 18.1 (Daft, 1989, p. 61). Smaller, community-based programs, especially those connected to informal systems of natural support, would exist in changing environments, and the resulting internal management system to cope with the environmental uncertainty will be looser, freer flowing, and adaptive. The organic management form would stress employee decision making and interaction rather than formalized policy and procedure (Koontz, O'Donnell, & Weihrich, 1986).

Community-based programs connected to the informal support service network will decentralize decision-making responsibility. Increased consumer autonomy and support service networks will decrease the relative role of the professional and increase the responsibilities of staff in geographically dispersed program settings, informal support providers, and

TABLE 18.1. Mechanistic and organic organization forms.

Mechanistic	Organic
1. Tasks are broken down into specialized, separate parts.	1. Employees contribute to the common task of the department.
2. Tasks are rigidly defined.	2. Tasks are adjusted and redefined through employee interactions.
3. There is a strict hierarchy of authority and control, and there are many rules.	3. There is less hierarchy of authority and control, and there are few rules.
4. Knowledge and control of tasks are centralized at the top of organization.	4. Knowledge and control of tasks are located anywhere in the organization.
5. Communication is vertical.	5. Communication is horizontal.

Note. From *Organization Theory and Design* (p. 61) by R. L. Daft, 1989, St. Paul, MN: West Publishing. Copyright 1989 by West Publishing. Reprinted by permission.

families. Professionals are already taking on new roles as orchestrators, coordinators, and facilitators of dialogue within support systems. Staffing patterns currently include parents and volunteers exercising leadership responsibilities (Kagan, Powell, Weissbourd, & Zigler, 1987).

The increasing body of knowledge about the medical, educational, and habilitative aspects of disability will preclude excellence in all areas of service. Information-based organizations will depend on teams of task and specialty focused staff (Cetron et al., 1988).

This decentralization and delegation of authority will occur only if there is a corresponding increase in management control and information-feedback systems. Managers can delegate only when there is a sufficient information-control system that allows them to monitor the delegated responsibilities. The management control system in the open system community-based option must be flexible, practical, and applicable to each individual manager. The management control system in place today relies on occasional observation, written logs, records, and documentation. It is more subjective than objective, and exceptions to expectation form the basis for action.

The management control systems of the future, especially in the decentralized service system, will be based on computerized information systems. Decision processes and management structures will be transformed as organizations move from using data to using information (data that have been analyzed) (Cetron et al., 1988). Managers will have access to habilitation program information to determine the effectiveness of programs. Staff and individuals with developmental disabilities will communicate, schedule, and report through integrated information systems. The future management control system will stress the measurement and correction of individual and group staff performance to ensure that organizational objectives (and the plans to attain them) are accomplished (Cain & Taber, 1987; Stewart, 1989).

Training Technology

The future of technology in an information society has begun. Futurists, for example, have examined the proliferation of electronic bulletin boards, information-sharing systems, and data bases such as the Library of Congress or the New York Stock Exchange. Projecting trends, Cain (1985) describes a "Net Console" as an integrated system of communication connected to the personal computer via satellite, cable, telephone line, or cellular radio. The home system will be linked to a global communication and data transmission matrix known as the "Net." Linked to the world grid, the user will have access to the vast richness of human knowledge and art. As a home–work–school learning station, the Net Console will include a number of computer-interface devices such as adaptive input devices, microphones, video cameras, videodisk recorders, biofeedback units, and key boards (Cain, 1985; Vail, 1980). In addition, the Integrated Services Digital Network (ISDN) will allow data to be transmitted in digital form without the expense of signal processing through modems. This will bring the smaller users into the communication system (Cetron et al., 1988).

SRI International Business Intelligence Project, a California think-tank operation, in 1986, identified some probable home uses of the Net Counsel, in the early 21st century. Some of those projections, listed as follows, can be quickly reinvented and applied to the field of developmental disabilities (Cain & Taber, 1987, p. 44).

Expert parent supervision systems that monitor activity of children, detect possible problems, and suggest alternative courses of action

Intelligent games that interact with multiple players, automatically change the parameters of play, and introduce new contingencies based on the levels of play

Expert systems for identifying problems in the home and directing the appropriate home repair

"Better systems to aid in identifying, overcoming, or compensating for specific learning or physical disabilities

Artificially intelligent computers that learn how to learn and can apply past experience to present circumstances will provide potentially powerful forms of support to people with developmental disabilities. The early 21st century should witness the elementary development of artificially intelligent natural language-analysis systems that will enable individuals with receptive or expressive language problems or with limited linguistic abilities to communicate in their own natural language system and let the computer translate into the language of the general population (Cain & Taber, 1987).

Artificial intelligence and expert systems could form the basis for most diagnostic work, evaluation and assessment, and programming in the next century. The data base for programming would contain the individual's assessment and individual program plan history, the full range of information from the health, education, and habilitation fields, and the collective knowledge of practitioners.

Robots coupled with artificial intelligence linked to the Net Console will be able to provide services ranging from environmental control, to mobility, to self-care. The ability of the robots to learn from experience, to communicate and be controlled through the natural language system of the user, and to perform delicate fine-motor tasks could potentially enable individuals to make significant strides in independence, productivity, and integration (Cain & Taber, 1987).

The new technology will have an impact on the training of staff, the roles and functions of staff and individuals with developmental disabilities, and staffing requirements for programs. Computer-assisted instruction, interactive videodisk, and satellite teleconferencing will provide instruction to new employees at minimal cost and disruption to the organization through the Net Counsel (Cain & Taber, 1987; Stewart, 1989). Job-simulation stations will facilitate the training process (Cetron et al., 1988).

More importantly, artificial intelligence, expert systems, robotics, and the Net Counsel will redefine roles of individuals with disabilities, staff, friends, and volunteers. People who support persons with disabilities will not be masters of content and technique. Rather, they will assist individuals with disabilities to access that information and support functions from the computer and the computer-assisted devices. The computer will address the specific learning and training needs of the new employee and the learning and habilitation needs of the individual with a developmental disability (Cetron, 1988). Software and artificial intelligence will perform a diagnostic prescriptive function for the employee facilitator and for the individual with the disability.

The technology for interactive training systems is presently available. The videodisk, for example, can incorporate existing media (printed text, color slides, graphics, or videotape) into a single medium while retaining the advantages of each. The 54,000 pages of video frames on the videodisk can be individually accessed as self-paced instruction, as programmed instruction, or as question and answer formats. Linking the computer with the videodisk allows multiple paths (based on individual needs and learning style) through information fields (Daynes, 1982; Kukla & Montenegro, 1981; Levine, 1982; Nugent, 1982). However, treading the path may be difficult. The development of interactive video is a complex process and can require up to 350 hours of production for each hour of computer-assisted instruction (Beausey, 1988; Lee & Zemke, 1987).

Because the "what to do" and the "how to do it" can be answered with the assistance of the computer, human resource development will become more focused on adult learning theory (Brookfield, 1986; Knowles, 1978; Wlodkowski, 1985). The emphasis on adult learning theory is consistent with the trends in technology, decentralized program sites, and organic management systems.

Modern adult learning theory rests on several assumptions, as articulated by Lindeman (1926, pp. 15–16):

1. Motivation to learn develops as adults experience interests and needs that learning will satisfy.
2. The adult orientation to learning is life-centered. The units for organizing adult learning are life situations, not subject matter.
3. Experience is the prime resource for adult learning. The primary methodology of adult education is the analysis of experience.
4. Because adults need to be self-directing, the role of the teacher is to facilitate mutual learning rather than transmit knowledge and evaluate their conformity with it.

5. Because individual differences increase with age, adult education should make allowances for variations in style, time, place, and pace of learning.

The human service agency in the year 2000 will mold the early 20th-century insights in adult education with the educational technology of the 21st century. The synthesis will be a midmanagement mentoring system based on adult learning theory supplemented by access to computer information.

Scarcity of entry-level staff and continued high turnover in the formal service system will cause organizations to place a premium on well-trained midlevel managers. The midlevel managers will, in turn guide entrylevel staff, and the education will be experientially based. The midlevel manager will serve as both supervisor and mentor, job-coach and learning facilitator.

The midlevel manager will perform a number of coaching functions. The functions will be job related and performed on a one-to-one basis. The multiple coaching functions support an organic management style and are consistent with adult learning theory. The four functions follow (Kinlaw, 1989, pp. 22–23):

1. Counseling—The midmanager assists the employee to better understand one's feelings and behavior. As counselor, the midmanager helps staff vent strong feelings and change points of view.
2. Mentoring—The midmanager enables the employee to understand the organization's culture, values, and norms. As mentor, the midmanager develops in staff the ability to do personal networking and managing one's career.
3. Tutoring—The midmanager aids the employee to gain the technical competence and develop a commitment to ongoing learning.
4. Confronting—The midmanager will increase the employee's ability to confront shortcoming in performance. The employee is assisted in identifying expectations, performance, and methods of self-evaluation.

This andragogical learning model is based on process as opposed to the content model of traditional education. The process model establishes a set of procedures for integrating individual needs, motivation, and goals with previous and current work experience (Knowles, 1978, 1984).

The process model of human resource development will more readily accommodate the diversity of the labor pool in the next century as well as the range of formal and informal support systems that will develop in response to individual needs. The process model suggests that the staff will participate in continued learning and analysis of the work situation as individuals with disabilities make greater use of technological supports in both the formal and informal service settings.

The process model may also be more appropriate for some forms of informal helping networks. When helpers within the individual's network provide assistance on the basis of established relationships, the costs associated with training, supervision, and recruitment are absent. Costs associated with these functions begin to rise when lay helpers unknown to the individual are employed. In a study of five types of helping networks, the costs associated with supervision, recruitment, and training of volunteer linking programs exceeded costs for similar functions in personal network, mutual aid, neighborhood helping, and community empowerment programs (Froland, Pancoast, Chapman, & Kimboko, 1981).

Human service programs serving persons with developmental disabilities did not adapt the new training technology during the 1970s and 1980s. Costs for hardware were expensive, and software programs were often marginal. In addition, employers often had access to inexpensive labor to replace staff. During the next century, there will be added incentives to use technology for training: lower cost and better, individualized instruction. However, the use of new technology will require the support and commitment of the opinion leadership in the field of developmental disabilities (Rogers, 1983). The diffusion of innovation will occur if state agency administrators and executive directors of organizations play the role of facilitators and change agents.

Conclusion

Emerging program models, the labor supply, and the adaption of new technology are interdependent. Technology can compensate for potential problems in the labor supply, and it can make major contributions to the independence, productivity, and integration of persons with disabilities. The technology of the information society can provide the management control systems that will enable decentralized and even informal support service programs to flourish. But history provides two cautions:

The not-for-profit human services sector has been conservative and traditional in its application of innovation. The leaders in the field of disability must make the case that people with disability have an equal and perhaps greater claim on the new technology than other citizens.

Technology must be incorporated to expand our value base for people with disabilities and not to supplant it. Lives filled with technology but void of values will be unfulfilled.

References

Asimov, I. (1984). Creativity will dominate our time after the concepts of work and fun have been blurred by technology. In L. Chiara & D. Lacey (Eds.), *Work in the 21st century: An anthology of writing on the changing world of work* (pp. 25–32). New York: Hippocrene Books.

Beauregard, R., & Indik, B. (1979). *A human service labor market: developmental disabilities.* New Brunswick, NJ: Rutgers University Center for Urban Policy Research.

Beausey, M. (1988). Videodisc development: No lone rangers, please. *Training: The Magazine of Human Resource Development, 25,* 65–68.

Beck, M. (1989). The geezer boom. *Newsweek: The 21st century family.* Winter/ Spring, pp. 62–71.

Benson, A. (1979). University affiliated facilities: A primary resource in improving services for developmentally disabled persons. Washington, DC: American Association of University Affiliated Programs.

Berger, P. L., & Neuhaus, R. J. (1977). *To empower people: The role of mediating structures in public policy.* Washington, DC: American Enterprise Institute for Public Policy Research.

Bird, C. (1984). Retirement will become obsolete in the improved work scheme of our 21st century economy. In L. Chiara & D. Lacey (Eds.), *Work in the 21st century: An anthology of writing on the changing world of work* (pp. 131–139). New York: Hippocrene Books.

Black, M., Cohn, J., Smull, M., & Crites, L. (1985). Individual and family factors associated with risk of institutionalization of mentally retarded adults. *American Journal of Mental Deficiency, 90*(3), 271–276.

Boulding, K. (1967). The boundaries of social policy, *Social Work, 12,* 3–11.

Brookfield, S. (1986). *Understanding and facilitating adult learning.* San Francisco, CA: Jossey-Bass.

Bruininks, R., Hill, B., Lakin, C., & White, C. (1985). *Residential services for adults with developmental disabilities,* (unpublished manuscript). Logan: Utah State University. Developmental Center for Handicapped Persons.

Cain, E. (1985). *The potential for advanced technology: Conference on computers for the handicapped,* (unpublished manuscript). Baltimore, MD: The Johns Hopkins University.

Cain, E., & Taber, F. (1987). *Educating disabled people for the 21st century.* Boston: Little, Brown.

Cappo, J. (1990). *FutureScope: Success strategies for the 1990s & beyond.* New York: Longman Financial Services Publishing.

Cetron, M. (1988). Class of 2000: The good news and the bad news. *The Futurist, 22,* 9–16.

Cetron, M., & Davies, O. (1989). *American renaissance: Our life at the turn of the 21st century.* New York: St. Martin's Press.

Cetron, M., Rocha, W., & Luckins, R. (1988, July–August). Into the 21 century: long-term trends affecting the United States. *The Futurist,* pp. 29–39.

Daft, R. (1989). *Organizational theory and design* (3rd ed.). St. Paul, MN: West Publishing.

Daynes, R. (1982, February 24–25). Experimenting with videodisc. *Instructional Innovator,* p. 44.

Froland, C., Pancoast, D., Chapman, N., & Kimboko, P. (1981). *Helping networks and human services.* Beverly Hills, CA: Sage Publications.

Garrard, S. (1982). Health services for mentally retarded people in community residences: Problems and questions. *American Journal of Public Health, 72,* 1226–1228.

Johnston, W., & Packer, A. (1987). *Workforce 2000: work and workers for the twenty-first century*. Indianapolis, IN: Hudson Institute.

Kagan, S., Powell, D., Weissbourd, B., & Zigler, E. (1987). Past accomplishments: Future challenges. In S. Kagan, D. Powell, B. Weissbourd, & E. Zigler (Eds.), *America's family support programs: Perspectives and prospects* (pp. 365–380). New Haven, CT: Yale University Press.

Kinlaw, D. (1989). *Coaching for commitment: Managerial strategies for obtaining superior performance*. San Diego, CA: University Associates.

Knowles, M. (1978). *The adult learner: A neglected species* (2nd ed.). Houston, TX: Gulf Publishing.

Knowles, M., & Associates. (1984). *Andragogy in action*. San Francisco, CA: Jossey-Bass.

Koontz, H., O'Donnell, C., & Weihrich, H. (1986). *Essentials of management*, 3rd ed. New York: McGraw-Hill.

Kramer, Ralph M. (1981). *Voluntary agencies in the welfare state*. Berkeley, CA: University of California Press.

Kukla, S., & Montenegro, M. (1981). *What's all this action about interaction. Westinghouse Technical Training Operations Group report*.

Lakin, C., Hill, B., White, C., & Wright, E. (1987). *Longitudinal change and interstate variability in the size of residential facilities for persons with mental retardation* (Brief report No. 28). Minneapolis: University of Minnesota, Minnesota University Affiliated Program.

Lee, C., & Zemke, R. (1987). How long does it take? *Training: The Magazine of Human Resources Development, 24*, 75–80.

Levine, C. (1982, January). Going interactive: A look at systems and applications. *Videography*, pp. 21–24.

Levitan, S., Mangum, G. L., & Marshall, R. (1972). *Human resources and labor markets*. New York: Harper & Row.

Lindeman, E. (1926). *The meaning of adult education*. New York: New Republic.

Norton, E. (1984). Minority workers tomorrow must tread a much different path than did today's middle class. In L. Chiara & D. Lacey (Eds.), *Work in the 21st century: An anthology of writings on the changing world of work* (pp. 65–76). New York: Hippocrene Books.

Nugent, R. (1982, March). Using videodisc technology. *Video Systems*, pp. 16–21.

Ostroff, J. (1989). An aging market. *American Demographics, 11*, 26–37.

President's Panel on Mental Retardation. (1962). A proposed program for national action to combat mental retardation. Washington, DC: Author.

Richardson, M., West, P., & Fifield, M. (1985). Preservice and professional training. In M. Fifield & B. Smith (Eds.), *Personnel training for serving adults with developmental disabilities* (pp. 67–83). Logan: Utah State University, Developmental Center for Handicapped Persons.

Rogers, E. (1983). *Diffusion of innovations* (3rd ed.) New York: The Free Press.

Rusch, F., & Hughes, C. (1988). Supported employment: Prompting employee independence. *Mental Retardation, 26*, 351–356.

Smull, M. (1989). *Crisis in the community*. Alexandria VA: National Association of State Mental Retardation Program Directors.

Smull, M., & Bellamy, G. (1991). Community services for adults with disabilities: Policy challenges in the emerging support paradigm. In L. Meyer, C. Peck, &

L. Brown (Eds.), *Critical issues in the lives of people with severe disabilities* (pp. 527–536). Baltimore: Paul H. Brookes.

Smull, M., Sachs, M., Cahn, L., & Feder, S. (1988). *Service requests: An overview*. Baltimore: Applied Research and Evaluation Unit: University of Maryland at Baltimore.

Schalock, R. L. (1983). *Services for developmentally disabled adults: Development, implementation, and evaluation*. Baltimore, MD: University Park Press.

Stewart, H. (1989). *Recollecting the future: A view of business, technology, and innovation in the next 30 years*. Homewood, IL: Dow Jones-Irwin.

Thurow, L. (1970). *Investment in human capital*. Belmont, CA: Wadsworth.

Thurow, L. (1975). *Generating inequality*. New York: Basic Books.

Vail, H. (1980). The home computer terminal: Transforming the household of tomorrow. In E. Cornish (Ed.), *Communications tomorrow* (pp. 125–130). Bethesda, MD: World Future Society.

White, C., Lakin, C., Hill, B., Wright, E., & Bruininks, R. (1988). *Persons with mental retardation in state operated residential facilities: Year ending June 30, 1987 with longitudinal trends from 1950 to 1987* (unpublished manuscript). Minneapolis: University of Minnesota, Center for Residential and Community Services.

Willer, B., Ross, M., & Intagliata, J. (1980). Medical school education in mental retardation. *Journal of Medical Education, 55*, 589–594.

Wlodkowski, Raymond J. (1985). *Enhancing adult motivation to learn: A guide to improving instruction and increasing learner achievement*. San Francisco, CA: Jossey-Bass.

19
Fiscal and Demographic Trends in Mental Retardation Services: The Emergence of the Family

GLENN T. FUJIURA and DAVID BRADDOCK

The nation's system of services for persons with mental retardation has undergone a fundamental transformation during the past two decades. Since 1967, the institutional census has been in steady decline as states have shifted away from reliance on traditional institutionally based service systems. In this same period, we have witnessed the collateral expansion of community-based service networks. Although there has been widespread commitment of state policies to these changes, segregated, large congregate-based care systems still dominate, both in terms of fiscal commitments and numbers of persons served (Braddock, Hemp, Fujiura, Bachelder, & Mitchell, 1990). The transformation is far from complete, and substantial challenges lie ahead as we enter the concluding years of the 20th century.

In this chapter, fiscal and demographic trends from the 1970s through the end of the 1980s are evaluated, and the contemporary character of the nation's system of care is critically assessed. Two central themes emerge from the analysis: (a) Despite the impressive advances in community services development, substantial additional growth in the national capacity will be required to meet current needs. Funding for this expansion, seen in the context of the national economy, may well depend on the continued advocacy of the needs and rights of citizens with mental retardation. (b) A considerable share of future need will emanate from the American family, a sector of the population not yet adequately served by the nation's formal systems of care. Our analysis of contemporary challenges confronting state service systems suggests that the family must be a principal component of policy initiatives for the future. To this end, special emphasis has been given to current developments in family support services, and the results of a recent survey of family support program initiatives are summarized in the concluding section.

A Recent History of Fiscal and Demographic Trends

The following discussion is based largely on a national and state-by-state survey of mental retardation and related developmental disabilities expenditures and programs (Braddock et al., 1990) and related studies (Braddock & Fujiura, 1991; Braddock, Fujiura, Hemp, Bachelder, & Mitchell, in 1991). The research has longitudinally tracked state and federal mental retardation services funding from 1977 through 1988.

The Changing Residential Services System: 1977 to 1988

In 1977, a decade after institutional populations peaked in the United States, 84 out of every 100 persons with mental retardation in residential programs were still located in large congregate facilities (Figure 19.1). They included 149,000 residents of state-operated institutions and an

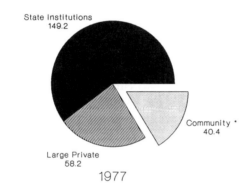

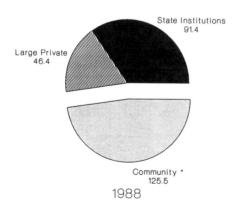

* 15-Bed or less facilities

FIGURE 19.1. Residential services: 1977 versus 1988 (in thousands of residents). From Braddock et al., 1990. Copyright 1990 by Brookes Publishing (POB 10624, Baltimore, MD 21285). Reprinted by permission.

additional 58,000 persons in 16+ bed, privately operated facilities. In that same year, approximately 40,000 persons with mental retardation resided in smaller, 15-bed or less, facilities (White, Lakin, Wright, Hill, & Menke, 1989). By 1988, the relative proportions were more nearly equal: 135,000 residents in large congregate facilities versus approximately 125,500 persons living in smaller residences (Braddock et al., 1990). The character of the nation's out-of-home residential system had been significantly recast during the 12-year period.

The Contraction of the Institutional System

The central dynamic for this change has been the reduction in size of the state-operated institutional system. The average daily census in these facilities, which stood at 149,000 in 1977, had dropped to 91,000 by 1988 (Figure 19.2). This represented a 39% decline and a dramatic decrease of 53% from the 1967 census of 195,000.

Two factors undergirded the declining census: (a) downsizing of institutional facilities, which had decreased in average size from 471 beds in 1977 to 315 beds by 1988, and (b) closures of institutions. In the most recent survey of institutional programs in the United States (Braddock et al., 1991), 44 completed and in-progress closures were identified. Nearly 90% of these closures occurred during the 1977 to 1988 period, and the trend appears likely to continue. Figure 19.3 graphically illustrates the accumulated closures (completed and in-progress) across the 25-year period of 1970 to 1995.

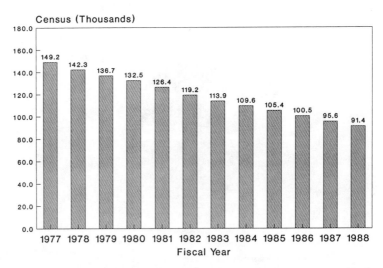

FIGURE 19.2. Average daily residents in state-operated institutions: fiscal year 1977 to 1988. From Braddock et al., 1990. Copyright 1990 by Brookes Publishing (POB 10624, Baltimore, MD 21285). Reprinted by permission.

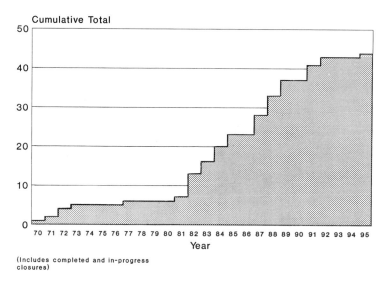

Year

(Includes completed and in-progress closures)

FIGURE 19.3. Cumulative institutional closures: fiscal year 1970 to 1995. From Braddock et al., 1990. Copyright 1990 by Brookes Publishing (POB 10624, Baltimore, MD 21285). Reprinted by permission.

There has been a parallel decline in the census of 16+-bed privately operated residential facilities during the 1977 to 1988 period, though not of a corresponding magnitude (20% versus 39% for institutional programs). Nearly 32,000 persons were served in facilities funded through the Intermediate Care Facilities for the Mentally Retarded (ICFs/MR) program in 1988 and another 14,500 in other large private facilities. Costs have spiraled; though the total numbers of residents have decreased by roughly 10,500, inflation-adjusted spending has increased by 296%.

Fiscal Trends

The decline of the large congregate residential services census and the corresponding expansion in community-based options is partially reflected in the relative balances of fiscal commitments made by states to the two service sectors. Total state and federal commitments to mental retardation services (excluding special education and federal income maintenance payments) have advanced from $3.5 billion in 1977 to $11.7 billion in 1988. The principal focus of this growth is apparent from inspection of Figure 19.4, which graphically displays the 12-year spending trend in inflation-adjusted dollars.

The increase in total outlays, which was an impressive 72% in inflation-adjusted dollars, largely represented the rapid increase in monies committed to the development of community services. However, spending on the large congregate care sector did not decrease in accord with the

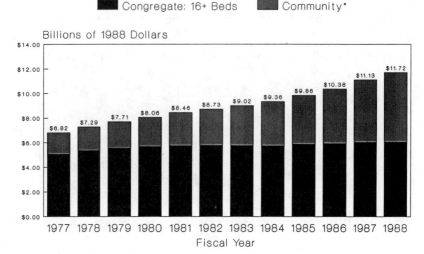

FIGURE 19.4. Adjusted mental retardation/developmental disabilities spending for congregate residential and community services, 1977 to 1988. From Braddock et al., 1990. Copyright 1990 by Brookes Publishing (POB 10624, Baltimore, MD 21285). Reprinted by permission.

declines in the census. Rather, it increased moderately, from an inflation-adjusted level of $5 billion in 1977 to $6.1 billion in 1988.

The juxtaposition of the 1977 residential counts and fiscal data to the most recently available data from 1988 illustrates two central trends of the 1980s: (a) the dramatic expansion of states' community service systems, both in terms of individuals served and monies expended, and (b) the rapid escalation of the costs of care within the large congregate residential services sector. In inflation-adjusted dollars, this latter system of services commanded 22% more funds in 1988 than in 1977, while providing services to 72,000 fewer persons (Figure 19.5). More dollars were supporting substantially fewer persons.

Challenges to State Service Systems

The fiscal and programmatic data underscore the impact of federal and state policies that have, in the aggregate, yielded significant gains during the past decade for persons with mental retardation. Yet, despite the real-dollar increases in fiscal commitments, the total number of individuals served in out-of-home residential facilities has grown by only 6%. Excluding nursing home placements, there were approximately 247,000 out-of-home residential placements in 1977; by 1988, the residential

1977 versus 1988

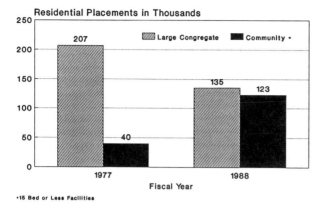

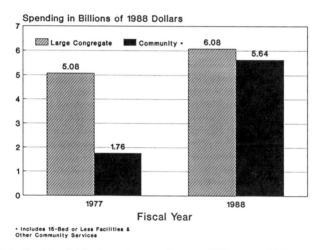

FIGURE 19.5. Residential beds and expenditures: 1977 versus 1988.

capacity of the nation had increased by only 16,000. While a considerable share of the decade's fiscal growth has been devoted to the development of nonresidential community services, clearly, the additional dollars have not purchased any substantial expansion of the nation's out-of-home residential capacity. Three implications of these trends are discussed in the next section.

The Large Congregate Bias

The aggregated national fiscal profile, which shows community service spending approaching parity with the level of funds committed to the large congregate sector, obscures the remarkable interstate variability in commitments to community services. There are wide disparities across state systems. Only 21 of the 51 states expended more on community services than on large congregate residential services. Eleven states expend less than one third of their total mental retardation services resources on community programs. The range of proportions is extreme, from a high of 78% in Michigan to a low of 16% in Mississippi.

With respect to the relative proportions of placements into small versus large residential settings, the 12-year trends and current status parallel the fiscal data. In 1977, the average rate of placements into 15-bed or less facilities was 16.6%, ranging from less than 1% in Oklahoma to 56% in Montana. By 1988, this placement average had increased to 51%, reflecting the dramatic growth in small facility options. However, these changes have manifested themselves unevenly across the nation. Oklahoma, Illinois, Louisiana, South Carolina, and Texas, states with the lowest rates of placements into 15-bed or less facilities in 1977, maintained an extensive large congregate service base into 1988. Mississippi and Missouri were virtually unchanged from their levels of 1977. In

TABLE 19.1. Community spending and 15-bed or less residential capacity as share of state total in 1988[a]

State	% Community funding	1988 Rank	% 15-Bed or less	1988 Rank
AK	66.6	5	83.5	2
AL	29.0	46	36.7	38
AR	28.4	47	29.5	45
AZ	59.0	8	80.0	5
CA	54.8	17	54.9	24
CO	71.1	3	72.3	9
CT	60.8	7	51.3	26
DC	66.6	6	72.8	8
DE	35.3	40	45.4	30
FL	44.8	27	51.5	25
GA	41.5	31	44.0	31
HA	42.2	30	71.1	10
IA	45.0	25	29.7	44
ID	51.0	21	38.0	37
IL	39.3	34	22.2	48
IN	46.1	22	56.0	23
KS	31.0	44	46.8	29
KY	41.1	32	36.0	39
LA	32.3	41	25.5	47
MA	45.0	26	59.7	18
MD	56.5	10	57.8	21
ME	55.1	15	60.4	16
MI	78.0	1	81.2	4
MN	55.3	14	61.9	15
MO	38.5	35	33.4	42
MS	15.7	51	12.2	51

contrast, states that have been fiscal leaders in community services, such as the District of Columbia, North Dakota, and Rhode Island, have radically transformed their systems, having placement rates below 10% in 1977 rising to 70% or more in 1988.

Nationally, less than half the state systems (25) have the majority of residential placements in small facilities; nine states serve fewer than one third of their residential population in these programs. Table 19.1 summarizes the proportional allocation of funds and residents in the community services sectors of each of the 50 states and the District of Columbia. There are many alternative models of community care, and the "large" versus "small" facility distinction is an imperfect descriptor of state systems. Nevertheless, it is a useful proxy for evaluating policy emphasis within a state. For the majority of state systems, the transformation to a community-based service system has just begun. Despite the considerable depopulation of states' institutional facilities, the nation's network of services is still predominantly a large congregate-based system.

TABLE 19.1. Continued

State	% Community funding	1988 Rank	% 15-Bed or less	1988 Rank
MT	58.8	9	78.2	7
NC	29.4	45	38.2	36
ND	55.6	13	78.8	6
NE	56.1	11	64.3	13
NH	72.6	2	83.0	3
NJ	40.0	33	32.4	43
NM	43.5	29	58.4	19
NV	43.7	28	59.8	17
NY	54.9	16	56.9	22
OH	51.9	20	40.5	35
OK	17.2	50	17.8	49
OR	36.8	37	57.9	20
PA	51.9	19	49.5	27
RI	69.2	4	85.2	1
SC	32.3	42	35.6	40
SD	52.4	18	67.4	12
TN	27.9	49	35.1	41
TX	28.1	48	17.6	50
UT	45.7	24	42.6	33
VA	31.4	43	27.3	46
VT	56.1	12	67.5	11
WA	35.3	39	48.8	28
WI	45.8	23	62.5	14
WV	37.6	36	42.8	32
WY	36.4	38	41.7	34

[a] Spending totals include 15-bed or less facilities and other community services.

The Adequacy of the Residential Supply

A second challenge, and perhaps a more basic concern, is the adequacy of the nation's residential capacity for meeting current and near future demand. Although it is impossible to characterize the parameters of supply and demand with great precision, a partial answer to the adequacy question may be found in comparing current capacity against secondary indices of service need.

Waiting List Data

Virtually every parent or relative of a person with mental retardation has encountered a waiting list. The Association for Retarded Citizens (ARC) conducted a telephone survey to quantify the scope of the problem in 1987 (Davis, 1987). The survey sample was composed of state ARC directors and/or state mental health and mental retardation and developmental disabilities agencies. Thirty-eight states regularly collected waiting list data or had conducted a recent evaluation of waiting lists. Estimates were obtained from those states not systematically assessing this information. Sixty-three thousand persons were estimated to be waiting for residential services. The number very likely underestimated the true extent of residential service need. First, the figure excluded six states for which estimates were unavailable, including California, the nation's most populous state. Second, waiting list data may represent only the subset of persons formally attempting to obtain service rather than the more inclusive population in need. Finally, waiting list data do not reflect those individuals currently in the residential service system but in need of alternative placements.

PL 100-203

PL 100-203 (OBRA, 1987), passed by Congress in 1987, included sections addressing the issue of quality of care for persons with mental retardation and developmental disabilities placed in nursing homes. The legislation specified that all states must have in place a pre-admission screening program to prevent admission of persons with mental retardation and developmental disabilities into nursing homes unless their primary need was nursing care. Of special significance to the larger issue of the nation's residential capacity, the legislation required states to furnish appropriate services to this population, either through "active treatment" within the facility or by movement of the resident to alternative care.

The size of this population and the extent to which states were planning to reduce its size were estimated in a recent study of nursing home placements and associated costs (Mitchell & Braddock, 1990). The study identified 50,606 persons with mental retardation living in nursing homes in 1988, an estimate within the range predicted by the sample-based surveys of the National Center on Health Statistics in 1977 and in 1985.

Thirty-four states provided a projection of the number of nursing home residents who would eventually be moved to alternative facilities. The estimate, 37% of all placements, was questioned by Mitchell and Braddock (1990) as being far too conservative. They cited past studies indicating that the vast majority of nursing home residents with mental retardation and developmental disabilities had been inappropriately placed (e.g., Anderson, Lakin, Bruininks, & Hill, 1987). Even if the 37% figure were accurate, then implementation of the provisions of PL 100-203 would result in another 19,000 persons attempting to enter the residential service system.

The Large Congregate Issue

Together, the waiting list and nursing home counts amount to over 81,000 persons with mental retardation in need of service options currently not available. This total represents the net growth in small residential bed capacity during the period of 1977 to 1988 and nearly one third of the nation's current mental retardation/developmental disabilities (MR/DD) residential services capacity. However, included on the supply side of this comparison were the 135,000 residents of public institutions and large private facilities. These are individuals also in need of family-scale community-based residential alternatives and in the long term, their numbers must be considered part of any future demand. Even if projected demand on community residential services were based only on past rates of movement from the large congregate sector, then thousands more per year could be added to the total count of persons in need of residential options.

Growth in the Context of National Resources

The third challenge is economic, reflecting the uncertain character of public financing in an era of fiscal conservatism and budgetary restraints. Maintenance of dual service systems, based in both the community and the institution, is an expensive proposition for the states. The large congregate residential system, though much constricted in capacity, has absorbed a relatively constant level of fiscal resources over the past 12 years. What gains we have witnessed in community services have been achieved through the infusion of *additional* funds dedicated to the field.

National Wealth

Spending for the community sector has grown over three times as fast as aggregate national wealth, that is, the total personal income of the United States. The higher rate of growth is graphically displayed in

Figure 19.6, where mental retardation services spending is expressed in terms of dollars spent per $1,000 of aggregate national wealth.

The two trendlines in the lower portion of Figure 19.6 represent spending per $1,000 of aggregate personal wealth broken out across the two major service sectors—large congregate services and community services. Their divergent slopes reflect the allocation of a majority of these additional resources to expansion of the community services sector. Since 1977, the state and federal governments' commitments to community-based mental retardation services have increased by an average of $.5 billion per year in inflation-adjusted 1988 dollars.

Governmental Expenditures

The fiscal trends are even more striking when viewed in relation to total expenditures by all levels of government. Community services funding has increased far more rapidly than total governmental expenditures. In 1977, $1.29 of each $1,000 of total governmental spending was devoted to community mental retardation services. By 1988, this share had more than doubled to $2.94. While absolute levels of spending are modest in terms of total governmental outlays, the rate of growth has been remarkable. In short, the contemporary status of community services has been achieved by the allocation of an increasing share of the nation's wealth and its governmental expenditures over these past 12 years.

The burden of this growth has been shared unequally by the federal,

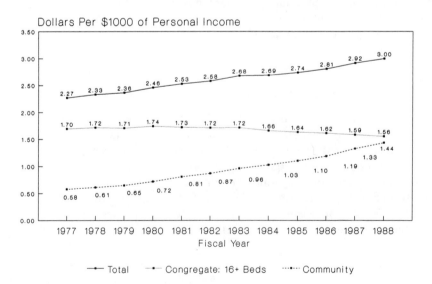

FIGURE 19.6. Mental Retardation/Developmental Disabilities spending per $1,000 of personal income, 1977 to 1988. From Braddock et al., 1990. Copyright 1990 by Brookes Publishing (POB 10624, Baltimore, MD 21285). Reprinted by permission.

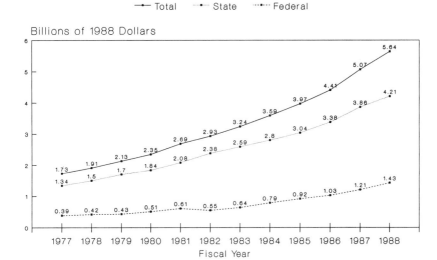

FIGURE 19.7. Adjusted federal versus state funding for community services: fiscal year 1977 to 1988. From Braddock et al., 1990. Copyright 1990 by Brookes Publishing (POB 10624, Baltimore, MD 21285). Reprinted by permission.

state, and local governments. Figure 19.7 graphically displays community services mental retardation funding from 1977 to 1988 in terms of state and federal funding. Despite the expanding federal presence in human services during the 1970s and 1980s, the states provided the majority of funds for community-based services. State and local source monies accounted for 75% of all community services funding in 1988, a ratio that has been relatively constant since 1977. *The expansion of the nation's community services base has been largely fueled by state revenues.*

It has primarily been the states that have set the agenda and allocated the resources for community services development over this past decade. Their response to the challenges of the coming decade will depend on their capacity to redress current inadequacies and, perhaps more importantly, on the depth of their commitments to the continued growth of community services. Capacity is an economic question, and while economic forecasting is an inexact science, it is likely that the growth of the American economy will slow in the near term from the rates seen in the 1980s. Slower economic growth will tighten state budgets. As we enter the 1990s, state budget surpluses are at their lowest levels in over a decade (Gettings & Smith, 1989; State Policy Research, 1990). The consequences of the slowdown are already being felt; austerity measures have been adopted throughout New England, a region of the country that has recently led the nation in fiscal commitments to community services. How services to persons with mental retardation will fare in this economic climate is unknown. Recent research has suggested the critical role advocacy has played in securing fiscal resources for community services

(Braddock & Fujiura, 1991); it is reasonable to assume that continued advocacy will be necessary to maintain the commitment of state leadership and government to the community services agenda.

Future Challenges: The Family Issue

To this point, we have summarized the major transformations that have occurred in the nation's mental retardation service-delivery system and described trends that reflect quite positively on the past decade's progress. Implicit in the presentation has been a concern that such rates of growth, though impressive, have left us with a system still plagued by inadequacies; an institutional or institution-like service system still dominates, while much community service need remains unmet. However, the single largest locus of mental retardation "services" in the nation—the American family—has yet to be considered.

Demographics

The vast majority of persons with mental retardation are supported at home by their families (Agosta & Bradley, 1985; Bruininks & Krantz, 1979; Wieck, 1985). Out-of-home services have historically been limited, and the family has always been the principal care option in the nation. Furthermore, the extent of this role has been reinforced in recent years as a consequence of statutorily mandated access to public education and state policies restricting institutional admissions (e.g., Agosta & Bradley, 1985). Despite the size of the family-based population and the high probability that it has grown in recent years as a consequence of public policy, little is known about the parameters of its size (e.g., Bruininks, 1979; Rowitz, 1984).

To establish an empirical context for the elaboration of these issues, it was necessary to derive population estimates, and conservative values were chosen. The intent of this analysis was not to derive precise population estimates but rather to more fully substantiate potential policy concerns for the coming decade. The following discussion of prevalence is restricted to those persons jointly classified as mentally retarded and developmentally disabled. The net effect of this restriction is to consider only that subset of individuals with mental retardation who are functionally limited. The restriction is imposed only to make possible a comparison of the known residential services population against those most likely to access it.

Estimates of the prevalence of developmental disabilities range between 1.20% and 1.65% (e.g., Administration on Developmental Disabilities [ADD], 1981; Boggs & Henney, 1979; Kiernan & Bruininks, 1986). For the purposes of the following exercise, we employed the ADD estimate of 1.2%, its projection of the *noninstitutionalized* population. Approximately 58.4% of the developmentally disabled population was projected to have mental retardation (ADD, 1981), which yields an estimated prevalence rate of .70% for persons jointly classified as mentally retarded and developmentally disabled in the general population. This estimate is consistent with the more conservative population estimates of the numbers of persons with levels of mental retardation in the severe to profound ranges (e.g., Baroff, 1982; McLaren & Bryson, 1987). Applying this rate to the general population of the United Sates in 1988 yields an estimated 1.7 million children and adults with mental retardation who are considered developmentally disabled.

The shape of the age distributions across this population for both 1970 and 1988 are graphically displayed in Figure 19.8. Age breakouts were based on U.S. Bureau of the Census data for 1970 and the 1988 population projections (U.S. Bureau of the Census, 1987). The age estimates

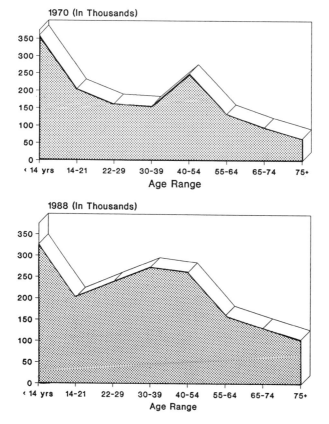

FIGURE 19.8. Age distributions of persons with mental retardation: 1970 versus 1988.

assumed that prevalence rates do not exhibit *significant* variations across ages; that is, the distribution of ages across the population with mental retardation parallel the distribution in the general population. Although there is some question about derived estimates at the older range of ages (e.g., Seltzer & Seltzer, 1985), the analysis employed rates derived from the general population. Our estimates at these older age ranges appear relatively conservative, falling well below the National Institute for Disability and Rehabilitation Research (LaPlante, 1988) estimates for the cohort aged 45+ years (.23% versus .38%) and slightly higher than the .1% derived by Jacobson, Sutton, & Janicki (1985) for those aged 55+ years (.16% in the present analysis).

Implications

Two conclusions can be drawn from inspection of Figure 19.8. First, that the nation's out-of-home residential system served only a small proportion of all persons with mental retardation in 1988. Total out-of-home placements in 1988, including nursing home placements, were 314,000 (Braddock et al., 1990), or less than 19% of all persons with mental retardation who have developmental disabilities. The balance of this population, over 1.38 million persons, were cared for by family members or friends. Though there are significant age-related variations in out-of-home placements—the distribution is narrow and skewed, with greater numbers of placements in the mid- to upper age ranges (Bruininks et al., 1983)—the total variance is small relative to the larger population and does not visibly affect the general shape of the family population distribution.

Figure 19.8 makes evident a second issue: that there are two very large cohorts, the school-age population and the post-war generation, the "baby-boomers." Should their families seek out-of-home residential options, the already overburdened residential system will be severely tested, a challenge not likely to be met in the near term. The impact of demographic pressure has been cited elsewhere in the literature, particularly in the area of aging and disabilities (e.g., Jacobson et al., 1985).

The American family is the largest "provider" of care in the nation. It has made relatively limited demands on the formal systems of care provided by the states (Moroney, 1979). However, the foregoing population estimates suggest that there may be impending demands that stem, in part, from governmental policies that have encouraged families to maintain their children at home and from the demographic impact of the post-war "baby-boom," currently in the care of aging parents. These cohorts are unprecedented in size, and their demands on the service system have not yet been fully realized.

A Look to the Future: Fiscal and Programmatic Status of Family Support

The needs of families caring for relatives with disabilities can be characterized as numerous, diverse, and generally ill served by the formal systems of care. That the care of one's child at home has represented a path of relative isolation, with little, if any, assistance from public agencies, is well-known; the concerns and needs of such families have been extensively documented (e.g., Agosta & Bradley, 1985; Bates, 1985; Bruininks & Krantz, 1979; Cohen, Agosta, Cohen, & Warren, 1989; Farber, 1968; Gallagher & Vietze, 1986). These issues will not be further elaborated on here. Suffice it to say that families have had limited options and minimal support and that this state of affairs is the result of public policies emphasizing the *substitution* of the family rather than its *enhancement* (Moroney, 1979). However, there are compelling reasons for shifting priority to family empowerments, reasons that range from American cultural values, which have emphasized the inviolability of the family unit, to more tangible rationales, such as the potential of supports to attenuate or delay out-of-home placements. This latter reason has stimulated interest among policy planners in the states (e.g., Knoll & Bersani, 1989; Parrott & Herman, 1987) and among researchers studying factors associated with caregiving ability (e.g., Engelhardt, Brubaker, & Lutzer, 1988; Kotsopoulus & Matathia, 1980). New models of service delivery, focused on the family and designed specifically for the enhancement of their caregiving capacities, have been developed across the nation in recent years. Some of the most exciting developments have occurred in the area of fiscal supports, and because of their relevance to the issue of near future demands on service systems, these are reviewed in detail in the next section.

The Family Support Survey of 1988

The Family Support Survey was based on data collected as part of the larger 18-month investigation of the fiscal and programmatic structure of states' mental retardation service-delivery systems (Braddock et al., 1990). The activities of the principal mental retardation services state agency were the primary focus of the study, though representatives of the state Medicaid and other social services agencies were frequently consulted. Published state executive budgets were collected directly from the states and evaluated for direct references to family support programs. The level of detail within these published documents was typically inadequate or required substantial amplification, and extensive interviews and written communication with financial management and program staff in the relevant agencies were necessary. The Wisconsin Developmental

Disabilities Council family support survey (Bates, 1985) served as an additional resource for information and state contacts.

The term *family support* encompasses many different forms of services across the states. State systems vary in both the types and methods of service delivery as well as guidelines for eligibility. In the absence of a common constellation of services, any method of definition and classification short of the inclusion of *all* services will necessarily fail to fully represent the true scope of a state's service system. Broadly speaking, any nonresidential service can be construed to be a form of support, and from this perspective, virtually all states provide some form of family support. In the survey however, a moderately restrictive set of definitions was employed. It was our intent to assess the level of state *policy effort* emanating from the principle mental retardation services agency. Thus, the survey of programs and related expenditures was constrained to discretely funded initiatives that had achieved *formal status*, either in the form of a line item in the state budget or in the agency's internal accounting and planning system. The program's *visibility* within the state bureaucracy was taken to be representative of its *priority*.

Family support consisted of any community-based service administered by the state mental retardation services agency providing for vouchers, direct cash payments to families, reimbursement, or direct payments to service providers that the state agency itself identified as family support. Examples of family support programs other than cash subsidy included respite care (a distinct category of data collection employed in the study), family counseling, equipment purchase, architectural adaptation of the home, in-home training, education, and behavior management services. In many states without a formal family support program initiative, there were a variety of relevant discretionary activities being carried out by local providers with state assistance.

Synopsis of findings

In their survey of family support services, Agosta, Jennings, and Bradley (1985) found some 62,000 families receiving support through state-government–sponsored family-support programs in 22 states. Wieck (1985) estimated expenditures at $50 million. In this most recent analysis, a discrete family support initiative—either cash subsidy, respite, or other family support—was identified in 42 of the 51 states. In these 42 states, an estimated 168,314 families were served, representing $171 million in total expenditures for 1988. With respect to total mental retardation services expenditures, the $171 million in discretely funded family support funds represented a mere 3% of all spending. Table 19.2 summarizes the state-by-state survey data.

Cash Subsidy Programs

Thirteen state MR/DD agencies were identified as having cash subsidy programs. Detailed information on the number of families served (5,275 nationally) and level of expenditure ($13.5 million) were available from 11 states. The subsidy programs fell into three basic categories:

1. Direct cash payments to families with no restrictions on the way the money was used
2. Direct cash payments tied to a tracking mechanism such as receipts or individual habilitation plans
3. Reimbursements after the family procures services on its own

It is noteworthy that only Michigan expended in excess of 1% of its total mental retardation services budget in 1988 for cash subsidies to families with a developmentally disabled member. In fact, Michigan's expenditure represented 70% of all cash subsidy expenditures identified in the study. Most states active in cash subsidy programs had only instituted programs within the past 1 to 3 years. The average annual cash subsidy expenditure per client in the U.S. in 1988 was $2,567. Virginia's program, the Family Support Project, was based in the state Department of Human Resources and was therefore excluded from the survey as a "non-MR" agency-based program. Families received up to $3,600 per year; approximately 201 families were served in Virginia in fiscal year 1988.

Nonsubsidy Support Programs

Considerably larger and more numerous programs providing respite care were identified in the states. Thirty-three states reported funds specifically budgeted for this activity. Total nationwide expenditures were $50.5 million for an estimated 50,369 clients. The largest programs were identified in California, Massachusetts, New Jersey, and Illinois. Other family support activities, ranging from family counseling to in-home behavior therapy programs, were reported in 30 states serving an additional estimated 102,181 families. The total national expenditure for the other family support category was $106 million.

Conclusion

In the period from 1977 to 1988, the nation increased its community services residential capacity by 83,000 beds, and spending grew by 541%. While this is a tangible manifestation of significant public policy commitments across the nation, it is sobering to consider what additional resources will be required to address and ameliorate current systemic

Table 19.2. Family support programs administered by state MR agencies in fiscal year 1988[a].

State	Cash subsidy		Respite care		Other family support		Total family support	
	Expenditures	Clients	Expenditures	Clients	Expenditures	Clients	Expenditures	Clients
AK	$0	0	$718,900	436	$0	0	$718,900	436
AL	$0	0	$250,000	341	$75,000	*	$325,000	*
AR	$0	0	$206,000	40	$0	0	$206,000	40
AZ	$0	0	$227,600	754	$3,748,300	1,027	$3,975,900	1,781
CA	$0	0	$10,791,546	10,754	$19,720,293	22,159	$30,511,839	32,913
CO	$0	0	$94,894	*	$195,000	65	$289,894	*
CT	$0	0	$836,228	*	$1,067,181	*	$1,903,409	1,492
DC	$0	0	$342,896	400	$150,186	30	$493,082	430
DE	$0	0	$71,818	266	$8,534	*	$80,352	266
FL	$5,100	12	$318,566	856	$10,961,568	*	$11,285,234	*
GA	$0	0	$311,562	*	$300,000	200	$611,562	1,056
HI	$0	0	*	*	*	*	$115,000	400
IA	$0	0	$0	0	$0	0	$0	0
ID	*	0	$71,500	250	$42,000	122	$113,500	372
IL	$0	0	$4,409,600	3,147	$7,905,900	8,903	$12,315,500	12,050
IN	*	*	$333,488	*	$37,054	*	$370,542	1,000
KS	$0	0	$0	0	$0	0	$0	0
KY	$0	0	$991,312	*	$1,741,645	*	$2,732,957	*
LA	$45,743	169	*	*	*	*	$45,743	169
MA	$0	0	$15,000,000	*	$3,900,000	*	$18,900,000	*
MD	$0	0	*	*	$4,050,136	2,008	$4,050,136	2,008
ME	$0	0	$197,306	500	$0	0	$197,306	500
MI	$9,429,251	3,288	*	*	$5,250,000	*	$14,679,251	*
MN	$1,062,700	410	*	*	$1,618,000	*	$2,680,700	*
MO	$0	0	$362,500	340	$174,155	160	$536,655	500
MS	$0	0	$0	0	$0	0	$0	0
MT	$0	0	$269,400	557	$2,575,000	1,198	$2,844,400	1,755
NC	$0	0	$1,070,200	1,369	$2,700	26	$1,072,900	1,395
ND	$460,100	255	$317,100	*	*	*	$777,200	*

State	$	No.	$	No.	$	No.	$	No.
NE	$0	0	$0	0	$0	0	$0	0
NH	$0	0	*	*	$0	*	$936,174	1,285
NM	$0	0	$187,770	224	$0	0	$187,770	224
NJ	$0	0	$5,357,000	*	$3,436,000	*	$8,793,000	*
NV	$162,200	70	*	*	$0	0	$162,200	70
NY	$0	0	$1,000,000	*	$15,536,000	*	$16,536,000	20,000
OH	$0	0	$0	0	$3,562,462	*	$3,562,462	*
OK	$0	0	$0	0	$0	0	$0	0
OR	$0	0	*	*	$0	0	$0	0
PA	$0	0	$300,000	100	$10,086,219	15,639	$10,086,219	15,639
RI	$320,000	75	$1,242,100	66	$1,080,000	*	$1,700,000	175
SC	$180,000	175	$0	0	$0	0	$1,422,100	241
SD	$0	0	$104,860	187	$0	0	$0	0
TN	$0	0	$1,272,276	498	$0	0	$104,860	187
TX	$1,000,000	267	$183,000	354	$7,370,580	2,884	$9,642,856	3,649
UT	$154,100	21	$0	0	$110,000	*	$447,100	*
VA	$0	0	$572,500	375	$0	0	$0	0
VT	$0	0	$1,900,000	*	$16,000	45	$588,500	420
WA	$0	0	$1,077,960	2,362	$566,094	*	$2,466,094	900
WI	$723,100	533	$114,850	*	$723,100	533	$2,524,160	3,428
WV	$0	0	$0	0	$0	0	$114,850	*
WY	$0	0	$0	0	$0	0	$0	0
Reporting states	$13,542,294	5,275	$50,504,732	24,176	$106,009,107	54,999	$171,107,307	104,781
U.S. total (imputed)	—	—	—	50,369	—	102,181	—	168,314

[a] An asterisk indicates that data were not available, and 0 indicates that a discrete family support activity was not identified. Alabama and North Dakota reported client-hours of service. These are not included in client data totals. Hawaii and New Hampshire reported total Family Support Expenditures only. Client data may include duplicate counts. Several states were able to report expenditures but not client data. In those instances, the imputed U.S. column totals for clients served in respite care, other family support, and total family support were imputed from the average expenditures per client for all reporting states.

Source: University of Illinois at Chicago University-Affiliated Program.

inadequacies. The 12-year increase in bed capacity is equal to the current total estimated need from the waiting list and nursing home data. It is a conservative estimate, and one that excludes those currently inappropriately placed in large congregate settings. Further expansion of the community system, while maintaining the institutional sector, dictates the commitment of substantial additional public funds. Rates of growth, exceeding those of the recent past, will be necessary to generate the funds needed to address these inadequacies. In the absence of massive infusions of federal monies, these additional resources must come from state and local revenues, from the governments that, to date, have raised the revenue and allocated the funds to drive the community services agenda. Critical challenges lie ahead as we enter an era likely marked by budgetary tensions and constraints on public spending growth.

The nation is not without options. Barring a catastrophic conclusion to the longest lasting economic expansion in our nation's history, fiscal commitments to community services will continue to increase impressively and the base of services will expand. Medicaid reform holds promise of attenuating the institutional bias of federal ICF/MR support, making available more resources to community service systems in the states. Nevertheless, it is likely that the discrepancy between service needs and service capacities will continue to be unacceptably large.

We conclude by summarizing the two central themes raised in our analysis. First, that no object of public policy is more central to the larger national portrait of services than the American family: the parents, grandparents, siblings and other relatives of persons with mental retardation who collectively represent the nation's largest alternative "system" of care. Our analysis of family support programs reveals important progress in the development of services, though the total allocations of discretely funded monies remains meager. New policy directions focused on the family must be considered, and included among these should be further development and expansion of support programs and additional economic empowerments through cash support subsidies and other entitlements. Family empowerment must be elevated to the level of a national priority.

Second, the impressive growth in services profiled in this chapter should be interpreted as a manifestation of goals accomplished but, more importantly, as a challenge for the new decade. The evolution of the nation's community services network is still underway, and maintenance of the momentum will continue to require additional resources. In this era of fiscal conservatism, the commitment of new resources will again depend on the vigorous individual and organizational advocacy that has spearheaded the community movement through the 1970s and 1980s.

References

Administration on Developmental Disabilities. (1981). Special report on the impact of the change in definition of developmental disabilities. Washington, DC: Author.

Agosta, J. M., & Bradley, V. J. (1985). *Family care for persons with developmental disabilities: A growing commitment.* Boston: Human Services Research Institute.

Agosta, J. M., Jennings, D., & Bradley, V. J. (1985). Statewide family support programs: National survey results. In J. Agosta & V. J. Bradley (Eds.), *Family care for persons with developmental disabilities: A growing commitment* (pp. 94–112). Boston: Human Services Research Institute.

Anderson, D., Lakin, K. C., Bruininks, R. H., & Hill, B. K. (1987). *A national study of residential and support services for elderly persons with mental retardation* (Report No. 22). Minneapolis: University of Minnesota, Department of Educational Psychology.

Baroff, G. (1982). Predicting the prevalence of mental retardation in individual catchment areas. *Mental Retardation, 20,* 133–135.

Bates, M. (1985). *State family support/cash subsidy programs.* Madison, WI: Wisconsin Council on Developmental Disabilities.

Boggs, E., & Henney, R. (1979). *A numerical and functional description of the developmental disabilities population.* Washington, DC: EMC Institute.

Braddock, D., & Fujiura, G. T. (1991). Politics, public policy, and the development of community services in the United States. *American Journal of Mental Retardation, 95,* 369–387.

Braddock, D., Fujiura, G. T., Hemp, R., Bachelder, L., & Mitchell, D. (1991). Current and future trends in state-operated mental retardation institutions. *American Journal of Mental Retardation, 95,* 451–462.

Braddock, D., Hemp, R., Fujiura, G. T., Bachelder, L., & Mitchell, D. (1990). *The state of the states in developmental disabilities.* Baltimore, MD: Brookes.

Bruininks, R. H. (1979). The needs of families. In R. H. Bruininks & G. C. Krantz (Eds.), *Family care of developmentally disabled members: Conference proceedings* (pp. 3–10). Minneapolis: University of Minnesota, Department of Educational Psychology.

Bruininks, R. H., Hauber, F. A., Hill, B. K., Lakin, K. C., McGuire, S. P., Rotegard, L. L., Scheerenberger, R. C., & White, C. C. (1983). *1982 national census of residential facilities: Summary report* (Brief No. 21). Minneapolis: Center for Residential and Community Services, University of Minnesota.

Bruininks, R. H., & Krantz, G. C. (1979). *Family care of developmentally disabled members: Conference proceedings.* Minneapolis: University of Minnesota, Department of Educational Psychology.

Cohen, S., Agosta, J., Cohen, J., & Warren, R. (1989). Supporting families of children with severe disabilities. *Journal of the Association for Persons With Severe Handicaps, 14,* 155–162.

Davis, S. (1987). *A national status report on waiting lists of people with mental retardation for community services.* Arlington, TX: Association for Retarded Citizens.

Engelhardt, J. L., Brubaker, T. H., & Lutzer, V. D. (1988). Older caregivers of adults with mental retardation: Service utilization. *Mental Retardation, 26,* 191–195.

Farber, B. (1968). *Mental retardation: Its social context and social consequences.* Boston: Houghton Mifflin.

Gallagher, J. J., & Vietze, P. M. (1986). *Families of handicapped persons.* Baltimore, MD: Brookes.

Gettings, R. M., & Smith, G. A. (1989). *Federal medicaid policies and services to Americans with developmental disabilities: Critical issues—difficult choices.* Alexandria, VA: National Association of State Mental Retardation Program Directors.

Jacobson, J. W., Sutton, M. S., & Janicki, M. P. (1985). Demography and characteristics of aging and aged mentally retarded persons. In M. P. Janicki & H. M. Wisniewski (Eds.), *Aging and developmental disabilities* (pp. 115–141). Baltimore, MD: Brookes.

Kiernan, W. E., & Bruininks, R. H. (1986). Demographic characteristics. In W. E. Kiernan & J. A. Stark (Eds.), *Pathways to employment for adults with developmental disabilities* (pp. 21–50). Baltimore, MD: Brookes.

Knoll, J., & Bersani, H. (1989). *A comparison of the costs of supporting children with severe disabilities in family and group care.* Syracuse, NY: Syracuse University, Research and Training Center on Community Integration.

Kotsopoulous, S., & Matathia, P. (1980). Worries of parents regarding the future of their mentally retarded adolescent children. *International Journal of Social Psychiatry, 26,* 53–57.

LaPlante, M. P. (1988). *Data on disability from the National Health Interview Survey, 1983–85.* Washington, DC: U.S. National Institute on Disability and Rehabilitation Research.

McLaren, J., & Bryson, S. E. (1987). Review of recent epidemiological studies of mental retardation: Prevalence, associated disorders, and etiology. *American Journal of Mental Retardation, 92,* 243–254.

Mitchell, D., & Braddock, D. (1990). Historical and contemporary issues in nursing home reform. *Mental Retardation, 28,* 201–210.

Moroney, R. M. (1979). Allocation of resources for family care. In R. H. Bruininks & G. C. Krantz (Eds.), *Family care of developmentally disabled members: Conference proceedings* (pp. 63–76). Minneapolis: University of Minnesota, Department of Educational Psychology.

Parrott, M. E., & Herman, S. E. (1987). *Family support subsidy program report: FY 1986–87.* Lansing, MI: Michigan Department of Mental Health.

Rowitz, L. (1984). The need for uniform data reporting in mental retardation. *Mental Retardation, 22,* 1–3.

Seltzer, M. M., & Seltzer, G. B. (1985). The elderly mentally retarded: A group in need of service. *The Journal of Gerontological Social Work, 8,* 99–119.

State Policy Research, Inc. (1990). *State policy reports* (Vol. 7, Issue 24). Alexandria, VA: Author.

United States Bureau of the Census. (1987). *Statistical abstract of the United States: 1988.* Washington, DC: U.S. Government Printing Office.

White C. C., Lakin, K. C., Wright, E. A., Hill, B. K., & Menke, J. M. (1989). *Populations of residential facilities for persons with mental retardation: Trends by size, operation and state, 1977 to 1987* (Brief report No. 32). Minneapolis: Center for Residential and Community Services: University of Minnesota.

Wieck, C. (1985). The development of family support programs. In J. Agosta & V. J. Bradley (Eds.), *Family care for persons with developmental disabilities: A growing commitment* (pp. 70–93). Boston, MA: Human Services Research Institute.

20
Future of National Data Bases

RICHARD K. EYMAN and JAMES F. WHITE

Interest in the use and construction of data banks in mental retardation has a long and varied history (Eyman & Committee, 1969). For example, in 1951 a Model Reporting area for Mental Health Statistics was organized by the Biometrics Branch, National Institute of Mental Health. This project represented the cooperative effort of hospital administrators and statisticians, representing 11 states, for the purpose of determining how statistics on the hospitalized mentally ill could be more uniform, comparable, and meaningful. The project was successful and expanded to include mental retardation and more states. Furthermore, as Best-Sigford, Bruininks, Lakin, Hill, and Heal (1982) noted, data on the level of retardation and ages of institutionalized and released residents were collected by the Bureau of the Census and the National Institute of Mental Health between 1922 and 1955, after which these data categories were dropped.

From 1961 to 1962, the President's Panel on Mental Retardation made 95 action recommendations as part of an intensive effort to learn and evaluate the nation's progress in combating mental retardation. Among 10 areas urgently found needing attention was a national mental retardation information and resource center. The center would serve as a central storage and dissemination point on mental retardation and mental retardation programs. It would gather, systematize, and furnish information on research, studies, programs, and services throughout the nation and in other countries, employing the most up-to-date facilities and techniques for information gathering, storage, evaluation, retrieval, exchange, and dissemination. Although such a center never really materialized, there were funded efforts to determine what was happening on a national level regarding the disposition of mentally retarded people.

For example, in 1963 the Western Interstate Commission for Higher Education and Pacific State Hospital (currently named Lanterman Developmental Center) initiated a joint data collection program among 19 institutions representing approximately 25,000 residents. At the time, the program was thought to have successfully developed and refined methods for collecting and processing large amounts of data across states.

This effort was followed in 1968 by the creation of an Ad Hoc Committee on the use and construction of data banks by Harvey Dingman, then president of the American Association on Mental Retardation (AAMR). This committee issued reports from time to time (Eyman & Committee, 1968, 1969, 1972) and continued to meet into the 1970s. Although committee reports reflected a great deal of optimism regarding state progress toward standardized data on mentally retarded people, Eyman (1973) noted that past failures regarding collection and evaluation systems can largely be laid to political, financial, or jurisdictional problems rather than technical ones.

Based on the optimism for new evaluation systems by some professionals in mental retardation in the 1970s and a new public law, PL 91-517, regarding Developmental Disabilities Services (DDS) and facilities construction amendments of 1970, the research group at the then Pacific Neuropsychiatric Center, UCLA, received funding from DDS to establish a model system capable of evaluating the costs and effectiveness of available services for the developmentally disabled people in Southern California and a sample of other western states (Grossman & Eyman, 1980). Although this effort was partially successful, it became evident that state autonomy, politics, and uncertain national interest in the plight of mentally retarded people were just a few of the problems that would eventually impede progress toward a national evaluation system regarding the care and treatment of people with mental retardation and developmental disabilities. Still, as long as institutions remained a significant placement for retarded people, there were continued efforts to survey these residents (Scheerenberger, 1975, 1976, 1977, 1978a, 1979, 1981).

The 1980s represented the era of deinstitutionalization, when the total population of state institutions for the mentally retarded dropped from about 195,000 residents in 1967 to 128,000 in 1980 and less than 100,000 in 1989 (Braddock, Hemp, & Fujiura, 1987). Hence, no longer can a data collection effort rely on information from institutional populations as a representative sample of mentally retarded people in the nation. There have been some studies on national samples of retarded people residing in community residential facilities in the late 1970s and 1980s (Bruininks, Hauber, & Kudla, 1980; Bruininks, Kudla, Hauber, Hill, & Wieck, 1981; Rotegard, Bruininks, & Lakin, 1982; Scheerenberger, 1980, 1981). Nevertheless, systematic investigations and data collection of the follow-up of community-placed clients are essentially nonexistent (Eyman, Borthwick, & Tarjan, 1984). Hence, evidence tends to still be based on institutional populations (Scheerenberger, 1978b, 1979, 1980) or anecdotal information from communities (Lakin, Krantz, Bruininks, Clumpner, & Hill, 1982).

A recent survey of state mental retardation directors revealed that a very small percentage of states currently have computerized data bases containing comprehensive information on all developmentally disabled clients whom they serve (Borthwick, 1988). It was also discovered in this survey that a number of states either do not include information on adaptive behavior in their computerized systems or are using nonstandard checklists with unknown reliability. This state of affairs prompted Rowitz (1989) to write:

Despite the increasing need for data about people with developmental disabilities for planning purposes, there is no evidence that any form of uniform data-reporting system is on the horizon for the next decade (also see Rowitz, 1984). This is unfortunate because it becomes difficult to make strong arguments for increases in federal spending for people with disabilities when we do not have reliable and valid data about this population. Some good data are being collected by a number of researchers around the United States, but decreases in federal monies for discretionary programs could affect these data bases in the future. (Rowitz, 1989, p. iii)

From this literature on historical trends regarding national data bases, there have been some insightful reasons provided for the decline of uniform data reporting systems since the 1970s in terms of federal spending for mental retardation. Like it or not, interest in national data reporting systems for mental retardation tend to be linked with interest in research on mental retardation. Braddock (1986) documented that federal support for mental retardation research and training activities has been steadily declining in real economic terms since about 1976. Braddock stated:

To describe this long-term decline as a crisis is an understatement and to attribute its cause solely to the present Administration or even to the recent deep recession is factually incorrect. Four consecutive presidential administrations (of both parties) dating back to budgetary decisions implemented during the first pre-sidential term of Richard M. Nixon have presided over the demise of mental retardation research and training as priorities of the federal government. In recent years mental retardation research and training activities have been fiscally de-emphasized, along with scientific research and training in general. The movement toward noncategorical research and training support in special education and vocational rehabilitation—like the general move toward block grants for financing services—has also contributed to diminished federal funding of MR/DD [mentally retarded and/or developmentally disabled] research and training activities. (Braddock, 1986, p. 487)

Given this state of affairs, data bases on the deposition and condition of MR/DD people will probably reflect state interests and need for such information. To this end, predictions on state attention to data on their handicapped residents across the nation will probably follow the evolution of the few states today who have such data systems operating.

Two states known to have aggressive data collection systems for MR/ DD clients are California and New York, although other states such as Colorado and Minnesota also have such systems. Of these two states, California has a more comprehensive tracking data system than New York (Borthwick, 1985). The reader should not interpret this assertion to mean that California spends more money for the care of MR/DD clients than New York or other states. Rather, Braddock, Hemp, and Fujiura (1987) found that in 1984, California ranked 33rd and New York ranked first in MR/DD spending as a share of personal income by state. Hence, the evolution of the California data system should be an interesting conservative predictor for other states, given that, unlike New York, California is far from the most altruistic state regarding expenditures for their MR/DD residents. Another advantage of using California as a model for prediction rests on past federal grant expenditures given to California institutions for the purpose of developing standardized data collection systems for states (Grossman & Eyman, 1980), which ultimately had a *minimal* influence on the data collection system currently ongoing in California. Thus, it cannot be argued that federally supported research on data bases subsidized the existing data system even though these research efforts were California based. The data system in California evolved for fiscal and accountability reasons likely to exist in all states.

The realization that most states will not install data reporting systems based on national interests in the problem of mental retardation or for necessarily humanitarian reasons does not preclude future hope for meaningful national data once the majority of states establish their own accountability systems. The eventual occurrence of computerized data systems in all states is inevitable, given the ubiquitous presence of computers and need for accountability in government. Moreover, the need for valid and accurate information about clients and the services they receive is reflected in state and federal law. This need has also been recognized by the agencies responsible for the provision of developmental services.

In the last two decades, major changes have taken place in the service-delivery system. Both the quantity and quality of services provided to clients have increased steadily. The major change in the focus of services has come about because of a marked shift away from the concept of a highly centralized service system provided by state hospitals. The direction is toward a more dispersed system that more and more, uses resources and personnel in the community. This community approach to services for the developmentally disabled relies on a certain amount of locally available generic services. Gaps in the service-delivery system are usually filled as resources are developed to improve the quality of life for the developmentally disabled.

In the State of California, some of these trends and changes have been expressed in law and in practice. The Lanterman Developmental

Disabilities Services Act declares that the state assume the responsibility for the developmentally disabled. The wide range of services required to accommodate the diverse conditions that occur in developmental disabilities needs to be recognized and addressed. Provision was made for a decentralized service system in the community. The act calls for both statewide and local planning through a state advisory council and 13 area boards. Another major change was the recognition of the need for consumer input, not just that of the professional and the general public. Therefore, the need for local services and the recognition of consumer rights to participate in planning was addressed.

The responsibility for planning and coordinating services to the developmentally disabled presumes the availability of adequate, accurate information. Two types of information are required to plan for and coordinate services. These are an assessment of needs and the quantity and quality of resources. The plans for services should be based on identified needs and allocation of resources. Once a plan has been developed and provided, there is a need to know the outcome or effects of the plan on the individual client and the direction and magnitude of change.

Evaluation is necessary for rational and meaningful planning. The Department of Developmental Services has the responsibility to implement and monitor the provisions of the Lanterman Act. The need for a client evaluation system, as outlined here, allows the department to plan remedial services and provides a mechanism of accountability. To administer the decentralized community service system and to assess the needs of the consumer with its attendant accountability was the impetus for the expenditure of money required to construct a comprehensive evaluation system.

The Department of Developmental Services has designed an evaluation system that uses the data collected by the Client Development Evaluation Report (CDER), in conjunction with information about costs and services to respond to a wide range of information requirements. The client data collection using the CDER began in 1979. The collection of data was in response to the demand by the Department of Finance for a comprehensive data system for planning, forecasting, and management information. Naturally, demographic data, client caseload projections, resource development, client needs assessment, federal and state program eligibility, and so on are all part of the management uses of these data.

The CDER consists of three components:

1. A unique client identification (UCI) number, which provides linkage to the client master file and to the uniform fiscal system file
2. A summary diagnostic element
3. An evaluation element

The UCI number is used to link to the client master file, where information on demographic characteristics—such as the location of clients, both geographically and within the service system, age, sex, ethnicity, employment status, educational program placement, and case management agency—are available. California is divided into 21 geographic regions, each one of which is served by a nonprofit agency called a regional center that serves as a clearing house for all client services. The operation of these regional centers is funded by the Department of Developmental Services under an annual contractual agreement.

The summary diagnostic section records information about types and levels of disabilities and surveys physical and psychological health. The cause of retardation and medical problems are coded using ICD-9-CM codes for accurate descriptions and universal use of these data elements.

Client evaluation element items record adaptive and maladaptive behaviors in six domains, or groupings:

1. Motor
2. Independent living and self-care items
3. Social
4. Emotional
5. Cognitive
6. Communication

Not all of the six domains are discrete, in the sense that behaviors represented in one domain are independent of behavior in the other domains. For example, some of the behaviors in the independent living domain involve motor skills measured in the motor domain. Each of the domains consist of measurements using a number of key indicators. Rating a person on these indicators provides a measure of level of functioning in each domain. Successive administration of the CDER at specified intervals, normally annually, provides a longitudinal measure of the magnitude and direction of developmental change.

Each item in the CDER evaluation element measures from a level of no ability to perform the function to completely independent functioning. This permits the evaluators to record observations of an individual's growth and development from a level of no skills through one where the individual has completely mastered the particular skill. This applies to skills acquired through the normal process of maturation as well as to skills acquired through specified intervention strategies.

To facilitate rating, most measurement items are written so that the rating is based on observed behavior. Each level of an item is written in behavioral terms, which in most cases are readily observable. However, in some instances, ratings are derived through the use of other methods or measures, usually those commonly used in clinical assessment.

The necessary linkage between the three data files is the UCI number, as indicated. This seven-digit numeric variable is assigned to each client at intake into the service system and remains with the client even though the client may move from one regional center to another. A central registry of the UCI numbers is maintained at department headquarters, and when an individual applies for service, the name and date of birth are checked with the registry to determine if the individual has had service in the past. Using this method aids in preventing duplicate provision of services.

The existence of comprehensive client data is the prime requisite for using a simulation model for forecasting and budgeting. California has developed a computerized forecasting model to project the client population over the next 10 years. The model is an example of what are sometimes called *stochastic entity simulation models.* These types of models simulate the behavior of social systems, in this case, the movement of individuals through the service-delivery system. The modeling is accomplished with the aid of random numbers, which can be used to imitate the probability distributions and describe the model system.

The primary usefulness of stochastic entity simulation models relates to policy analysis. Because the model is actually a computer representation of the population and movement of clients who receive services, it can be used to "play out" changes in department policy, new legislation, or demographic trends of the client population.

The existence of a centralized comprehensive client data system provides the motivation for using a simulation model for budget forecasting, client population growth, changing population characteristics, and service use.

Each regional center maintains its own client data system. This system includes the CDER, the client master file, and the Uniform Fiscal system files. These data systems are used primarily for cost accounting in the daily operation of each regional center. Some of California's regional centers have constructed a client management information system composed of the three basic data files linked together to extract and analyze detailed client data. These Management Information Systems (MIS) can be used to find the least restrictive environment for client placement in that community facilities data are part of the MIS and can be used to match client characteristics to the characteristics of groups of clients in the community facilities. Many centers have used their MIS to partially automate the client Individual Program Plan (IPP). Service providers can be linked to client objectives, and the service use can be monitored and analyzed. This use of data can aid in resource development and can help identify areas of service need and conversely areas of service proliferation.

All additions and changes in the regional center client data files are transmitted to the Department of Developmental Services each week. In this manner, the department has all client data and is the focal point for statewide data and information. Evaluation data on clients in the State Developmental Centers (formerly State Hospitals) are used to allocate staffing to the programs in each center and are also used to identify the changing mix of client characteristics that are an outgrowth of efforts in deinstitutionalization.

The ever increasing use of personal computers and the increasing speed and capacity of these devices seem to be a solution for the smaller states, which could use them for a client data system. Because there is no uniform system of data collection, the basics of a data system appear to be:

1. Client characteristics to include adaptive behavior
2. Use of client services
3. Cost of services
4. A file of service-provider data

From these files, a very good statewide data base can be constructed.

One can approach the concept of collecting client evaluation data in a modular way. If we assume that six domains of functioning are adequate to provide a comprehensive measure of adaptive and maladaptive behaviors, we can then construct a questionnaire with three levels of precision.

Five questions in each domain can be constructed to provide a measure of general functioning. Each of these five questions can be expanded into two or three more questions, each of which will provide a secondary level of precision in describing a more specific measure of that skill. Again, each of these items can be expanded into two or three more questions, which form the tertiary level of precision. Standard levels of functioning can be created for each client based on level of retardation, age range, and living arrangement, and can be applied to the five primary questions. If an individual scores below the standard skill level, then the 10 or 15 questions of the secondary level can be completed. The tertiary level need only be completed for those items of specific skill that fall far below the standards set or to gain a level of precision on certain types of clients.

The modular approach to evaluation is very cost-effective and, even at its most general level, can be used to construct IPPs and at the same time provide data for management information use. By completing the secondary and tertiary levels of items for clients whose level of functioning is materially below or above the standard levels defined, the instrument becomes more flexible and specific in its scope.

With advances in optical scanning, it won't be long before data input becomes fast and accurate and will solve the current problem of time and cost of input. Many data base management software systems are available, and many can be customized to suit different situations.

The future of national data bases depends on each state constructing at least a basic data gathering system for use in that state. These systems need not be too complex or detailed but should consist of client diagnostic data, adaptive behavior data, and the type and cost of services. Such a system would go a long way to aid in the construction of a national data file.

The push to collect client data arises out of the need for client services and its attendant cost. The availability of money for services may in time require objective cost data and a stringent means of accountability. It may be that methods of accountability consist of the transmission of data in machine-readable form rather than on printed output. In any case, the information age will require more detailed data than formerly and will reward the users who can stay in step with technology in hardware and in software.

The question, then, is when and how this progress will take place. California's data system was largely dictated by the more than 80,000 clients being served in dispersed community programs and institutions that are funded through the Department of Developmental Services. Because community reimbursements must be based on appropriate services rendered to a particular individual, a computerized system was not optional in the sense of accounting for expenditures when a large number of people are involved. It is not unrealistic to predict that in the near future all states will have some type of computerized data system in place to account for their expenditures. Because the cost of services largely depends on the clients' problems, sooner or later, diagnostic and adaptive and maladaptive behaviors will need to be measured. Hence, the evolution of the data system in California cannot be looked on as an unusual occurrence.

The eventual emergence of computerized data systems for developmentally disabled people will not reflect the idealism of the 1960s but rather accountability requirements of the 1990s. Nor will these data bases be standardized or otherwise necessarily similar. Nevertheless, it is possible to still extract meaningful information from diverse data systems if special projects are undertaken.

For example, during the funding period for the Individualized Data Base (IDB) project (Grossman & Eyman, 1980), 11 states annually reported scores on a version of the AAMR Adaptive Behavior Scale (as well as diagnostic and service data), demonstrating the potential usefulness of a computerized, standardized reporting system. However, it became clear that the challenge was to make data compatible across states and agencies by accommodating idiosyncratic state procedures without the need for mandating special procedures and instruments. In fact, different adaptive behavior measurements could also probably be accommodated if sufficient reliability is present. For example, California uses a client evaluation form that was found to be compatible to the AAMR adaptive behavior scale.

The real challenge of the 1990s is to reestablish interest in research and demonstration projects dealing with the developmentally disabled. Political interest in the problems of these people has been declining, as noted earlier. Computer technology, fiscal accountability, and awareness of liability for the care of handicapped persons will eventually force all states to adopt fairly comprehensive data systems. However, the existence of these data bases will not ensure that questions concerning the welfare of the people comprising such data systems will be addressed. In other words, the recommendations put forward from 1961 to 1962 by the President's Panel on Mental Retardation regarding the provision of information services, programs, outcomes, and so on that clients experience will require a more complete set of data than state data systems by themselves will be likely to provide.

References

Best-Sigford, B., Bruininks, R. H., Lakin, K. C., Hill, B. K., & Heal, L. W. (1982). Resident release patterns in a national sample of public residential facilities. *American Journal of Mental Deficiency*, *87*, 130–140.

Borthwick, S. A. (1985). *The California data base experience*. Paper presented at the annual meeting of the American Psychological Association, Los Angeles, CA.

Borthwick, S. A. (1988). Maladaptive behavior among the mentally retarded: The need for reliable data. In J. Stark, F. Menolascino, M. Albarelli, & V. Grey (Eds.), *Mental health in people with mental retardation: Diagnosis, treatment, and service programs* (pp. 29–40). New York: Springer-Verlag.

Braddock, D. (1986). From Roosevelt to Reagan: Federal spending for mental retardation and developmental disabilities. *American Journal of Mental Deficiency*, *90*, 479–489.

Braddock, D., Hemp, R., & Fujiura, G. (1987). National study of public spending for mental retardation and developmental disabilities. *American Journal of Mental Deficiency*, *92*, 121–133.

Bruininks, R. H., Hauber, F. A., & Kudla, M. J. (1980). *National survey of community residential facilities: A profile of facilities and residents in 1977*. Minneapolis: Department of Psychoeducational Studies, University of Minnesota.

Bruininks, R. H., Kudla, M. J., Hauber, F. A., Hill, B. K., & Wieck, C. A. (1981). Recent growth and status of community based residential alternatives. In R. H. Bruininks, C. E. Meyers, B. B. Sigford, & K. C. Lakin (Eds.), *Deinstitutionalization and community adjustment of mentally retarded people* (AAMD Monograph No. 4, pp. 14–27). Washington, DC: American Association on Mental Deficiency.

Eyman, R. K. (1973). Program evaluation and data reporting systems. *Mental Retardation*, *11*, 48–49.

Eyman, R. K., Borthwick, S. A., & Tarjan, G. (1984). Current trends and changes in institutions for the mentally retarded. In N. Ellis & N. Bray (Eds.), *International review of research in mental retardation* (Vol. 12, pp. 178–203). Orlando, FL: Academic Press.

Eyman, R. K., & Committee (1968). Report of the Ad Hoc Committee on the use and construction of data banks in mental retardation. *American Journal of Mental Deficiency*, *73*, 355–369.

Eyman, R. K., & Committee (1969). Use and construction of data banks in mental retardation: Second report of the AAMD Ad Hoc Committee. *American Journal of Mental Deficiency*, *74*, 441–447.

Eyman, R. K., & Committee (1972). Report of the AAMD Ad Hoc Committee on the use and construction of data banks. *Mental Retardation*, *10*, C9–C10.

Grossman, H. J., & Eyman, R. K. (1980). *Individualized data base project* (DHHS Grant No. 54-71117/9, Final Project Report). Washington, DC: Administration on Developmental Disabilities, DHHS Office of Human Development.

Lakin, K. C., Krantz, G. C., Bruininks, R. H., Clumpner, J. L., & Hill, B. K. (1982). One hundred years of data on populations of public residential facilities for mentally retarded people. *American Journal of Mental Deficiency*, *87*, 1–8.

Rotegard, L. L., Bruininks, R. H., & Lakin, K. C. (1982). *Epidemiology of mental retardation and trends in residential services in the United States*. Washington, DC: NICHD Conference.

Rowitz, L. (1984). The need for uniform data reporting in mental retardation. *Mental Retardation*, *22*, 1–3.

Rowitz, L. (1989). Trends in mental retardation in the 1990's. *Mental Retardation*, *27*, iii–vi.

Scheerenberger, R. C. (1975). *Current trends and status of public residential services for the mentally retarded, 1974*. Madison, WI: National Association of Superintendents of Public Residential Facilities for the Mentally Retarded.

Scheerenberger, R. C. (1976). *Public residential services for the mentally retarded, 1976*. Madison, WI: National Association of Superintendents of Public Residential Facilities for the Mentally Retarded.

Scheerenberger, R. C. (1977). *Current trends and status of public residential facilities for the mentally retarded, 1976*. Madison, WI: National Association of Superintendents of Public Residential Facilities for the Mentally Retarded.

Scheerenberger, R. C. (1978a). Public residential services for the mentally retarded, 1977. In N. R. Ellis (Ed.), *International review of research in mental retardation* (Vol. 9, pp. 187–208). New York: Academic Press.

Scheerenberger, R. C. (1978b). *Public residential services for the mentally retarded, 1977*. Minneapolis: University of Minnesota, Department of Psycho-educational Studies.

Scheerenberger, R. C. (1979). *Public residential services for the mentally retarded, 1979*. Madison, WI: National Association of Superintendents of Public Residential Facilities for the Mentally Retarded.

Scheerenberger, R. C. (1980). *Community programs and services*. Madison, WI: National Association of Superintendents of Public Residential Facilities for the Mentally Retarded.

Scheerenberger, R. C. (1981). Deinstitutionalization: Trends and difficulties. In R. H. Bruininks, C. E. Meyers, B. B. Sigford, & K. C. Lakin (Eds.), *Deinstitutionalization and community adjustment of mentally retarded people* (AAMD Monograph No. 4, pp. 3–13). Washington, DC: American Association on Mental Deficiency.

Epilogue

21
Predictions for the 1990s and Beyond

Louis Rowitz

Throughout this book, we have reviewed in depth 19 major trends in the field of mental retardation. These trends will impact the field throughout the 1990s and into the next century. At a systems level, the authors believe that the trends will affect the lives of people with mental retardation and other developmental disabilities in a significant manner. Although the trends have been presented separately, there is interaction between them. Synergistic effects will also be a product of the interaction. At the microlevel, a number of predictions can be made for each trend. This final chapter will summarize these 130 predictions.

Trends on Conceptual Issues

The first set of trends related to issues in diagnosis and paradigms of disability, ethics, and conceptions about quality of life. These trends were overarching in that they clearly have an impact on all the other trends that were discussed. Predictions based on conceptual issues also tend to be extremely controversial in that they are based on theoretical models that may still need further testing. Predictions made about conceptual issues were as follows:

1. The 1990s will continue to see many types of diagnoses related to mental and physical handicap included under the general rubric of developmental disabilities—the "homogenization of deviance."

2. The use of cognitive models to define mental retardation initially will increase in contrast to psychomedical models of diagnosis. The cognitive model is oriented to learning and motivation, which it defines in a positive rather than a negative way, whereas the psychomedical model tends to be more negative.

3. Movement away from discriminatory categorization and educational program placement will continue. Some of the book's contributors would argue that this will not be an easy task.

4. The 1990s will continue to see the dominance of the psychomedical model because much federal and state legislation is based on it.

5. By the year 2000, multiparadigm models will begin to predominate in the screening and assessment of children with disabilities. Cultural diversity concerns will be addressed more directly.

6. By the year 2000, psychometric assessment will include only standardized measures of achievement, and intelligence will no longer be measured. Many psychometricians will argue against the demise of the intelligence test.

7. The medical models of diagnosis, assessment, and screening will continue for the more severe forms of disability. In fact, the medical model will reemerge as the primary diagnostic model in mental retardation because mental retardation will be defined primarily by biological dysfunction.

8. With the dominance of the medical model paradigm for severe disorders, the prevalence rate for many nonbiologically based forms of learning disability will shrink as people with social forms of learning disability are no longer labeled.

9. The 1990s will see changes relative to the importance of power relations, individual rights, and personal autonomy. By the year 2000, values related to human development and community priorities will begin to predominate in the areas of social policy, and ethical decisions based on power relationships will diminish. If this prediction comes to pass, prediction 10 will also occur.

10. The 1990s will see an evolution in thinking about the development of an ethical community that will culturally redress inequalities that were produced by genetic, environmental, or other conditions that have been destructive to the human development process. The ethical community will promote the purpose of service interventions to enhance the sense of community and to enhance the human development process. In addition, service programs will be oriented to strengthen the ability of families of people with disabilities including mental retardation to master skills to help all family members to adjust. The ethical community will enhance individual development and protect the rights of all family members.

11. The 1990s will bring an increase in interest in the issue of quality of life. There will be further clarifications of the dimensions of this issue. There will also be criticism of the use of quality of life as a measure or as a social standard.

12. Quality of life concerns will be international in scope during the 1990s.

13. Research into quality of life issues and the ways in which quality of life is affected by changing social and economic conditions will occur well into the 21st century.

Trends on Family and Life Course

During the 1980s, there has been increasing interest in family issues in mental retardation from a clinical as well as a research perspective. Part of the reason for this resurgence of interest relates to the increase in the life span of people with mental retardation and the increasing possibility that the individual with mental retardation will spend his or her life in the community rather than a public residential institution. The major trends in this section relate to the critical issues in family life as we enter the 1990s and as we look at major increases in the number of older individuals with mental retardation as we look forward to the year 2000 and beyond. Predictions made about family, life-course, and life-span issues are as follows:

14. As family research continues to define predictive factors that affect marital and family problems and adjustment, it will be discovered that the problems that occur in "ordinary" families will be similar to the families of people with mental retardation. These predictive factors will be strongly associated with ecological concerns as well as time-specific concerns.

15. During the 1990s, research will continue to show that race, socio-economic status, and marital status have differential effects on the lives of women who work outside the home and will show how their lives are affected by the presence of a child who is disabled.

16. During the 1990s, more children will grow up in one-parent house-holds, usually headed by the mother. The income of the divorced or never married mother will be significantly lower than the income of the two-parent family households or the income of the father in the divorced family situation. The 1990s will see a major increase in research on differential care arrangements of single parents.

17. Systematic research will be undertaken related to the role of the mental retardation service community in helping families with a child with mental retardation be more "ordinary."

18. More research and service interventions will occur with siblings who may be adversely affected by the presence of a disabled brother or sister. Sibling concerns will be life-span oriented. There will be growing concern about sibling caretakers who may often take over for their parents after the parents die. The process of the sibling taking over responsibility of their sibling with a disability will be a major research concern.

19. The historical family paradigm that will be prevalent by the year 2000 will stress the values of personal rights, self-expression, and autonomy.

20. In the year 2000 and beyond, family caregiving will be significantly affected by the fact that the American population will be aging. Changing demographics in other parts of the world will also affect family caregiving concerns. Increases in the life span of people with mental retardation will

lead to concerns about caregiving throughout the life span. The ratio of older to younger caregivers has been shifting toward older caregivers and will continue to shift into the 21st century.

21. With the trend toward increasing proportions of older families, there will be pressure for family-support programs for older families in particular. This will mean that programs to support younger families are at risk of budgetary cuts.

22. The dependency ratio will continue to become less favorable. Parents will have life-span caregiving responsibilities. As pointed out in prediction 16, the burden may be greater for women, who may be caregiving without a husband present.

23. Life-span research will significantly increase throughout the 1990s with a growing concentration of research on later life. Longitudinal research will be strongly recommended even though funding of this research is limited.

24. More research on adolescents with mental retardation will occur in the 1990s. This research will compare adolescents with and without mental retardation.

25. On the basis of demographic information on births, increasing life span for people with disabilities, and information related to poverty, there will be a higher prevalence of adolescents with mental retardation living in community settings by the year 2000. Specific poverty factors that will affect this population include teenage pregnancy and parenthood concerns, low educational attainment, and substance abuse.

26. In contrast to prediction 3, the 1980s trend toward delabeling and mainstreaming of individuals with IQ scores in the 55 to 70 range will reverse during the 1990s. The trend toward early classification and service provision that has occurred as a result of U.S. federal legislation will increase labeling. This reversal will clearly impact on the lives of adolescents with mental retardation who have IQ scores below 70.

27. As a follow-up to prediction 25, the presently relatively drug-free adolescent population with mild mental retardation may reverse because mainstreaming and community integration programs encourage close associations between adolescents with and without mental retardation.

28. During the 1990s, there will be increasing evidence of problems in community adjustment for adolescents with all levels of mental retardation. In addition, problems will arise, and programs will need to be modified to address adolescents who will remain dependent as adults.

29. With increases in the life span of people with mental retardation, major demands for service will be made on the aging service network well into the 21st century.

30. During the 1990s, state developmental disabilities councils will continue to appoint council members from the aging services field to deal with problems related to aging and developmental disabilities.

31. Major competition will occur during the 1990s related to the issue of intergeneration equity in service-delivery competition for scarce resources.

32. Intragenerational equity issues related to segregated or integrated senior services will be discussed and affect service policy.

33. A life-course policy and service-related concern will relate to the older person with mental retardation and their still older parents.

34. Attempts to consolidate day and residential services for age-similar dependent populations with similar problems, which were administered by different human services agencies in the 1980s, will occur during the 1990s.

35. Retirement programs for seniors with mental retardation will be developed. Transition supports will evolve for this population.

36. Alternative residential options will need to be developed for frail older persons with mental retardation or other disabilities.

37. Education and health-promotion programs will be developed for all older Americans, regardless of disability.

38. Community organizations will build partnerships and cooperative agreements to address common problems. The partnership model will also involve people with disabilities and also lifelong caregivers of these people. Agency linkages will have to evolve if comprehensive service models are to be implemented.

Trends on Health and Service

With an increase in the chances of a person spending his or her entire life in community settings comes a concern for the health-care needs and other service needs of this population. As with all people who spend their lives in a community, the problems will be similar. On the scientific level, breakthroughs in genetics and successful prevention activities will positively impact on all of society as well as on future generations. On the negative side, the potential spread of infection with human immuno-deficiency virus (HIV) will affect the lives of many as yet unborn children. All people, regardless of disability, may be affected by mental health-related problems. Early intervention programs may positively affect the lives and potential of toddlers and young children. Finally, a policy that stresses community living over institutional living for people with mental retardation will eventually change the configuration of the service-delivery system. The following predictions reflect some of these concerns:

39. During the 1990s, HIV will become the most common infectious cause of developmental disability. This will be partially affected by the increase in HIV infection in adolescent girls and the possibility of adoles-

cent pregnancy. Infection will occur through either intravenous drug use or sexual contact.

40. HIV cures seem unlikely during the early 1990s, although improved treatment interventions will be developed.

41. The 1990s will see the development and implementation of programs that will coordinate services between health providers, mental retardation service providers, educational service programs, and other social service providers. New linkages will be made to agencies serving substance abusers, pregnant teenagers, and minority infants from poor families.

42. Interdisciplinary team treatment models will increase for working with HIV persons with developmental disabilities. Life-span service programs will also be developed. Because parents will continue to work if they are able during the 1990s, increases in day-care programs for these children with HIV infection will need to be developed.

43. Public fears about infectivity will continue, with potential discrimination possible against HIV mothers and their children.

44. Because the mothers with HIV-infection are at high risk of developing AIDS and may die, problems related to children with HIV infection and mental retardation and no parents will become a visible service and community problem.

45. DNA markers for all of the major genetic causes of mental retardation will be available by the end of the first decade of the 21st century, either by linkage analysis or demonstration of the abnormality in the gene itself.

46. Major technical advances will diminish the cost of the "unit of detection" of a preventable genetic cause of severe mental retardation. More money will need to be spent on therapies by the year 2000. More effective therapies will be found. A lack of money may slow down the development of these advances.

47. Multivitamin and folic acid supplementation in early pregnancy will reduce the prevalence of neural tube defects during the 1990s and beyond.

48. Large-scale screening for genetic disorders associated with mental retardation will become feasible at affordable costs during the 1990s.

49. By the year 2005, national and international research will determine the three billion base pairs that comprise the human genome. This will greatly increase the knowledge base about the genetic causes of mental retardation.

50. The 1990s will see the continued refinement of high-resolution cytogenetic techniques and the partial automation of these techniques through computer-assisted technology.

51. Breakthroughs on chorionic villus sampling for the early prenatal diagnosis of cytogenetic abnormalities indicate that first-trimester prenatal

diagnosis is accurate and carries minimal risk to mother and fetus. This sampling technique will be used more extensively in the 1990s.

52. During the 1990s and beyond, there will be an increasing need for more trained technically qualified personnel. Cost will be a major factor here.

53. Research on dual diagnosis and the problems generated for people with mental retardation and mental illness will triple by the year 2000.

54. During the 1990s, there will be a major shortage of mental health workers who are willing to work with individuals with dual-diagnosis problems.

55. There will be major efforts during the 1990s to improve and refine the diagnostic procedures related to people with mental retardation and mental illness. Part of the reason for this increased effort will relate to eligibility concerns that will affect funding. Improvements in classification of people with a dual diagnosis will improve epidemiologic work and lead to better estimates of prevalence.

56. By the year 2000, the application of the dual diagnosis of mental retardation and mental illness will increase significantly.

57. Major breakthroughs will occur during the 1990s in neuroanatomy, which will improve our knowledge base on basic neuroanatomic systems, which will lead to treatments that will eventually reduce the manifestations of mental retardation and mental illness.

58. Model programs will proliferate by the mid-1990s. Model service centers will be established throughout the country during the 1990s. This will also be affected by funding priorities, which could slow down the process.

59. By the year 2000, we will know more about how the brain functions. This will lead to more efficient pharmacologic methods.

60. Efforts will be made in the 1990s by various professional, government, and consumer groups to establish standards of health care for adults with mental retardation.

61. During the 1990s, primary health care for persons with mental retardation will predominantly be provided by general community-based physicians.

62. There will be widespread use of the problem-oriented record and also portable health and habilitative services records that will accompany the person on his or her medical visits.

63. Case-management services for adults with mental retardation will expand during the 1990s. Many case managers will be nurses.

64. More medical education in mental retardation will need to occur during the 1990s.

65. There will be an increase in the development of computer-based resource or medical referral systems similar to New England INDEX to assist families with a family member who is disabled.

66. Prevention issues will be prominent throughout the 1990s with a major emphasis on the prevention of secondary disability in people with mental retardation.

67. The development of health-promotion programs for people with disabilities will increase (see prediction 37).

68. Funding of medical services for people with mental retardation throughout the life course will be a problem during the 1990s and beyond. Medicaid coverage is clearly not sufficient, and many individuals are denied coverage. There will be an expansion in the managed care system for people with disabilities by the year 2000.

69. Most children with mental retardation who have special health-care needs will receive most of their medical care through the generic health-care system. These services will be family centered, community based, and coordinated systematically.

70. Because of federal legislation on the right to education of all people with disabilities, the schools will continue to provide therapeutic services during the next decade. The provision of direct nursing and medical supports in the school will increase gradually.

71. The number and proportion of children living in poverty with poorly educated mothers will increase steadily over the next three decades. Poverty contributes to both prenatal and perinatal problems that make normal development less probable, as has been pointed out in several other predictions.

72. It will probably be shown in the 1990s that the traditional model of a center-based program on a daytime schedule or a home-visit program is inadequate because more mothers are working. The 1990s will see an expansion of a combination of early intervention and day-care services.

73. Changes in legislation related to early childhood programs will result in an increase in family involvement in program-service planning for their children with disabilities. Parents will also be recipients of some of these services, which will be provided in conformity with an Individualized Family Service Plan.

74. New methods for family assessment will be developed during the 1990s. Family-focused programs will be much more common by the year 2000.

75. The family-empowerment movement will be enhanced during the 1990s because parents will be part of the multidisciplinary team that guides service delivery to all family members (see preceding predictions about families).

76. New service models for early intervention for infants and toddlers will evolve during the next two or three decades. Creative financing of these programs will be necessary.

77. With the aging of our population including both parents and people with disabilities (see predictions 29 to 38), it is likely that there will be increasing pressure during the 1990s and beyond for higher rates of

placement in residential institutions. This pressure will be accompanied by an adult focus in residential services in contrast to a child focus in the past.

78. The 1990s will see an increased emphasis on permanency planning activities where families will make life-time plans for their offspring with mental retardation.

79. There will be more large institutional closings during the 1990s, and deinstitutionalization initiatives will continue. However, resources to support community-based programs will still be a major funding problem.

80. Interstate variability in the access to community services will continue during the 1990s.

81. The shift from institutional to community-based settings will not only be a shift in the locus of service but it will also be a shift from publicly to privately provided services.

82. Foster care programs will be difficult to maintain in the 1990s because of high rates of out of home employment by women.

83. The total size of the mental retardation residential care system will be about 315,000 by the year 2000 with only 31,500 living in state institutions. Large private and local governmental institutions (16 or more people) will house more people than those facilities operated by the state. Major placements will be in small community residences.

84. During the 1990s, there will be a concern about finding a balance between the requirements of developmental training and the right to have a reasonably typical home life. It has been shown that the best place for teaching needed community living skills is in a community setting.

85. A major programmatic concern of the 1990s will be to help people with mental retardation and other developmental disabilities who are living in the community to develop social skills that will help them make friends and maintain social relationships. These programs will attempt to lessen the social isolation of people with disabilities. There will be an enhanced appreciation of the importance of relationships with peers with and without mental retardation.

86. The promotion of the community residence as a "home" will occur. Choice in the selection of a home will be promoted. There will be an increasing separation of the housing component from other residential support services. People with mental retardation and other developmental disabilities will be able to buy and get financing for their own home.

Trends in Service and Policy Issues

The final set of trends relate to services and their policy implications. Much discussion has occurred since the end of World War II on the vocational needs of people with mental retardation and other disabilities.

Some of the early discussions and programs related to vocational training and programs in institutional settings or sheltered workshops in the community. Throughout the 1980s, major changes occurred in our approach to work-related issues for people with disabilities. The 1980s saw the expansion of the supported and competitive employment movement. With greater numbers of people with mental retardation living in the community, the next decade and the next century will present many new policy and service considerations. The issue of technology and how technological advances will affect the lives of people with disabilities is a critical concern for the 1990s.

A major issue with strong policy implications relates to the law. Legal protection of people with mental retardation will remain important throughout the 1990s. A number of predictions will be presented that will be affected by the vagaries of the legal and legislative process of the next decade. Other policy concerns relate to shortages of staff to work in the field of mental retardation. Fiscal and demographic issues will also have major policy implications. Finally, the issue of uniform data reporting systems will impact on the way money is spent.

The following predictions address some of the issues raised by this final group of trends:

87. During the 1990s, there will continue to be a shortage of entry-level skilled jobs for which persons with mental retardation will be eligible. These direct-service staff shortages will continue and will be a factor in developing and implementing a variety of integrated employment models. About 4,000 jobs will be available during the 1990s, and more will become available in the new century. Jobs in the supported employment area at the secondary and postsecondary level will also be readily available and need to be filled.

88. The 1990s will see an expansion of the move toward integrated employment and also efforts to identify 18- to 21-year-old people with mental retardation as high-priority candidates for vocational services.

89. Transition planning will be a major priority in the vocational field during the 1990s. Interagency collaboration and sharing of resources will occur relative to job placement as people with mental retardation plan to leave school. Attempts will be made by agency personnel to work more closely with the schools to bring about more successful transition programs.

90. More linkages will be made between schools and business and industry to promote job placement. Business and industry will more directly reflect the content of vocational curricula. More business and industry sites will be used for on-site training.

91. The movement away from segregated day programming to integrated employment services will continue, although the process will be a slow one.

92. New service programs will be developed for secondary school teachers so that they can provide systematic instruction in community-

based settings, learn skills related to communication with adult service agencies, and be able to coordinate transition services.

93. More preservice and inservice training programs will be developed for teachers and agency personnel on transition and its various dimensions.

94. Future research will focus on integrated employment and on the improvement of strategies to facilitate the match between individual choice and the actual level of participation.

95. A number of communities will establish business advisory boards to help in the development of vocational training programs.

96. Assistive technologies will expand in the 1990s in the areas of communication, self-care, and other personal self-help devices. Major technology advances will lead to changes in the life-style of all people with disabilities. Training programs will need to be modified as technology advances.

97. Advancing technologies will give teachers and therapists more powerful and easy-to-program therapy and education aids. Programming will use English-like languages so that teachers and therapists will be able to create their own tools in an expeditious manner.

98. By the year 2000, speech recognition will have evolved to the point where it will become usable by people with disabilities in a broader way.

99. Advances in graphic animation will aid teachers and therapists as well as people with disabilities.

100. By the year 2000, major enhancing and extending aids will be available to people with mental retardation. These aids will help strengthen individual skills.

101. Reminder aids will also be available, such as an electronic pocket notebook that can be used by people with disabilities.

102. Companion and tool technologies will be emerging by the year 2000. These technologies will extend or enhance the individual's cognitive abilities. More artificial intelligence techniques will be used with people with mental retardation.

103. The 1990s will see the implementation of the Americans With Disabilities Act of 1990, which is an antidiscrimination act.

104. Although Congress has defended the rights of people with disabilities, changes in the composition of the U.S. Supreme Court toward a more conservative perspective may lead to the erosion of judicially declared rights by the year 2000.

105. The 1990s will see continued consensus on the goals, if not the procedures, for saving the lives of infants with life-threatening conditions.

106. Legal cases in the 1990s will ensure that all children will receive effective instruction and placement in the least restrictive educational environment in their home communities.

107. The 1990s will see the further implementation of programs related to the right to habilitation at the state and local level. Habilitation rights will need to be demonstrated in community-based situations.

108. During the 1990s, reform laws on guardianship and alternatives to guardianships will be formulated in many countries. By the year 2000, plenary guardianship may become a relic as a result of the fact that people with disabilities can legally avoid excessive protection and undue restriction of rights.

109. Normalization policy will govern most countries in the 1990s. As pointed out in several of the preceding predictions, community living is the ultimate goal of most programs. The 1990s will see more class action suits in the United States to close institutions and implement rights to community living arrangements.

110. The 1990s will see many more judicial and legislative discussion and laws related to zoning and nondiscriminatory housing opportunities.

111. During the 1990s, protection and advocacy programs will be oriented to the protection of people with disabilities from abuse and neglect in community settings.

112. The 1990s will see many states develop statutes related to capital punishment for people with mental retardation. These statutes will preclude the death penalty for persons with mental retardation.

113. A number of states will pass laws related to medical choices of adults who are incompetent as a result of the Cruzan decision. This issue relates to whether substitute decision makers are possible when an individual with mental retardation cannot make rational medical choices.

114. With legal barriers to full citizenship disappearing, the individual will need support and community acceptance to enjoy its benefits. Client choice and training to make these choices will be a high priority during the 1990s.

115. The 1990s will see a growing international movement to eradicate discrimination on the basis of disability.

116. In the 21st century, staffing and training models will reflect the intersection of labor supply, the range of program models that define employment responsibilities and wages, and the use of available teaching and training technologies.

117. In adult services, there will continue to be shortages of occupational therapists, speech pathologists, and other allied health professionals who are trained to work in the developmental disabilities field. As pointed out in several preceding predictions, there will be a shortage of specially trained physicians.

118. Changes in national labor force demographics will affect the field of developmental disabilities. The work force will be older and will include more women and more immigrants, of whom many will not speak English well. In-service and other job-training programs will become more complex, which is due to the need to provide culturally normative habilitative programs.

119. Increased competition for skilled labor in an information- and service-based economy will mean that skilled labor personnel will have

multiple job choices with varying salary options during the 1990s. Jobs in the mental retardation and other developmental disabilities fields will be harder to fill relative to other information- or service-based jobs.

120. Technology driven by efficiency and cost savings alone will lead to a process of dehumanization of human services.

121. Some experts predict an expansion in institutional placements in some states because of possible limitations in funding for community programs. This, however, is a minority view. Most experts believe that the 1990s will continue to see a downsizing of the institutional facility system as well as the continued closure of institutions.

122. During the 1990s, we will see the limits of present models of community care. There will need to be a shift from community-based residential living, which uses paid staff, to community-based networks of support, which rely on community people not in the mental retardation field. Increases in volunteerism will thus occur in the 1990s.

123. In the future, the management control system, which will be based on the more decentralized volunteer system, will have computerized information systems. Future management systems will stress measurement and correction of individual and group staff performance to ensure that organizational objectives are met.

124. Declines in the census of 16- and more bed privately operated residential facilities will occur during the 1990s. In addition, the movement of people with mental retardation out of nursing homes into alternative residential facilities will continue well into the 1990s (see prediction 83).

125. The continued expansion of the nation's community services base will remain largely funded by state rather than federal revenues (see prediction 80). Potentially slow economic growth may affect this continued expansion. Continued advocacy will be needed if we want to maintain the commitment of state legislatures to the community services agenda. Medicaid reform, if it occurs, will alleviate the funding problems somewhat by increasing federal financial participation in the area of residential services.

126. The American family, as pointed out in several predictions, will remain the largest provider of care over the next decade and beyond. Family-support program initiatives will continue during the 1990s, because these programs tend to prevent or significantly delay out of home placements.

127. The 1990s will see an increasing need for state and local mental retardation public agencies to create data bases that will allow for better health care and social services planning for populations with mental retardation. With data, it will be possible to design more efficient preventive and supportive care protocols.

128. Mental retardation data bases will primarily be state based rather than federally based during the 1990s. These data bases will be oriented toward state needs for data rather than national data needs. All states will

develop computerized data bases during the 1990s if they already do not have them.

129. National data files will be constructed out of data collected at the state level.

130. Data bases will be tied to community-based systems of care rather than institutionally based systems, as in the past.

The Future

In this book, we have reviewed 19 major trends in the field of mental retardation for the 1990s and also presented 130 predictions for the field of mental retardation based on these major trends. Although most of the trends have related to the United States, they also have international implications. We are in a major period of change. The new millennium causes us to evaluate where we are presently and where we want to go in the new century. It is important to constantly review the field and to monitor the predictions in terms of accuracy or a need to reformulate them on the basis of societal or political changes. The future is ours to mold. People with mental retardation will help us in this process.

Indexes

Author Index

Subject Index